Dermatitis: Clinical Theory and Aspects

Dermatitis: Clinical Theory and Aspects

Edited by Heidi Mueller

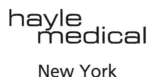

New York

Hayle Medical,
750 Third Avenue, 9th Floor,
New York, NY 10017, USA

Visit us on the World Wide Web at:
www.haylemedical.com

ISBN: 978-1-63241-448-9

Cataloging-in-Publication Data

Dermatitis : clinical theory and aspects / edited by Heidi Mueller.
     p. cm.
Includes bibliographical references and index.
ISBN 978-1-63241-448-9
1. Skin--Inflammation. 2. Atopic dermatitis. 3. Skin--Diseases. 4. Skin--Inflammation--Diagnosis.
I. Mueller, Heidi.
RL231 .D47 2017
616.5--dc23

Table of Contents

Preface

The purpose of the book is to provide a glimpse into the dynamics and to present opinions and studies of some of the scientists engaged in the development of new ideas in the field from very different standpoints. This book will prove useful to students and researchers owing to its high content quality.

Dermatitis is the disease of the skin. The symptoms include rashes, blisters, itchiness, etc. This book on dermatitis discusses the genetic and environmental factors that cause dermatitis. Corticosteroids and immunosuppressants are common medications that are available for the treatment of dermatitis. Clean environment and hygiene is a vital factor in the prevention and alleviation of various dermatological diseases such as eczema, cradle cap and discoid eczema. Topics included in this text aim to advance research in the field of dermatitis diagnosis and therapy. Different approaches, evaluations, methodologies and advanced studies on dermatitis have been included in this book. For all those who are interested in this field, this book can prove to be an essential guide.

At the end, I would like to appreciate all the efforts made by the authors in completing their chapters professionally. I express my deepest gratitude to all of them for contributing to this book by sharing their valuable works. A special thanks to my family and friends for their constant support in this journey.

Editor

Additive Effect between IL-13 Polymorphism and Cesarean Section Delivery/Prenatal Antibiotics Use on Atopic Dermatitis: A Birth Cohort Study (COCOA)

So-Yeon Lee[1], Jinho Yu[2], Kang-Mo Ahn[3], Kyung Won Kim[4], Youn Ho Shin[5], Kyung-shin Lee[6], Seo Ah Hong[2], Young-ho Jung[2], Eun Lee[2], Song-I Yang[2], Ju-hee Seo[7], Ji-Won Kwon[8], Byoung-Ju Kim[9], Hyo-Bin Kim[9], Woo-Kyung Kim[9], Dae Jin Song[10], Gwang Cheon Jang[11], Jung Yeon Shim[3], Soo-Young Lee[12], Ja-Young Kwon[13], Suk-Joo Choi[14], Kyung-Ju Lee[15], Hee Jin Park[15], Hye-Sung Won[16], Ho-Sung Yoo[6], Mi-Jin Kang[6], Hyung-Young Kim[17], Soo-Jong Hong[2]*

1 Department of Pediatrics, Hallym University College of Medicine, Anyang, Korea, 2 Childhood Asthma Atopy Center, Asan Medical Center, Seoul, Korea, 3 Department of Pediatrics, Sungkyunkwan University of School of Medicine, Seoul, Korea, 4 Department of Pediatrics, College of Medicine, Yonsei University, Seoul, Korea, 5 Department of Pediatrics, CHA University of School of Medicine, Seoul, Korea, 6 The Asan Institute for Life Science, Seoul, Korea, 7 Department of Pediatrics, Korea Cancer Center Hospital, Seoul, Korea, 8 Department of Pediatrics, Seoul National University Bundang Hospital, Seongnam, Korea, 9 Department of Pediatrics, Inje University College of Medicine, Seoul, Korea, 10 Department of Pediatrics, Korea University Guro Hospital, Seoul, Korea, 11 Department of Pediatrics, National Health Insurance Corporation Ilsan Hospital, Goyang, Korea, 12 Department of Pediatrics, Ajou University School of Medicine, Suwon, Korea, 13 Department of Obstetrics and Gynecology, Yonsei University College of Medicine, Seoul, Korea, 14 Department of Obstetrics and Gynecology, Samsung Medical Center, Sungkyunkwan University School of Medicine, Seoul, Korea, 15 Department of Obstetrics and Gynecology, Pochon CHA University College of Medicine, Seoul, Korea, 16 Department of Obstetrics and Gynecology, Asan Medical Center, University of Ulsan College of Medicine, Seoul, Korea, 17 Department of Pediatrics, Kosin University College of Medicine, Busan, Korea

Abstract

Background: Although cesarean delivery and prenatal exposure to antibiotics are likely to affect the gut microbiome in infancy, their effect on the development of atopic dermatitis (AD) in infancy is unclear. The influence of individual genotypes on these relationships is also unclear. To evaluate with a prospective birth cohort study whether cesarean section, prenatal exposure to antibiotics, and susceptible genotypes act additively to promote the development of AD in infancy.

Methods: The Cohort for Childhood of Asthma and Allergic Diseases (COCOA) was selected from the general Korean population. A pediatric allergist assessed 412 infants for the presence of AD at 1 year of age. Their cord blood DNA was subjected to interleukin (IL)-13 (rs20541) and cluster-of-differentiation (CD)14 (rs2569190) genotype analysis.

Results: The combination of cesarean delivery and prenatal exposure to antibiotics associated significantly and positively with AD (adjusted odds ratio, 5.70; 95% CI, 1.19–27.3). The association between cesarean delivery and AD was significantly modified by parental history of allergic diseases or risk-associated IL-13 (rs20541) and CD14 (rs2569190) genotypes. There was a trend of interaction between IL-13 (rs20541) and delivery mode with respect to the subsequent risk of AD. (*P* for interaction = 0.039) Infants who were exposed prenatally to antibiotics and were born by cesarean delivery had a lower total microbiota diversity in stool samples at 6 months of age than the control group. As the number of these risk factors increased, the AD risk rose (trend p<0.05).

Conclusion: Cesarean delivery and prenatal antibiotic exposure may affect the gut microbiota, which may in turn influence the risk of AD in infants. These relationships may be shaped by the genetic predisposition.

Editor: Muriel Moser, Université Libre de Bruxelles, Belgium

Funding: This research was supported by a fund (2008-E33030-00, 2009-E33033-00, 2011-E33021-00, 2012-E33012-00) from the Research of Korea Centers for Disease Control and Prevention. The funders had no role in study design, data collection and analysis, decision to publish, or preparation of the manuscripts.

Competing Interests: The authors have declared that no competing interests exist.

* E-mail: sjhong@amc.seoul.kr

Introduction

Although cesarean delivery and prenatal exposure to antibiotics are likely to affect the gut microbiome in infancy [1,2], their effect on the development of atopic dermatitis (AD) in infancy is unclear [3–6].

Microbes are recognized by the innate immune system using pattern recognition receptors (PRRs). cluster-of-differentiation (CD)14 is, together with Toll-like receptor(TLR)4, involve in the recognition and signal transduction of bacterial endotoxin, a major component of the bacterial cell wall of gram negative bacteria. Downstream affects of CD14/TLR receptor activation on antigen presenting cells include the release of cytokines, such as IL-10, and IL-12 [7]. Interleukin (IL)-13 is a cytokine typically produced during Th2 responses and plays a crucial role in atopy and allergic diseases [8].

Several studies show that polymorphisms in the immune system-related genes IL-13 and CD14 associate with AD [9–11]. However, the results from cross-sectional and case-control studies on the influence of these gene polymorphisms on the development of AD in different populations are inconsistent [12–14]. They may reflect differences between the studies in terms of environmental factors that modify genetic associations.

Early microbial contact (i.e., during fetal life and infancy) has been suggested to be involved in the initiation and perpetuation of the aberrant immune activation and responsiveness that plays a central role in the pathogenesis of allergic diseases. This may be particularly true for AD, which appears early in life. Individual immune system-related genotypes may also shape the responsiveness to gut microbes during fetal life and infancy.

It was hypothesized that prenatal exposure to antibiotics and cesarean delivery may affect the gut microbiota in early infancy, which is an important period in the development of the immune system. It was also hypothesized that these prenatal risk factors may be modified by the genetic background. This is the first study to assess how cesarean section birth, prenatal antibiotic exposure, and IL-13 and CD14 risk alleles interact in the development of AD in infancy.

Methods

Ethics Statement

This study was approved by the institutional review board of the Asan Medical Center (IRB No. 2008-0616), the Samsung Medical Center (IRB No. 2009-02-021), the Severance Hospital (IRB No. 4-2008-0588) and the CHA Medical Center (IRB No. 2010-010). Written informed consent was confirmed by each IRB and obtained from the parents of each infant.

Study Population

The Cohort for Childhood Origin of Asthma and Allergic Diseases (COCOA) was composed of the general Korean population after recruiting healthy pregnant women who delivered at four hospitals in a metropolitan city (Seoul). The recruitment period commenced in December 2007. A modified questionnaire of the International Study of Asthma and Allergies in Childhood (ISAAC) was completed by the parents at 36 weeks gestational age [15]. The delivery mode and other prenatal variables were extracted from the maternal and neonatal medical records shortly after delivery. The presence of AD was clinically diagnosed by pediatric allergy specialists using the criteria of Hanifin and Rajka [16] when the infants were followed up at the hospital at 12 months of age.

Of the 534 12-month infants who were enrolled, 122 infants dropped out. At the time the present study was conducted, 412 of the infants met the inclusion criteria: age>1 year, examined for the presence of AD at 12 months by pediatric allergy specialists, and completion of the 12 month questionnaire by the parents.

DNA Collection and SNP Genotyping

Genomic DNA was extracted from the cord blood mononuclear cells of each child and genotyped for the IL-13 rs2569190 and CD14 rs1927911 polymorphisms by using the TagMan fluorogenic 5′ nuclease assay (ABI, Foster City, CA, USA). The endpoint fluorescent readings were performed on an ABI 7900 HT Sequence Detection System (ABI, Foster City, CA, USA).

Duplicate samples and negative controls were included to ensure genotyping accuracy.

Microbial Analysis

Fecal samples were obtained from 11 of the 412 infants in this study at the age of 6 months. Of these, six had both prenatal antibiotic exposure and were delivered by cesarean section, while the remaining five were delivered vaginally and were not exposed to antibiotics prenatally. These infants were selected randomly. The fecal sampling and DNA extraction methods have been described in detail elsewhere [17].

Statistical Analysis

The means and standard deviations or frequencies and percentages of general characteristics were presented for overall study population.

The multivariable logistic regression models were used to estimate odd ratios (OR) and corresponding 95% confidence intervals (95% CI) for comparison of AD at infancy occurrence risk by relevant covariates. The following covariates were considered as potential confounders: gestational age at birth, sex, pre-pregnancy maternal body-mass index (BMI), maternal age at delivery, maternal education level, prenatal exposure to smoke, prenatal exposure to pets, presence of older siblings, and parental allergic disease history. The regression models included a priori potential confounding co-variables which are known risk factors of infant AD established in the literature, and significant variables identified from initial univariate analyses (p<0.2). Data from subjects were divided into 4 groups based on environmental factors (delivery mode and prenatal exposure to antibiotics) and genetic background (parental history of allergic diseases and genotypes) and logistic regression were used to estimate aORs.

Finally, we tested for trends regarding the effect of the number of risk factors (early life environmental factors and genetic polymorphisms) on the development of AD in infancy. P-value for trends was determined using the general linear model for continuous variables.

All statistical tests were two-sided significance levels of p value less than 0.05. Statistical analyses were done with IBM SPSS Statistics 20.0 (IBM SPSS Statistics, Inc., Chicago, IL).

Results

Study Population Characteristics

The study included 412 infants (229 boys and 183 girls) and their families (Table 1). In total, 9.9% of all infants were exposed to antibiotics prenatally and 32.5% were born by cesarean delivery. Moreover, 47.7% of the infants had at least one parent with a history of allergic diseases and 28.2% were diagnosed with AD at 12 months of age.

Relationship between AD in Infancy and Delivery Mode and/or Prenatal Antibiotic Exposure

In multivariable regression analyses, cesarean section increased the odds or AD in infancy by 1.84 (95% CIs 0.95–3.56; p = 0.07) and prenatal antibiotic exposure did not increased (data not shown). The combination of cesarean section and prenatal antibiotic exposure significantly increased the odds of AD in infancy (adjusted OR [aOR] 5.70, 95% CIs 1.19–27.3, p = 0.03). Stool analysis at 6 months of age in 11 randomly selected infants revealed that the total microbiota of the infants with prenatal antibiotic exposure and cesarean delivery was less diverse than the total microbiota of the control infants (Fig. S1).

Table 1. Characteristics of the participating infants.

Individual characteristics	Number (n/d)*	Percentage (%) or mean ± SD
Male gender	229/412	55.6
Gestational age at birth, weeks		39.2±1.2
Maternal education level		
Low	300/393	76.3
High[†]	93/393	23.7
Mother's age at delivery, years		32.3±3.5
Pre-pregnancy maternal body-mass index		20.8±2.7
Prenatal smoking		
No	150/384	39.1
Passive	234/384	60.9
Prenatal exposure to pets	11/381	2.9
Prenatal exposure to antibiotics	38/384	9.9
Mode of delivery		
Vaginal	210/311	67.5
Cesarean section	101/311	32.5
History of parental allergic diseases	178/373	47.7
Older sibling(s)	138/390	35.4
Atopic dermatitis ever	116/412	28.2

*n, number of children with each characteristic; d, the total number of children with information available on this characteristic.
[†]graduated from graduate school.

Effect of Parental Allergic Disease History, Delivery Mode, and/or Prenatal Antibiotic Exposure on the Development of AD in Infancy

Table 2 and table S1 show how the development of AD in infancy related to cesarean section birth and/or prenatal antibiotic exposure when there was an allergic genetic background (defined as one or both parents having a history of allergic disease). In multivariable regression analyses, cesarean section significantly increased the odds of AD in infants when there was a history of parental allergic diseases (aOR 3.46, 95% CI 1.43–8.39, p<0.01, Table 2). Also, cesarean section significantly increased the odds of AD in infants than vaginal delivery in subjects with parental allergic history (aOR 2.83, 95% CI 1.03–7.73, p-value = 0.04, data not shown).

However, prenatal antibiotic exposure did not significantly elevate the odds of AD in infants when there was a parental allergic disease history (Table S1).

When the three factors (parental allergic disease history, cesarean delivery, and prenatal antibiotic exposure) were each defined as risk factor of AD in infancy, multivariable regression analysis revealed that the more risk factors there were, the higher the likelihood that the infant would be diagnosed with AD at the age of 1 year (aOR 10.62, 95% CI 1.28–88.37, p = 0.03; Table 3).

Additive Effects between Cesarean Delivery or Prenatal Antibiotic Exposure and IL-13 or CD14 Gene Polymorphisms on Infant AD Risk

The distributions of two polymorphisms of the IL-13 and CD14 were in Hardy–Weinberg equilibrium. The genetic polymorphisms IL-13 rs20541 and CD14 rs2569190 themselves did not significantly influence the risk of AD in infancy (data not shown). However, compared to vaginally delivered infants with the IL-13 rs20541 GG genotype, vaginally delivered infants with the IL-13 rs20541 GA+AA genotypes tended to have a higher risk of infant AD (aOR 2.37, 95% CIs 0.96–5.84; p = 0.06; Table 4). The

Table 2. Combined effects of mode of delivery and parental history of allergic diseases on the development of atopic dermatitis (AD) at 1 year of age.

Parental history of allergic diseases/Delivery mode	Number (%) of AD	OR (95% CI)	p-value	aOR (95% CI)*	p-value
Negative parental history/Vaginal delivery	25 (23.6)	1.00		1.00	
Negative parental history/C-section delivery	12 (24.5)	1.21 (0.59–2.50)	0.60	1.40 (0.57–3.47)	0.47
Positive parental history/Vaginal delivery	25 (30.9)	2.14 (1.19–3.83)	0.01	1.44 (0.69–3.01)	0.33
Positive parental history/C-section delivery	23 (48.9)	2.69 (1.36–5.29)	<0.01	3.46 (1.43–8.39)	<0.01

*Adjusted for gestational age at birth, sex, pre-pregnancy maternal body-mass index, maternal age at delivery, maternal education level, prenatal exposure to smoke, prenatal exposure to pets, and presence of older sibling(s).

Table 3. Additive effects of mode of delivery, prenatal antibiotic exposure, and parental history of allergic diseases on the development of atopic dermatitis (AD) at 1 year of age.

Number of risk factors[†]	Number (%) of AD	OR (95% CI)	p-value	aOR (95% CI)*	p-value
Risk (0)	20 (21.3)	1.00		1.00	
Risk (1)	35 (28.9)	1.51 (0.80–2.83)	0.20	1.83 (0.89–3.73)	0.10
Risk (2)	22 (42.3)	2.71 (1.30–5.68)	0.01	3.10 (1.28–7.51)	0.01
Risk (3)	5 (62.5)	6.17 (1.36–28.03)	0.02	10.62 (1.28–88.37)	0.03
Trend P-value			0.001		0.001

*Adjusted for gestational age at birth, sex, pre-pregnancy maternal body-mass index, maternal age at delivery, maternal education level, prenatal exposure to smoke, prenatal exposure to pets, and presence of older sibling(s).
[†]Risk factors were: parental history of allergic diseases, prenatal use of antibiotics, and cesarean delivery.

infants who had the GG genotype had a significantly higher risk of AD if they were delivered by cesarean section (aOR 3.85, 95% CI 1.25–11.83, p = 0.02). This effect of cesarean section was even more pronounced in infants who had the GA+AA genotypes (aOR 4.70, 95% CIs 1.43–15.40; p = 0.01).

With regard to the CD14 genotypes, compared to vaginally delivered infants with the CD14 rs2569190 TT genotype, infants with the TT genotype who were born by cesarean section tended to have a higher risk of AD (aOR 3.11, 95% CIs 0.80–12.12, p = 0.10). This effect of cesarean section became significant in infants who had the CD14 rs2569190 TC+CC genotypes (aOR 3.56, 95% CI 1.12–11.36, p = 0.03; Table 3). Combined effect between CD14 rs2569190 and delivery mode has a significant trend P-value (P = 0.02).

With regard to prenatal antibiotic exposure, multivariable regression analysis revealed that there was a statistically significant trend for an association between this factor and IL-13 rs20541 genotype (trend p-value<0.05, data not shown). This trend was not observed for the CD14 rs2569190 genotype.

Additive Effects between Unfavorable Genotypes and One or Two Environmental Risk Factors on the Development of AD in Infancy

The subjects were divided into four groups according to the number of risk factors, namely the presence of unfavorable IL-13 rs20541 or CD14 rs2569190 genotypes, prenatal antibiotic

exposure, and cesarean delivery. The risk of AD in each group was then assessed relative to the group who had none of the three risk factors (Fig. 1 and Table S2). In terms of the IL-13 rs20541 genotype, the aOR for AD rose as the number of risk factors increased (one risk factor: aOR 2.59, 95% CIs 1.04–6.45; two risk factors: aOR 5.09, 95% CIs 1.57–16.52; three risk factors: aOR 9.56, 95% CIs 0.81–112.97; trend p-value<0.01). Although the statistical power to conduct analyses with the CD14 rs2569190 genotype was limited, the AD risk also rose as the number of risk factors increased (trend p-value 0.03, Table S2). Thus, unfavorable genotypes and exposure to prenatal environmental risk factors appeared act addictively in increasing AD risk in infancy.

Discussion

This prospective birth cohort study showed for the first time that the impact of important intestinal microbiota-shaping risk factors (the delivery mode and prenatal antibiotic exposure) on the early development of AD can be modified by the genetic background (functional IL-13 and CD14 gene variants) in a additive fashion. The present study also showed that cesarean delivery and prenatal antibiotic exposure may affect the gut microbiota diversity in infants.

Although cesarean section and prenatal antibiotic exposure did not associate independently with an increased AD risk in infancy, infants who were delivered by cesarean section and had been exposed prenatally to antibiotics were more likely to have AD than

Table 4. Combined effects of IL-13 or CD14 genetic variations and delivery mode on the development of atopic dermatitis (AD) at 1 year of age.

IL-13 rs20541/Delivery mode	Number (%) of AD	OR (95% CI)	p-value	aOR (95% CI)*	p-value
GG/Vaginal delivery	17 (22.7)	1.00		1.00	
GA+AA/Vaginal delivery	27 (26.7)	1.24 (0.61–2.54)	0.55	2.37 (0.96–5.84)	0.06
GG/C-section delivery	15 (45.5)	2.84 (1.19–6.81)	0.02	3.85 (1.25–11.83)	0.02
GA+AA/C-section delivery	13 (43.3)	2.61 (1.06–6.43)	0.04	4.70 (1.43–15.40)	0.01
CD14 rs2569190/Delivery mode					
TT/Vaginal delivery	13 (23.6)	1.00		1.00	
TC+CC/Vaginal delivery	28 (26.7)	1.18 (0.55–2.51)	0.68	1.34 (0.53–3.44)	0.54
TT/C-section delivery	9 (42.9)	2.42 (0.84–7.03)	0.10	3.11 (0.80–12.12)	0.10
TC+CC/C-section delivery	17 (43.6)	2.50 (1.03–6.06)	0.04	3.56 (1.12–11.36)	0.03

*Adjusted for gestational age at birth, sex, pre-pregnancy maternal body-mass index, maternal age at delivery, maternal education level, prenatal exposure to smoke, prenatal exposure to pets, presence of older sibling(s), and parental history of allergic diseases.

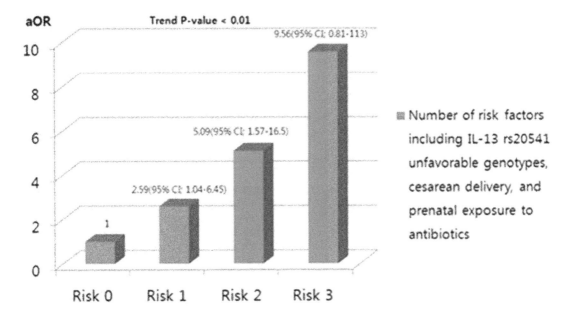

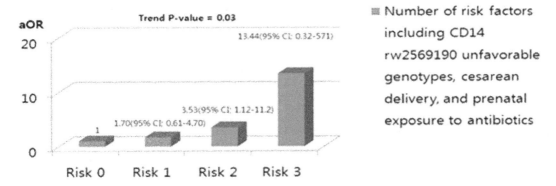

Figure 1. Additive effects of unfavorable IL-13 or CD14 genotypes, prenatal antibiotic exposure, and delivery mode on the development of atopic dermatitis in infancy. (A) IL-13 rs20541 genotype. (B) CD14 rs2569190 genotype. aOR, odds ratio adjusted for gestational age at birth, sex, pre-pregnancy maternal body-mass index, maternal age at delivery, maternal education level, prenatal exposure to smoke, prenatal exposure to pets, presence of older sibling(s), and parental history of allergic diseases.

those who were born vaginally and had not had prenatal antibiotic exposure. This trend was particularly notable in infants who carried risk-associated genotypes or whose parents had an allergic disease history. The present study confirms that the influence of cesarean section and prenatal antibiotic exposure on the development of AD should be assessed in the context of individual genetic susceptibility (e.g., parental allergic disease history). Another study reported a similar observation: Norwegian children who were born by cesarean section and had a maternal history of allergy had a 9-fold higher likelihood of food allergy than those

who were born by vaginal delivery and had no maternal history of allergy [18].

In early life, the intestinal microbial composition changes markedly. A previous study showed that the mode of delivery significantly influences the microbiota composition of the intestine of neonates [19]. Interestingly, previous studies have also shown that the intestinal microbiota of cesarean section-born infants is similar to the microbiota of infants born to mothers who received antibiotics during late pregnancy and/or while breastfeeding [20,21]. Other studies also reported that in cesarean delivered infants, there was a delay in fecal colonization and low numbers of *Bacteroides fragilis* [22,23]. Moreover, in the first year of life, infants delivered by cesarean section do not catch up to vaginally delivered infants in terms of colonization by *Bacteroides* and *Escherichia coli* [24]. Hence, cesarean section and prenatal antibiotic exposure may promote the suboptimal development of the microbiota in infancy to similar extents. The present study showed that infants who had been exposed to antibiotics prenatally and were born by cesarean delivery had lower total microbiota diversity in the stool at 6 month of age than infants who did not have prenatal exposure to antibiotics and were born by vaginal delivery. The two groups did not differ significantly in terms of any of the dominant bacterial genera probably because of the small sample size. Thus, the findings of the present study support the notion that prenatal antibiotic exposure and delivery mode may affect the gut microbiota.

Although the gut microbiota is believed to play an intermediate role in the causal pathway between mode of delivery and AD, only one study has assessed this role directly [25]. That study showed that mode and place of delivery affect the gut microbiota at 1 month of age, especially in terms of *Clostridium difficile* colonization, and that this subsequently influences the risk of atopic manifestations at the age of 6–7 years. That study also showed that gut microbiota composition and mode and place of delivery both mainly associated with the development of allergic diseases in children with a positive family history of atopy. The present study demonstrated for the first time that not only cesarean delivery but also prenatal exposure to antibiotics play an important role in the development of AD in infancy, particularly in infants carrying IL-13 and CD14 genetic susceptibility alleles.

The present study showed that while cesarean section itself may influence the development of AD in infancy, this effect was enhanced in infants carrying the IL-13 rs20541 GA+AA genotypes. IL-13 rs20541 is a single nucleotide polymorphism (SNP) in the coding region of the IL-13 gene. In our previous study, children with the IL-13 GA+AA polymorphisms were found to be at increased risk of allergic rhinitis if they were exposed to mold in the home during their first year of life [26], and were associated with susceptibility of asthma [27]. For this reason, and because the combined effects between cesarean section or prenatal antibiotic exposure and IL-13 SNPs had not yet been examined, the IL-13 rs20541 SNP was selected for our study.

The present study also supports the notion that the C allele of the CD14 SNP rs2569190 confers a risk of AD in infants who are born by cesarean section. In rodents, oral exposure to lipopoly-saccharides during vaginal birth activates gut epithelial cells [28]. By contrast, gut epithelial activation is not found in mice born by cesarean section. The Allergy and Endotoxin (ALEX) Study [29] supported the endotoxin switch theory that the C allele of CD14 rs2569190 confers risk at low endotoxin exposure whereas the T allele confers risk at high endotoxin exposure. Thus, infants with the C allele of CD14 SNP rs2569190 may be at higher risk of AD if their endotoxin exposure is low because their microbiota is undeveloped due to cesarean delivery and prenatal antibiotic exposure.

The strengths of the present study include its prospective nature and its population-based design. This is the first study to assess how cesarean section, prenatal antibiotic exposure, and gene susceptibility alleles interact in the development of AD in infancy while adjusting for other prenatal environment factors. We acknowledge that it also has some limitations. The main limitations are the relatively smaller sample size compared to those in similar studies. Our findings should be confirmed by larger studies. In addition, this study focused on only two well-known candidate genes that are involved in Th1/Th2 balance. It remains likely that other, as-yet unknown but important, genes can also regulate the influence of cesarean section and prenatal antibiotic exposure on the development of AD in infancy. However, IL-13 and CD14 genes are good candidate genes in terms of allergic susceptibility and innate immunity since several studies have shown that IL-13 rs1295685 and CD14 rs20541 play an important role in the development of allergic diseases in Korean children [26,27,30]. Another possible limitation is that the diet history of the infants in this study was not considered. As a result, the present study focused largely on the prenatal environmental factors that may influence the development of AD in infancy. We showed the limited results of difference of gut microbiota in small population because it is very difficult to find the pregnant women who had used antibiotics during pregnancy.

Conclusions

We found that cesarean section, prenatal antibiotic exposure, and unfavorable risk alleles acted additively to promote the development of AD in infancy. The present findings suggest that further studies that evaluate the effect of gut microbiota on AD in the context of individual genetic variation are warranted. The type of information yielded by such studies might enable physicians in the future to provide more personalized medical care and advice to mothers that will reduce the risk of AD in their children.

Acknowledgments

The authors thank DongSan Lee for organizing the data. We would also like to express our gratitude to Dong-in Seo and Hyeung-Jong Yang for their comments and support. The authors thank Hee-Sook Kim for laboratory support. We also thank Sung-Ok Kwon, Se-Young Oh, Cheol Min Lee, Soo-Young Oh, Kyung-Sook Lee, and Yee-Jin Shin for their participation in the study. Finally, we would like to thank Ho Kim and Kim Clara Tammy for their support in statistical analysis.

Author Contributions

Conceived and designed the experiments: So-Yeon Lee JY KMA KWK YHS HBK WKK DJS GCJ JYS Soo-Young Lee JYK SJH. Performed the experiments: JY KMA KWK YHS SJC KJL HJP HSW YHJ EL SIY JHS JWK BJK. Analyzed the data: KSL SAH HSY MJK HYK. Contributed reagents/materials/analysis tools: KSL SAH. Wrote the paper: So-Yeon Lee KSL SAH SJH.

References

1. Adlerberth I, Lindberg E, Åberg N, Hesselmar B, Saalman R, et al. (2006) Reduced enterobacterial and increased staphylococcal colonization of the infantile bowel: an effect of hygienic lifestyle? Pediatr Res 59: 96–101.
2. Antonopoulos DA, Huse SM, Morrison HG, Schmidt TM, Sogin ML, et al. (2009) Reproducible community dynamics of the gastrointestinal microbiota following antibiotic perturbation. Infec Immun 77: 2367–2375.
3. Pistiner M, Gold DR, Abdulkerim H, Hoffman E, Celedón JC (2008) Birth by cesarean section, allergic rhinitis, and allergic sensitization among children with a parental history of atopy. J Allergy Clin Immunol 122: 274–279.
4. Laubereau B, Filipiak-Pittroff B, von Berg A, Grübl A, Reinhardt D, et al. (2004) Caesarean section and gastrointestinal symptoms, atopic dermatitis, and sensitization during the first year of life. Arch Dis Child 89: 993–997.

5. Dom S, Droste JHJ, Sariachvili MA, Hagendorens MM, Oostveen E, et al. (2010) Pre-and post-natal exposure to antibiotics and the development of eczema, recurrent wheezing and atopic sensitization in children up to the age of 4 years. Clin Exp Allergy 40: 1378–1387.

6. MaKeever TM, Lewis SA, Smith C, Hubbard R (2002) The importance of prenatal exposures on the development of allergic disease: a birth cohort study using the west midlands general practice database. Am J Respir Crit Care Med 166: 827–832.

7. Vercelli D (2003) Innate immunity: sensing the environment and regulation the regulators. Curr Opin Allergy Clin Immunol 3: 343–346.

8. Wills-Karp M (2004) Interleukin-13 in asthma pathogenesis. Immunol Rev 202: 175–190.

9. Namkung JH, Lee JE, Kim E, Kim HJ, Seo EY, et al. (2011) Association of polymorphisms in genes encoding IL-4, IL-13 and their receptors with atopic dermatitis in a Korean population. Exp Dermatol 20: 915–919.

10. He JQ, Chan-Yeung M, Becker AB, Dimich-Ward H, Ferguson AC, et al. (2003) Genetic variants of the IL13 and IL4 genes and atopic diseases in at-risk children. Genes Immun 4: 385–389.

11. Litonjua AA, Bracken MB, Celedón JC, Milton DK, Bracken MB, et al. (2005) Polymorphisms in the 5' region of the CD14 gene are associated with eczema in young children. J Allergy Clin Immunol 115: 1056–1062.

12. Arshad SH, Karmaus W, Kurukulaaratchy R, Sadeghnejad A, Huebner M, et al. (2008) Polymorphisms in the interleukin 13 and GATA binding protein 3 genes and the development of eczema during childhood. Br J Dermatol 158: 1315–1322.

13. Sengler C, Haider A, Sommerfeld C, Lau S, Baldini M, et al. (2003) Evaluation of the CD14 C-159T polymorphism in the German Multicenter Allergy Study cohort. Clin Exp Allergy 33: 166–169.

14. Weidinger S, Novak N, Klopp N, Baurecht H, Wagenpfeil S, et al. (2006) Lack of association between toll-like receptor 2 and toll-like receptor 4 polymorphisms and atopic eczema. J Allergy Clin Immunol 118: 277–279.

15. Kim HB, Ahn KM, Kim KY, Shin YH, Seo JH, et al. (2012) Cord blood cellular proliferative response as a predictive factor for atopic dermatitis at 12 months. J Korean Med Sci 27: 1320–1326.

16. Hanifin JM, Rajka G (1980) Diagnostic features of atopic dermatitis. Acta Derm Venereol Suppl (Stockh) 92: 44–47.

17. Kim BS, Kim JN, Yoon SH, Chun J, Cerniglia CE (2012) Impact of enrofloxacin on the human intestinal microbiota by comparative molecular analysis. Anaerobe 18: 310–320.

18. Eggesbø M, Botten G, Stigum H, Nafstad P, Magnus P (2003) Is delivery by cesarean section a risk of food allergy? J Allergy Clin Immunol 112: 420–426.

19. Hooper LV (2004) Bacterial contributions to mammalian gut development. Trends Microbiol 12: 129–134.

20. Fallani M, Young D, Scott J, Norin E, Amarri S, et al. (2010) Intestinal microbiota of 6-week-old infants across Europe. Geographic influence beyond delivery mode, breast-feeding, and antibiotics. JPGN 51: 77–84.

21. Adlerberth I, Strachan DP, Matricardi PM, Ahrné S, Orfei L, et al. (2007) Gut microbiota and development of atopic eczema in 3 European birth cohorts. J Allergy Clin Immunol 120: 343–350.

22. Orrhage K, Nord CE (1999) Factors controlling the bacterial colonization of the intestine in breastfed infants. Acta paediatr 88: 47–57.

23. Gronlund MM, Lehtonen OP, Eerola E, Kero P (1999) Fecal microflora in healthy infants born by different methods of delivery: permanent changes in intestinal flora after cesarean delivery. J Pediatr Gastroenterol Nutr 28: 19–25.

24. Adlerberth I, Lindberg E, Aberg N, Hesselmar N, Saalman R, et al. (2006) Reduced enterobacterial and increased staphylococcal colonization of the infantile bowel: an effect of hygienic lifestyle? Pediatr Res 59: 96–101.

25. van Nimwegen FA, Penders J, Stobberingh EE, Postma DS, Koppelman GH, et al. (2011) Mode and place of delivery, gastrointestinal microbiota, and their influence on asthma and atopy. J Allergy Clin Immunol 128: 948–955.

26. Kim WK, Kwon JW, Seo JH, Kim HY, Yu J, et al. (2012) Interaction between IL13 genotype and environmental factors in the risk for allergic rhinitis in Korean children. J Allergy Clin Immunol 130: 421–426.

27. Kim HB, Kang MJ, Lee SY, Jin HS, Kim JH, et al. (2008) Combined effect of tumor necrosis factor-alpha and interleukin-13 polymorphisms on bronchial hyperresponsiveness in Korean children with asthma. Clin Exp Allergy 38: 774–780.

28. Lotz M, Gutle D, Walther S, Ménard S, Bogdan C, et al. (2006) Postnatal acquisition of endotoxin tolerance in intestinal epithelial cells. J Exp Med 203: 973–984.

29. Eder W, Klimecki W, Yu L, von Mutius E, Rieder J, et al. (2005) Opposite effects of CD14/-260 on serum IgE levels in children raised in different environments. J Allergy Clin Immunol 116: 601–607.

30. Hong SJ, Kim HB, Kang MJ, Lee SY, Kim JH, et al. (2007) TNF-a(-308 G/A) and CD14(-159 T/C) polymorphisms in the bronchial responsiveness of Korean children with asthma. J Allergy Clin Immnol 119: 398–404.

2

Filaggrin Gene Defects Are Independent Risk Factors for Atopic Asthma in a Polish Population: A Study in ECAP Cohort

Joanna Ponińska[1], Bolesław Samoliński[2], Aneta Tomaszewska[2], Filip Raciborski[2], Piotr Samel-Kowalik[2], Artur Walkiewicz[2], Agnieszka Lipiec[2], Barbara Piekarska[2], Jarosław Komorowski[2], Edyta Krzych-Fałta[2], Andrzej Namysłowski[2], Jacek Borowicz[2], Grażyna Kostrzewa[1], Sławomir Majewski[3], Rafał Płoski[1]*

1 Department of Medical Genetics, Medical University of Warsaw, Warsaw, Poland, 2 Department of Prevention of Environmental Hazards and Allergology, Medical University of Warsaw, Warsaw, Poland, 3 Department of Dermatology and Venereology, Medical University of Warsaw, Warsaw, Poland

Abstract

Background: FLG null variants of which 2282del4 and R501X are the most frequent in Caucasians are established risk factors for atopic dermatitis (AD) with an effect probably mediated through impairment of epidermal barrier. Among subjects with AD FLG defects are also consistently associated with asthma and allergic rhinitis (AR) but it is less clear to what extent these associations are also present independently from skin disease. The aim of the present study was to evaluate the role of 2282del4 and R501X in predisposing to these allergic phenotypes in a Polish population.

Methodology: 2282del4 and R501X were typed among 3,802 participants of the Epidemiology of Allergic Diseases in Poland (ECAP) survey, a cross-sectional population-based study using ECRHS II and ISAAC questionnaires, and ambulatory examination.

Principal Findings: The FLG null variants were associated with AD (OR = 2.01, CI: 1.20–3.36, P = 0.007), allergic rhinitis (in particular persistent form, OR = 1.69, CI:1.12–2.54, P = 0.011), and asthma (in particular atopic asthma, OR = 2.22, CI:1.24–3.96, P = 0.006). Association with atopic asthma (but not persistent allergic rhinitis) was also present in the absence of AD, (OR = 2.02, CI: 1.07–3.81, P = 0.027) as well as in the absence of AD and history of broadly defined inflammatory skin disease (OR = 2.30, CI: 1.07–4.93, P = 0.03). Association to atopic asthma would have not been found if diagnosis was made by questionnaire only (OR = 1.15, CI: 0.58–2.32, P = 0.8). We did not observe an association between FLG variants and allergic sensitizations (P = 0.8) or total IgE. (P = 0.6).

Conclusions/Significance: In a Polish population FLG 2282del4 and R501X carriage increases risk for development of AD and atopic asthma (also in the absence of AD or history thereof). This suggests that interventions aimed at restoring epidermal barrier may have a general role in asthma prophylaxis/treatment.

Editor: Jacques Zimmer, Centre de Recherche Public de la Santé (CRP-Santé), Luxembourg

Funding: The work was financed by grants from Polish Ministry of Science and Higher Education, Ministry of Health grant nr 6P052005C/06572, and Warsaw Medical University grant nr 1WY/NK1W/2009. The funders had no role in study design, data collection and analysis, decision to publish, or preparation of the manuscript.

Competing Interests: The authors have declared that no competing interests exist.

* E-mail: rploski@wp.pl

Introduction

Filaggrin gene (*FLG*) is strongly expressed in the granular cells of the epidermis leading to production of a large precursor protein profilaggrin. In the process of differentiation profilaggrin is proteolytically cleaved into functional filaggrin peptides which bind and collapse the keratin cytoskeleton and subsequently are degraded into hydrophilic amino acids forming the natural moisturizing factor. The N-terminal domain of profilaggrin is likely to have an additional function as it specifically localizes to the nucleus. All these processes are critical for creation of epidermal barrier with appropriate mechanical and biochemical properties [1].

FLG null variants are strong risk factor for AD [2,3]. In Caucasians two such variants are particularly common: 2282del4

and R501X with originally reported carrier rates in general population of ~2 and 6%, respectively [2]. Both variants result in a complete loss of processed filaggrin due to premature termination codons within the first *FLG* repeat. Whereas several new *FLG* variants have been reported they are substantially less prevalent and qualitatively different with some residual function [4].

Among subjects with AD *FLG* defects are associated with other allergic disease such as asthma and allergic rhinitis (AR) however, it is less clear to what extent these associations are present independently from skin disease [5]. Two meta-analyses concluded that there was no association between *FLG* null variants and asthma among subjects without AD although the ORs from pooled estimates suggested a trend in the direction of association

[5,6]. Regarding association with AR in the absence of AD two studies reported conflicting results: Weideinger et al. [7] found an effect whereas Marenholz et al. did not [8].

Our purpose was to examine in a Polish population association of the 2282del4 and R501X *FLG* loss-of-function variants with AD, asthma and allergic rhinitis.

Materials and Methods

Ethics Statement

The study was approved by Ethical Committee of Medical University of Warsaw. All ECAP subjects gave an informed written consent including specific consent to genetic testing. Written consent for anonymous use of DNA was also obtained from subjects undergoing paternity tests whose samples were used to verify population prevalence of R501X.

Subjects

The study was based on participants of Epidemiology of Allergic Diseases in Poland (ECAP, www.ECAP.pl) living in major metropolitan areas of Poland (Katowice, Wrocław, Lublin, Gdańsk, Warszawa, Poznań and Białystok). ECAP is a continuation of the European Community Respiratory Health Survey II (ECRHS II) and International Study of Asthma and Allergy in Childhood (ISAAC). ECAP includes randomly selected population aged 20–44 y.o. (ECRHS standard) as well as 6–7 y.o. and 13–14 y.o. (ISAAC standard). The recruitment was done by a randomization procedure based on the personal identity number (PESEL). Out of the 25262 subjects who were approached by pollsters, 9446 refused participation (response rate −62.6%). In the present analysis two of the questionnaire's answers were used (i) "Have you ever had asthma?", (ii) "Have you ever had eczema, atopic dermatitis or other inflammatory skin condition".

Those who completed questionnaire were invited for an ambulatory examination. Four thousand thirty eight subjects (25.5%) have taken up the offer. The examination included medical history, physical examination, spirometry, PNIF (Peak Nasal Inspiratory Flow) and skin prick tests with 15 allergens: hazel, alder, birch, grasses/grain, rye, Artemisia, plantain, Alternaria, Cladosporium, molds I (Alternaria tenuis, Botrytis cinerea, Cladosporium herbarum, Culvularia lunata, Fusarium moniliforme, Helminthosporium), molds II (Aspergillus fumigatus, Mucor mucedo, Penicillium notatum, Rhizopus nigricans, Serpula lacrymans, Pullularia pullulans), Dermatophagoides pteronyssinus, Dermatophagoides farinae, dog, cat, negative control, histamine.

Concentration of total IgE in serum was determined with reagents of the Phadia CAP System [9] (N = 3440) or the Allergopharma-ELISA-Test [10] (N = 712). The obtained data were presented in IU/ml (international units per mililitre).

The clinical diagnoses of asthma (atopic or non atopic), intermittent allergic rhinitis (i.e. with symptoms present <4 days a week or for <4 consecutive weeks), persistent allergic rhinitis, (i.e. with symptoms present >4 days a week and for >4 consecutive weeks) and atopic dermatitis were based on the International Global Initiative for Asthma (GINA) guidelines [11], ARIA criteria [12,13], and criteria of Hanifin and Rajka [14], for asthma, allergic rhinitis and atopic dermatitis, respectively. In addition a history of food allergy, drug allergy, insect bite allergy, urticaria, Quincke's oedema or other chronic diseases was obtained. During the examination blood samples were collected.

While analyzing associations between *FLG* variants and allergic disorders comparisons were performed against a group of healthy controls (N = 1865), defined as individuals without any allergic disorder or other chronic disease (including ichtyosis vulgaris)

based on performed clinical workup and history. Family history of atopy or other disease(s) was not an exclusion criterion.

Due to faulty blood sample collection (wrong labeling, degradation) the final genetic analysis was carried in 94% of those who underwent medical exam, i.e. 3802 subjects: 951 children 6–7 y.o. (47.6% females), 1054 children 13–14 y.o. (49.2% females) and 1797 adults (60.7% females).

Genetic analysis

Genomic DNA was extracted from whole blood. Typing for 2282del4 was performed by sizing of fluorescently labeled PCR product on ABI 3130 sequencer, typing for R501X was done by PCR-RFLP with *NlaIII* restrictase (1639 samples) or TaqMan allelic discrimination assay (2323 samples). One hundred sixty samples were typed for R501X by both methods with complete concordance. All these methods were described previously [2,8,15]. During typing every positive sample was repeated by reanalysis of DNA from the original stock. Whole screening was blinded to diagnoses.

Statistical analysis

In the analysis heterozygous and homozygous genotypes were pooled. Statistical significance of differences in genotype frequency among analyzed groups was assessed with chi square test or Fisher's exact test as appropriate. The strength of association was estimated by calculating Odss Ratio (OR) with 95% confidence interval (CI). Given the reports on the role of the *FLG* null variants in predisposing to AD, asthma and AR no correction for multiple testing was applied. Deviation from Hardy-Weinberg equilibrium was assessed by a Chi-square test with one degree of freedom. Total IgE concentration was log transformed to achieve normal distribution and presented means are geometric means (i.e. back transformed). In the analysis of *FLG* status vs. total IgE the adjustment for test-method, sex and age was performed by univariate ANOVA.

In our study we could detect the following effects with the power of 0.8 at alpha = 0.05: asthma–OR = 2.0, allergic rhinitis–OR = 1.7, atopic dermatitis–OR = 2.3 and allergic sensitization–OR = 1.5.

Calculations were performed with *Statistica* package.

Results

The FLG R501X variant is rare in a Polish population

While analyzing the 3802 subjects from ECAP cohort we identified 3629 wild type, 140 heterozygous and three homozygous 2282del4 genotypes (carriage rate: 3.76%, CI: 3.20–4.41) as well as 30 heterozygous R501X genotypes (carriage rate: 0.8%, CI: 0.55–1.12). There were no compound heterozygotes. In order to verify relatively low frequency of R501X vs. 2282del4 variant in a Polish population we also tested 510 samples randomly selected from an anonymous bank containing DNA isolated for the purpose of paternity tests [16]. We found 19 samples positive for 2282del4 (carriage rate: 3.79%, CI: 2.44–8.85) and five positive for R501X (carriage rate: 1.0%, CI: 0.43–2.31). The distribution of *FLG* variants did not deviate from Hardy-Weinberg equilibrium in either cohort (P = 0.5 in both cases).

Associations between FLG variants and studied phenotypes

When analyzing distribution of combined *FLG* variants we found an association with AD (OR = 2.01, P = 0.007), asthma (OR = 1.70, P = 0.024) and AR (OR = 1.43, P = 0.046, Table 1). Analysis of individual variants showed statistically significant associations between 2282del4 and AD (OR = 1.92, P = 0.022), asthma (OR = 1.97, P = 0.005), and AR (OR = 1.47, P = 0.047, Table 1).

Further analysis indicated that the statistically significant associations between 2282del4 or combined genotype and asthma as well as AR were limited, respectively, to atopic asthma (AA) and persistent AR (pAR, Table 1).

We noted that when subjects were stratified according to the answer to the question: 'Have you ever had asthma' the frequency of *FLG* variants was statistically significantly increased only among those who were diagnosed with asthma by a physician during the present study but who were not aware of having the disease as judged by questionnaire data (OR = 1.81, P = 0.03 and OR = 3.53, P = 0.00005, for the comparison of combined genotype frequency vs. healthy controls, for all asthma and AA, respectively, Table 2). Had the study been based solely on questionnaire data, only a trend for association between combined *FLG* variants and asthma would have been found (OR = 1.15, P = 0.83, Table 2).

In ECAP cohort there was no association between *FLG* variants and allergic sensitizations or total IgE concentration. The prevalence of the combined genotype was 4.7% (78/1676) vs. 4.5% (95/2126) among those with a positive skin-prick test to at least one allergen and the remaining group, respectively (OR = 1.04, CI:0.77–1.42, P = 0.8). Mean concentration of total IgE was 9.08 (CI: 7.38–11.17) vs. 9.62 (CI: 9.20–10.06) for those with and without *FLG* defects, respectively (P = 0.6, analysis adjusted for test-method, sex and age category).

The association between FLG null variants and atopic asthma (AA) is also found among those without atopic dermatitis (AD) or history thereof

Although the OR for AA conferred by 2282del4 or the combined genotype was higher among those with than those without AD (OR = 4.37 vs. OR = 2.23, and OR = 3.61 vs. OR = 2.02, respectively) the associations were statistically significant in both subgroups (P<0.03, Table 3). Analysis of pAR showed similar trends although the statistical significance of these associations among those without AD was borderline (P = 0.049 and P = 0.053, for 2282del4 and combined *FLG* variants, respectively (Table 4).

The frequency of the combined genotype showed a trend for increase among subjects who were not diagnosed with AD but

who reported history of an inflammatory skin condition in the questionnaire (OR = 1.38, CI: 0.96–2.0, P = 0.08, comparison vs. healthy controls). Thus, we were interested whether the observed associations between *FLG* variants and AA among those without AD could be caused by an association among those with a history of AD or other inflammatory skin disease. However, this was not apparent since there was an association between 2282del4 or combined genotype and AA also among subjects without AD according to both clinical diagnosis and self reported history of an inflammatory skin condition: 7.1% (7/99) vs. 3.1% (55/1790), OR = 2.40 (CI: 1.06–5.42), P = 0.03 and 8.1% (8/99) vs. 3.7% (66/1790), OR = 2.30 (CI: 1.07–4.93), P = 0.03, for 2282del4 and combined genotype, respectively.

Since the chances of AD resolution increase with age we also analyzed the association between AA and *FLG* variants among those without AD in the youngest age group (i.e. children 6–7 y.o.). Among those with AA the prevalence of 2282del4 and the combined genotype was 12.9% (4/31) which was higher than among controls (OR = 4.53, CI: 1.54–13.38, P = 0.018 and OR = 3.74, CI: 1.28–10.98, P = 0.032, for 2282del4 and the combined genotype, respectively).

Conversely, analysis of pAR did not show associations with *FLG* variants among those without AD according to both the questionnaire and clinical diagnosis: 3.8% (13/340) vs. 3.1% (55/1790), OR = 1.25 (CI: 0.68–2.32, P = 0.5), and 4.7% (16/340) vs. 3.7% (66/1790), OR = 1.29 (CI: 0.74–2.26, P = 0.4) for prevalence of 2282del4 and the combined genotype among pAR and healthy controls, respectively.

Discussion

While studying a population based cohort of subjects we observed that the *FLG* defects conferred an increased risk for development of AD, AR (in particular pAR) and asthma (in particular AA). Whereas both associations were particularly strong among subjects with AD, the association with AA remained after exclusion of subjects with current AD even when analysis was limited to the youngest age group, i.e. a group with the lowest chance of complete resolution of skin disease. Association between AA and *FLG* variants was also present among those without current AD or history of AD or other inflammatory skin disease.

The association between *FLG* defects and AA in the absence of AD contrasts with conclusions of two recent meta-analyses

Table 1. Prevalence of *FLG* variants according to clinical diagnosis.

| Diagnosis | n | 2282del4 | | | R501X | | | 2282del4 or R501X | | |
		n (%)	OR (95%CI)	P	n (%)	OR (95%CI)	P	n (%)	OR (95%CI)	P
Atopic Dermatitis	271	16 (5.9)	1.92 (1.09–3.39)	0.022	4 (1.5)	2.31 (0.74–7.22)	0.14	20 (7.4)	2.01(1.20–3.36)	0.007
Asthma										
All	414	25 (6.0)	1.97 (1.22–3.18)	0.005	1 (0.2)	0.37 (0.05–2.89)	0.3	26 (6.3)	1.70 (1.07–2.69)	0.024
Atopic	186	14 (7.5)	2.49 (1.36–4.56)	0.002	1 (0.5)	0.84 (0.11–6.46)	0.9	15 (8.1)	2.22 (1.24–3.96)	0.006
Non-atopic	228	11 (4.8)	1.55 (0.8–3.0)	0.19	0	NA	0.2	11 (4.8)	1.28 (0.67–2.46)	0.5
Allergic Rhinitis										
All[1]	1114	51 (4.6)	1.47 (1.01–2.15)	0.047	8 (0.7)	1.22 (0.49–3.04)	0.7	59 (5.3)	1.43 (1.01–2.04)	0.046
persistent	591	33 (5.6)	1.81 (1.17–2.8)	0.007	4 (0.7)	1.05 (0.34–3.28)	0.9	37 (6.3)	1.69 (1.12–2.54)	0.011
intermittent	497	17 (3.4)	1.08 (0.63–1.88)	0.7	4 (0.8)	1.37 (0.43–4.31)	0.59	21 (4.2)	1.31 (0.69–1.86)	0.63
Healthy controls	1865	59 (3.2)			12 (0.6)			71 (3.8)		

[1]In 24 subjects allergic rhinitis could not be classified as intermittent or persistent; NA not applicable; All comparisons vs. healthy controls.

Table 2. Prevalence of the *FLG* variants vs. concordance between diagnosis of asthma (all kinds or atopic asthma) by a physician (i.e. diagnosed during the present study) and individual awareness of having asthma (all kinds) according to questionnaire data.

Diagnosis:			2282del4	R501X	2282del4 or R501X	OR (CI) P *
Physician	Questionnaire	N	n (%)	n (%)	n (%)	
All asthma						
+	+	127	7 (5.5)	0	7 (5.5)	1.47 (0.68–3.22) 0.34
+	-	269	17 (6.3)	1 (0.4)	18 (6.7)	**1.81 (1.07–3.07) 0.03**
Atopic asthma						
+	+	61	2 (3.3)	0	2 (3.3)	0.86 (0.23–3.25) 0.9
+	-	116	12 (10.3)	1 (0.9)	13 (11.2)	**3.53 (1.86–6.72) 0.00005**
Asthma (all) by questionnaire irrespective of physician's diagnosis		206	9 (4.4)	0	9 (4.4)	1.15 (0.58–2.32) 0.83
Healthy controls		1865	59 (3.2)	12 (0.6)	71 (3.8)	

* Calculated for the comparison of the frequency of the combined genotype (2282del4 or R501X) vs. healthy controls. Cells with P values <0.05 are **boldfaced**; Questionnaire data were not available in 18 subjects with asthma including 9 with AA.

although it should be noted that both these studies reported trends in the direction of association (OR = 1.11 and OR = 1.30) [5,6].

On one hand, some cases of resolved AD might have been missed in our study due to lack of patients'/parents' recall. Recall errors regarding history of allergic diseases have been demonstrated [17] and are likely to exist also in our cohort. On the other hand, the discrepancy with pervious studies [5,6] might also be caused by population specific genetic, environmental and/or life style factors as well as methodological issues. In our cohort the association between *FLG* null variants and asthma (in particular AA) was found preferentially (exclusively?) among those who were not aware of having the disease. This suggests that AA associated with *FLG* defects in the absence of AD may have a subtle phenotype being particularly difficult to diagnose by family practitioners. Notwithstanding the precise reasons for the discussed discrepancies, our results indicate that in a Polish population *FLG* defects represent a risk factor for asthma, irrespective of apparent skin disease or history thereof which it is possible to elicit in a clinical setting.

Interestingly, association between *FLG* defects and asthma without eczema has also been found in a cohort of Danish children prospectively followed from birth [18]. Furthermore, similar longitudinal follow-up methodology which should maximize the diagnosis rate was also employed in a study of German cohort where a relatively distinct trend towards an association was found (OR = 2.47, P = 0.11) [8]. Further evidence implicating epidermal barrier function in asthma pathogenesis came recently from a large genome-wide study showing that a locus with a likely function in keratinocytes (*RORA*) was among ten loci most strongly associated with this disease [19]. These findings suggest that at

least in some cohorts epidermal barrier defects may play a role in asthma pathogenesis among those without AD.

In contrast to studies in other populations [5,6] we did not observe an association between *FLG* null variants and allergic sensitization(s) as judged by analysis of skin prick test results or concentration of total IgE. This result is consistent with recent observations in a Danish cohort where the risk of sensitization among *FLG* defect carriers increased only after onset of asthma and/or eczema [18] and suggests that the effect of *FLG* null variants on AD or AA development is not likely to be primarily mediated through allergic sensitization.

The association between *FLG* variants and AD confirms the findings in other populations [3,6]. However, the association found in our study had only moderate statistical significance and effect size. This is consistent with suggestions that *FLG* variants are associated with severe forms of AD which are more readily ascertained in hospital based studies [20–23].

Our results also add to data on differences in population specific prevalence of *FLG* variants. We showed that in a Polish population the prevalence of the R501X variant (~1%) was distinctly lower than the prevalence of ~6% reported for Irish and Scottish populations [2]. An intermediate R501X frequency in German population (~2.5% as estimated from pooled data of Stemmler et al. [24] and Weidinger et al. [20]) suggests a clinal variation in prevalence of this variant in Europe.

In conclusion, we show that in a Polish population *FLG* null variants 2282del4 and R501X are risk factors for AD, and independently from it, for AA. A methodological observation is that in a Polish population AA associated with *FLG* defects may

Table 3. Distribution of the *FLG* variants in subjects with atopic asthma (AA) stratified by diagnosis of atopic dermatitis.

Atopic dermatitis		2282del4			R501X			Combined genotype		
	n	n (%)	OR (CI)	P	n (%)	OR (CI)	P	N (%)	OR (CI)	P
-	162	11 (6.8)	2.23 (1.15–4.33)	0.015	1 (0.6)	0.96 (0.12–7.42)	0.97	12 (7.4)	2.02 (1.07–3.81)	0.027
+	24	3 (12.5)	4.37 (1.27–15.07)	0.011	0	NA	0.69	3 (12.5)	3.61 (1.05–12.38)	0.029

All comparisons vs. healthy controls (Table 1), NA: not available.

Table 4. Distribution of the *FLG* variants in subjects with persistent allergic rhinitis (pAR) stratified by diagnosis of atopic dermatitis.

Atopic dermatitis	n	2282del4			R501X			Combined genotype		
		n (%)	OR (CI)	P	n (%)	OR (CI)	P	n (%)	OR (CI)	P
-	523	26 (5.0)	1.6 (1.0–2.57)	0.049	4 (0.8)	1.19 (0.38–3.71)	0.76	30 (5.7)	1.54 (0.99–2.38)	0.053
+	68	7 (10.3)	3.51 (1.54–8.01)	0.001	0	NA	0.51	7 (10.3)	2.9 (1.28–6.57)	0.008

All comparisons vs. healthy controls (Table 1), NA: not available.

have a subtle phenotype being difficult to diagnose by a questionnaire.

Kuna (Łódź), Barbara Rogala and Radosław Gawlik (Katowice) for help in carrying out the study.

Acknowledgments

We would like to thank Andrzej Emeryk (Lublin), Ewa Niżankowska-Mogilnicka (Kraków), Andrzej Fal (Wrocław), Wojciech Silny (Poznań), Anna Bodzenia-Łukaszyk (Białystok), Ewa Jassem (Gdańsk), Anna Bręborowicz (Poznań), Jurek Kruszewski, Marek Kulus (Warszawa), Piotr

Author Contributions

Conceived and designed the experiments: RP BS SM JP. Performed the experiments: JP GK. Analyzed the data: RP JP BS. Contributed reagents/materials/analysis tools: AT FR PS-K AW AL BP JK EK-F AN JB. Wrote the paper: RP BS JP SM.

References

1. O'Regan GM, Sandilands A, McLean WHI, Irvine AD (2008) Filaggrin in atopic dermatitis. Journal of Allergy and Clinical Immunology 122: 689–693.
2. Palmer CNA, Irvine AD, Terron-Kwiatkowski A, Zhao Y, Liao H, et al. (2006) Common loss-of-function variants of the epidermal barrier protein filaggrin are a major predisposing factor for atopic dermatitis. Nat Genet 38: 441–446.
3. Baurecht Hr, Irvine AD, Novak N, Illig T, Buhler B, et al. (2007) Toward a major risk factor for atopic eczema: Meta-analysis of filaggrin polymorphism data. Journal of Allergy and Clinical Immunology 120: 1406–1412.
4. Sandilands A, Terron-Kwiatkowski A, Hull PR, O'Regan GM, Clayton TH, et al. (2007) Comprehensive analysis of the gene encoding filaggrin uncovers prevalent and rare mutations in ichthyosis vulgaris and atopic eczema. Nat Genet 39: 650–654.
5. van den Oord RAHM, Sheikh A (2009) Filaggrin gene defects and risk of developing allergic sensitisation and allergic disorders: systematic review and meta-analysis. BMJ 339: b2433.
6. Rodriguez E, Baurecht H, Herberich E, Wagenpfeil S, Brown SJ, et al. (2009) Meta-analysis of filaggrin polymorphisms in eczema and asthma: Robust risk factors in atopic disease. Journal of Allergy and Clinical Immunology 123: 1361–1370.
7. Weidinger S, O'Sullivan M, Illig T, Baurecht Hr, Depner M, et al. (2008) Filaggrin mutations, atopic eczema, hay fever, and asthma in children. Journal of Allergy and Clinical Immunology 121: 1203–1209.
8. Marenholz I, Nickel R, Ruschendorf F, Schulz F, Esparza-Gordillo J, et al. (2006) Filaggrin loss-of-function mutations predispose to phenotypes involved in the atopic march. Journal of Allergy and Clinical Immunology 118: 866–871.
9. Johansson GOS (1998) Clinical Workshop. IgE antibodies and the Pharmacia CAP System in allergy diagnosis. Lidkoping: Landstroms. 48 p.
10. Debelic M, Wahl R (1996) In vitro tests: immunoglobulins E and G. In: Fuchs E, Schulz KH, eds. Manuale allergologicum IV. Deisenhofen, Germany: Dustri-Verlag Dr Karl Feistle. pp 1–27.
11. Global Initiative for Asthma (2009) Global Strategy for Asthma. Management and Prevention NHLBI/WHO Workshop Report. http://www.ginasthma.com.
12. Bousquet J, van Cauwenberge P, Khaltaev N (2001) Allergic rhinitis and its impact on asthma. J Allergy Clin Immunol 108: S147–S334.
13. Bousquet J, Khaltaev N, Cruz AA, Denburg J, Fokkens WJ, et al. (2008) Allergic rhinitis and its impact on asthma (ARIA) 2008 update (in collaboration with the World Health Organization, GA(2)LEN and AllerGen). Allergy 63: 8–160.
14. Hanifin JM, Rajka G (1980) Diagnostic features of atopic dermatitis. Acta Derm Venereol (supl) 92: 44–47.
15. Smith FJ, Irvine AD, Terron-Kwiatkowski A, Sandilands A, Campbell LE, et al. (2006) Loss-of-function mutations in the gene encoding filaggrin cause ichthyosis vulgaris. Nat Genet 38: 337–342.
16. Mueller-Malesinska M, Nowak M, Ploski R, Waligora J, Korniszewski L (2001) Epidemiology of 35delG mutation in GJB2 gene in a Polish population. Journal of Audiological Medicine 10: 136–141.
17. Kulig M, Bergmann R, Edenharter G, Wahn U (2000) Does allergy in parents depend on allergy in their children? Recall bias in parental questioning of atopic diseases. Multicenter Allergy Study Group. J Allergy Clin Immunol 105: 274–278.
18. Bonnelykke K, Pipper CB, Tavendale R, Palmer CN, Bisgaard H (2010) Filaggrin gene variants and atopic diseases in early childhood assessed longitudinally from birth. Pediatr Allergy Immunol 21: 954–961.
19. Moffatt MF, Gut IG, Demenais F, Strachan DP, Bouzigon E, et al. (2010) A Large-Scale, Consortium-Based Genomewide Association Study of Asthma. New England Journal of Medicine 363: 1211–1221.
20. Weidinger S, Rodriguez E, Stahl C, Wagenpfeil S, Klopp N, et al. (2006) Filaggrin Mutations Strongly Predispose to Early-Onset and Extrinsic Atopic Dermatitis. J Invest Dermatol 127: 724–726.
21. Brown SJ, Sandilands A, Zhao Y, Liao H, Relton CL, et al. (2007) Prevalent and Low-Frequency Null Mutations in the Filaggrin Gene Are Associated with Early-Onset and Persistent Atopic Eczema. J Invest Dermatol 128: 1591–1594.
22. Barker JNWN, Palmer CNA, Zhao Y, Liao H, Hull PR, et al. (2006) Null Mutations in the Filaggrin Gene (FLG) Determine Major Susceptibility to Early-Onset Atopic Dermatitis that Persists into Adulthood. J Invest Dermatol 127: 564–567.
23. Henderson J, Northstone K, Lee SP, Liao H, Zhao Y, et al. (2008) The burden of disease associated with filaggrin mutations: A population-based, longitudinal birth cohort study. Journal of Allergy and Clinical Immunology 121: 872–877.
24. Stemmler S, Parwez Q, Petrasch-Parwez E, Epplen JT, Hoffjan S (2006) Two Common Loss-of-Function Mutations within the Filaggrin Gene Predispose for Early Onset of Atopic Dermatitis. J Invest Dermatol 127: 722–724.

3

Cowhage-Induced Itch as an Experimental Model for Pruritus. A Comparative Study with Histamine-Induced Itch

Alexandru D. P. Papoiu[1,9], **Hong Liang Tey**[1,9], **Robert C. Coghill**[2], **Hui Wang**[1], **Gil Yosipovitch**[1,2,3*]

1 Department of Dermatology, Wake Forest University School of Medicine, Winston-Salem, North Carolina, United States of America, 2 Department of Neurobiology and Anatomy, Wake Forest University School of Medicine, Winston-Salem, North Carolina, United States of America, 3 Department of Regenerative Medicine, Wake Forest University School of Medicine, Winston-Salem, North Carolina, United States of America

Abstract

Background: Histamine is the prototypical pruritogen used in experimental itch induction. However, in most chronic pruritic diseases, itch is not predominantly mediated by histamine. Cowhage-induced itch, on the other hand, seems more characteristic of itch occurring in chronic pruritic diseases.

Objectives: We tested the validity of cowhage as an itch-inducing agent by contrasting it with the classical itch inducer, histamine, in healthy subjects and atopic dermatitis (AD) patients. We also investigated whether there was a cumulative effect when both agents were combined.

Methods: Fifteen healthy individuals and fifteen AD patients were recruited. Experimental itch induction was performed in eczema-free areas on the volar aspects of the forearm, using different itch inducers: histamine, cowhage and their combination thereof. Itch intensity was assessed continuously for 5.5 minutes after stimulus application using a computer-assisted visual analogue scale (COVAS).

Results: In both healthy and AD subjects, the mean and peak intensity of itch were higher after the application of cowhage compared to histamine, and were higher after the combined application of cowhage and histamine, compared to histamine alone ($p < 0.0001$ in all cases). Itch intensity ratings were not significantly different between healthy and AD subjects for the same itch inducer used; however AD subjects exhibited a prolonged itch response in comparison to healthy subjects ($p < 0.001$).

Conclusions: Cowhage induced a more intense itch sensation compared to histamine. Cowhage was the dominant factor in itch perception when both pathways were stimulated in the same time. Cowhage-induced itch is a suitable model for the study of itch in AD and other chronic pruritic diseases, and it can serve as a new model for testing antipruritic drugs in humans.

Editor: Lucienne Chatenoud, Université Paris Descartes, France

Funding: The current work was supported by NIH (NIAMS) award 5R01AR055902 to Dr. Gil Yosipovitch. The funders had no role in study design, data collection and analysis, decision to publish, or preparation of the manuscript.

Competing Interests: The authors have declared that no competing interests exist.

* E-mail: gyosipov@wfubmc.edu

⑨ These authors contributed equally to this work.

Introduction

Histamine has been the prototypical pruritogen used in experimental itch induction for many decades [1,2]. However, in many chronic pruritic conditions, such as atopic dermatitis (AD), the histaminergic pathway does not seem to play the major role since antihistamines are known to be largely ineffective. Some of the characteristics of itch which are common in chronic pruritus, such as itch occurring without a flare and also the mechanically-induced itch, cannot be attributed to the histaminergic pathway.

The rationale of this study was to evaluate and establish a new model of itch in humans, which relates to the PAR-2 pathway.

The PAR-2 receptors have been implicated in the pathophysiology of itch and of atopic eczema. Cowhage spicules provide an exogenous route to stimulate PAR-2 receptors in the skin and to elicit itch. Cutaneous application of spicules of the plant cowhage (*Mucuna pruriens var. pruriens*) produces itch without axonal reflex flare [3–5]. Cowhage-induced itch is also usually accompanied by a burning and/or pricking sensation [6,7], which appear to correspond to the nociceptive and burning sensations that accompany itch in atopic dermatitis [8,9]. Cowhage stimulates nerve fibers distinct from those activated by histamine, and these are polymodal C- neurons that can transmit mechanical and other noxious signals, in addition to itch [10,11]. The active ingredient of cowhage is mucunain, a cysteine protease, which binds to proteinase-activated receptors-2 and 4 (PAR-2 and PAR-4) [12]. Furthermore, it was previously found that the epidermis and cutaneous nerve fibers of AD patients express elevated levels of PAR-2 [13]. Other endogenous proteases binding to PAR-2, such as cathepsin S, mast cell tryptase and kallikrein [14] may play an important role in mediating pruritus in AD. Therefore, the active ingredient in cowhage, mucunain, acting as an exogenous PAR-2 ligand, may provide a model to study itch in AD and other chronic pruritic diseases.

As cowhage has not been employed in previous clinical or translational studies, we aimed to test the validity of cowhage as an experimental itch model, and contrast it with histamine, in AD patients and healthy controls. We also planned to investigate if there was a summation effect when both agents are administered simultaneously to induce itch.

Materials and Methods

Subjects and setting

Fifteen healthy individuals and fifteen AD patients were recruited at the Wake Forest University Health Sciences Department of Dermatology, Winston-Salem, North Carolina, USA. This clinical research involving human participants has been approved by the Internal Review Board of Wake Forest University Heath Sciences. Informed consent has been obtained in all cases and the investigation has been conducted according to the principles expressed in the Declaration of Helsinki. The diagnosis of AD was made using the Hanifin and Rajka criteria [15]. The severity of disease was assessed using the Eczema Area and Severity Index (EASI) [16]. The assessment was performed for all subjects at a screening visit, prior to experimental itch induction, by the same investigator (AP). AD subjects had to present a baseline itch intensity of minimum 3 out of 10 on a Visual Analog Scale (VAS) in order to qualify, and an eczema-free area on the volar aspect of either forearm. The AD group included 8 males and 7 females, average age 32.6 ± 11.2 years (age range 21 to 54), while the healthy group was comprised of 7 males and 8 females, average age 30.9 ± 6.0 years (age range 19 to 41).

Subjects were required to cease all systemic antipruritic medications, including antihistamines, at least 1 week prior to the study. No topical agents were allowed to be applied to their forearms for at least 1 week, but these could be used on other parts of the body.

Itch induction

Itch stimuli were applied alternatively to the volar aspect of the forearms in the following sequence: histamine (right forearm), cowhage (left forearm), and cowhage and histamine together (right forearm). Between itch inductions, a break was taken to allow previous itch sensations to completely subside. The combination of the two stimuli was administered on the right forearm in an area 10 cm away from the area where histamine was first applied. Histamine and cowhage were delivered on eczema-free areas. A 1% solution of histamine dissolved in 2% methylcellulose gel (Sigma, St. Louis, USA) was delivered using a current of 200 μA through a round iontophoresis electrode, 14 mm in diameter, for 30 seconds (Perimed PF 3826 Perilont Power device; Perimed, Sweden) as we previously reported [2]. Itch intensity was assessed continuously for 5.5 minutes subsequently.

After the itch sensation from histamine iontophoresis had completely subsided, an eczema-free area on the other forearm was used for cowhage application. A number of 40 to 45 cowhage spicules were counted under the microscope, picked-up by a microtweezer and were applied within a 4 cm^2 circular area on the skin. The spicules were gently rubbed for 45 seconds onto the subjects' skin with a circular motion to facilitate contact; a cotton cloth was used to demarcate the area to prevent any stray spicules from stimulating surrounding skin. (A previous study had reported that 1 spicule was sufficient to induce a significant itch, and furthermore, there was no difference in sensation intensity when 1 or 7 spicules were inserted over a small area [6]). Subjects were instructed to ignore the initial stinging or pricking sensations and rate only the itch sensation *per se*. After 5.5 minutes, during which itch intensity was continuously reported, the spicules were removed using adhesive tapes (3M, St.Paul, MN).

When itch sensation induced by cowhage completely subsided, an area on the contralateral forearm (10 cm away from the area that was used for histamine's single application previously) was chosen for application of both histamine and cowhage. Histamine was administered for 30 seconds by iontophoresis as described above. Immediately thereafter (approximately 1 minute later), cowhage was applied to an adjacent site (1 cm away). Itch intensity was assessed continuously for another 5.5 minutes. Subjects were instructed to rate the itch sensation from both stimuli together after the application of cowhage was finalized.

Quantitative psychophysical assessment

Subjects used a computerized visual analogue scale (COVAS, Medoc, Ramat-Yishai, Israel) for continuous reporting of itch intensity for a duration of 5.5 minutes. The COVAS allows rating of itch intensity on a 100 mm scale that ranges from "no itch" at one end to "unbearable itch" at the other. The subjects can slide an indicator between the two ends to reflect the intensity of their sensations and the values were continuously registered by a computer throughout the experimental period. Visual analog scales have long been used to assess various sensations and have been shown to exhibit ratio-scale properties for psychophysical ratings [17] (Price et al. 1994) and to be more reproducible than verbal descriptor scales [18] (Rosier et al. 2002). Continuous ratings over time acquired via computerized VAS closely mirror post-stimulus retrospective ratings [19] (Koyama et al. 2004). We have adapted the VAS and the COVAS use for ratings of itch perception and have demonstrated that these scales are 1) sensitive to manipulations which can reduce itch, 2) capable of assessing changes in itch intensity over time, and 3) able to distinguish differences between acute and chronic itch [20,21].

Statistical analysis. COVAS data were sampled at 9 Hz. Custom written programs in IDL (ITT Visual Information Solutions, Boulder, CO) were used to extract the peak itch rating as well as ratings at 30 seconds intervals. These programs were also used to calculate the average itch over time, and to calculate group averages.

Using JMP software we examined the entire perception (intensity ratings) curves for the full duration, identified the peak value and calculated the means. Peak and mean itch intensity ratings were analyzed using a two factor analysis of variance (ANOVA, JMP Software: SAS, Cary, NC) assessing effects of itch stimulus (cowhage, histamine, and cowhage+histamine) within subjects, and effects of disease state (healthy vs. atopic patients) across subjects, as well as the interaction between these factors. Orthogonal comparisons were used to determine differences between pairs of itch stimuli.

Time courses of itch were analyzed at 30 seconds intervals using a three factor analysis of variance (ANOVA), assessing the effects of time and itch stimulus within subjects, and the effects of disease status across subjects. As above, orthogonal comparisons were used to determine differences between pairs of itch stimuli, compared to the reference value, set for time point = 30 seconds.

Separate linear regression analyses were employed for each itch stimulus in order to determine if the evoked itch intensity was significantly influenced by the severity of AD, as evaluated by EASI scores.

Results

Differences in mean and peak itch intensity ratings for itch induced by cowhage, histamine and their combination

Itch intensity measured by COVAS ratings over time in AD patients and healthy subjects are shown in figures 1 and 2. In both groups, the mean and peak COVAS ratings were significantly influenced by the itch stimulus (main effect of stimulus: mean rating p<0.0001, peak rating: p<0.0001). Both peak and mean itch ratings were higher following cowhage application versus following histamine application (both p<0.0001), but were not significantly different between the combined application of cowhage and histamine, compared to cowhage alone (contrast of mean ratings: p=0.89; for peak ratings: p=0.29). Although AD patients appeared more sensitive to all stimuli, there was no significant main effect of disease status on itch ratings (mean rating: p=0.77; peak rating: p=0.36).

Continuous itch response curves reveal a different pattern of variation over time between AD and healthy subjects

Analysis of the time course of perceived itch intensity from continuous ratings revealed that itch intensity varied significantly across (over) time (analyzed as a main effect time: p<0.0001, Fig. 1, 2). Ratings gradually rose following the application of the itch stimuli, and then, after reaching a peak, tapered down slowly over time. In healthy participants, itch increased faster (following a steeper slope) and started to subside quicker than in atopic dermatitis patients. This pattern of time dependency was different in AD patients vs. healthy subjects (interaction of time×disease status, p=0.0025). AD patients exhibited a slower onset of itch than healthy subjects; also, their itch decreased very slowly after it

reached peak values. As in the case of the peak and mean (average intensity) ratings, a significant main effect of itch stimulus was detected in the time course data (p<0.0001), and this effect did not vary with disease status (drug×disease status interaction: p=0.91).

The Relationship between EASI scores and perceived itch intensity ratings in AD subjects

For histamine-induced itch, the mean COVAS ratings were positively correlated to the EASI scores ($r^2 = 0.32$, p=0.02), and the peak COVAS ratings also were positively correlated to the EASI scores ($r^2 = 0.54$, p=0.0016). The COVAS ratings for cowhage-induced itch and for the itch induced by cowhage and histamine in combination showed no linear relationship with disease severity as evaluated by EASI scores (Table 1).

Discussion

Histamine is the classic, best known mediator of itch which has been used as the standard experimental pruritogen in numerous studies in the past decades. However, a novel, distinct pathway for itch transmission, which is stimulated by cowhage has been elucidated in recent years. The spicules of this tropical plant release upon skin contact a cysteine protease, mucunain, that binds to PAR2/4 receptors [12] which leads to stimulation of cutaneous polymodal C-fibers [10]; this pathway is distinct from the neuronal circuits transmitting histamine itch, and synapses in a separate subset of spinothalamic secondary neurons [22]. In chronic pruritic diseases of which AD is the most common, the histaminergic pathway does not appear to be the most relevant circuit (antihistamines are ineffective for chronic itch relief). However, cowhage induces an itch associated with burning and pricking sensations, commonly observed in AD, and it works via PAR-2 [12] receptors, which display an increased expression in atopic skin. These findings support the hypothesis that PAR-2 mediated itch pathway may represent the relevant pathway predominantly stimulated in AD.

This study showed that the response to cowhage was reproducible, reliable and consistent in both healthy and AD

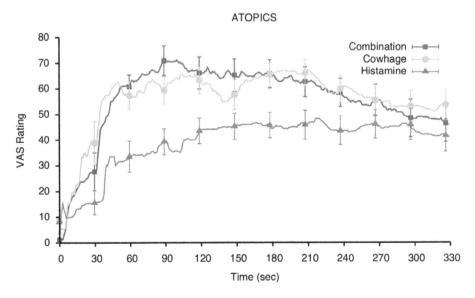

Figure 1. Time course of continuous itch intensity ratings (on a visual analog scale of 0 to 100 mm) in atopic dermatitis subjects, following itch induction with histamine, cowhage and their combination. A significant difference in time course and in the magnitude of response is observed between cowhage and histamine-induced itch (p<0.0001).

HEALTHY

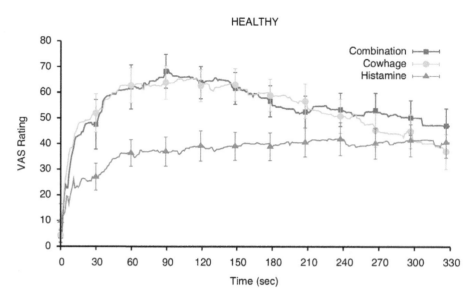

Figure 2. Time course of continuous itch intensity ratings (on a visual analog scale of 0 to 100 mm) in healthy subjects, following itch induction with histamine, cowhage and their combination. A significant difference in time course and in the magnitude of response is apparent between cowhage and histamine-induced itch (p<0.0001).

subjects. We found that a rather minimal dose of cowhage, approximately 45 spicules, equivalent to 45 μg of material (maximally containing about 90 ng of mucunain) induced a more intense itch sensation compared to histamine, at a dose of 6 mg histamine (base) that was contained in the chamber of the drug delivery electrode. Delivery experiments revealed that the number of cowhage spicules inserted upon rubbing, as examined under regular or polarizing light by magnifying lens at 5× magnification (Fig. 3), represents about a third of the total spicules applied, therefore the actual dose of mucunain deliverable by spicules can be estimated at 15–30 ng.

The co-stimulation of histaminergic and cowhage-itch pathways did not results in a summation of itch intensity. The combination of the stimuli induced an itch that was much more intense than using histamine alone, but it was not significantly more intense compared to itch induced by cowhage alone. This suggests that the major contributor of perceived itch sensation is cowhage, when both pathways are stimulated concurrently.

We propose that cowhage could be used a suitable model to induce experimental itch. Cowhage-itch more closely resembles the characteristics of pruritus in chronic conditions and induces a more intense sensation compared to histamine. Cowhage-induced itch appears as the dominant component of itch perception when these two pathways are stimulated simultaneously. From a therapeutic standpoint, drugs capable to inhibit cowhage itch pathway appear promising to pursue for the treatment of chronic pruritus. Cowhage induce itch could offer a new paradigm to test antipruritics in humans.

Table 1. EASI scores of the severity of disease in atopic dermatitis subjects included in the study.

Sbj. #	EASI score	Age	Gender
1	15.0	36	m
2	3.8	25	m
3	12.2	22	f
4	3.8	30	f
5	1.1	24	f
6	0.8	54	f
7	12.9	20	f
8	5.2	40	m
9	3.0	21	f
10	9.3	34	m
11	22.5	41	m
12	2.3	24	f
13	17.3	46	m
14	49.0	49	m
15	16.2	23	m
AVG	11.6	32.6	

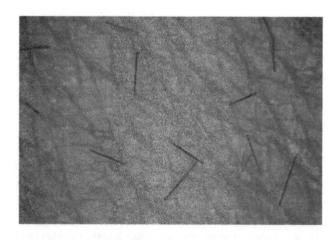

Figure 3. An image of cowhage spicules inserted into the skin by gentle rubbing, under polarizing light at 5× magnification.

We also investigated the potential correlation of the EASI scores, a validated, objective measure of the severity of atopic eczema [16], with the subjective perception of itch intensity in AD subjects. Interestingly, ratings of histamine induced itch were correlated to the EASI scores, while the perceived intensity of cowhage induced itch was not. Although we do not have a definitive explanation for the lack of correlation between EASI scores and the perception of itch induced with cowhage, we note note that clinical features such as lichenification, excoriations, pigmentation and disease extension on body areas (included in this scoring) may have a limited ability to reflect the subjective expression of itch severity in patients [23]. Histamine induced itch causes a neurogenic inflammation, therefore the mechanisms underlying the inflammatory processes involved in the pathophysiological manifestation of atopic dermatitis (factored into the EASI score) may share a common link with the histamine induced response, while the itch induced via PAR-2 pathway may not, since it does not evoke a neurogenic response [10].

Previous studies have shown that AD patients exhibited higher intensity ratings for histamine induced itch than in healthy subjects, suggesting that AD subjects present a hypersensitization of the itch response [20,24]. In this study, we found only a trend for a higher intensity of itch perception in AD subjects. However, when analyzing itch intensity fluctuation over time, AD patients displayed a significantly prolonged itch response compared to healthy subjects for both stimuli, supporting the notion that AD involves a neuronal hypersensitization at peripheral and/or central levels, in similarity with chronic pain [25].

Conclusion

Cowhage induced a much more intense itch sensation compared to histamine and it was the dominant player in itch induction when both pathways were activated at the same time. Cowhage-induced itch could serve as a suitable model for the study of itch in AD and other chronic itch diseases.

Acknowledgments

Authors kindly thank Dr. Ethan A. Lerner from the Cutaneous Biology Research Center, Massachusetts General Hospital, Charlestown, MA, for generously supplying the cowhage spicules for this study.

Author Contributions

Conceived and designed the experiments: GY AP. Performed the experiments: AP HW HLT. Analyzed the data: AP RC GY HLT. Contributed reagents/materials/analysis tools: RC HLT. Wrote the paper: AP HLT GY RC HW. Designed figures: RC AP.

References

1. Melton FM, Shelley WB (1950) The effect of topical antipruritic therapy on experimentally induced pruritus in man. J Invest Dermatol 15: 325–332.
2. Ishiuji Y, Coghill RC, Patel TS, Oshiro Y, Kraft RA, et al. (2009) Distinct patterns of brain activity evoked by histamine-induced itch reveal an association with itch intensity and disease severity in atopic dermatitis. Br J Dermatol 161: 1072–1080.
3. Shelley WB, Arthur RP (1955) Studies on cowhage (Mucuna pruriens) and its pruritogenic proteinase, mucunain. AMA Arch Derm 72: 399–406.
4. Shelley WB, Arthur RP (1957) The neurohistology and neurophysiology of the itch sensation in man. AMA Arch Derm 76: 296–323.
5. Johanek LM, Meyer RA, Hartke T, Hobelmann JG, Maine DN, et al. (2007) Psychophysical and physiological evidence for parallel afferent pathways mediating the sensation of itch. J Neurosci 27: 7490–7497.
6. LaMotte RH, Shimada SG, Green BG, Zelterman D (2009) Pruritic and nociceptive sensations and dysesthesias from a spicule of cowhage. J Neurophysiol 101: 1430–1443.
7. Sikand P, Shimada SG, Green BG, LaMotte RH (2009) Similar itch and nociceptive sensations evoked by punctate cutaneous application of capsaicin, histamine and cowhage. Pain 144: 66–75.
8. Dawn A, Papoiu AD, Chan YH, Rapp SR, Rassette N, et al. (2009) Itch characteristics in atopic dermatitis: results of a web-based questionnaire. Br J Dermatol 160: 642–644.
9. T-J Goon A, Yosipovitch G, Chan YH, Goh CL (2007) Clinical characteristics of generalized idiopathic pruritus in patients from a tertiary referral center in Singapore. Int J Dermatol 46: 1023–1026.
10. Namer B, Carr R, Johanek LM (2008) Separate peripheral pathways for pruritus in man. J Neurophysiol 100: 2062–2069.
11. Schmelz M. Itch and pain (2010) Neurosci Biobehav Rev 34: 171–176.
12. Reddy VB, Iuga AO, Shimada SG, LaMotte RH, Lerner EA (2008) Cowhage-evoked itch is mediated by a novel cysteine protease: a ligand of protease-activated receptors. J Neurosci 28: 4331–4335.
13. Steinhoff M, Neisius U, Ikoma A, Fartasch M, Heyer G, et al. (2003) Proteinase-activated receptor-2 mediates itch: a novel pathway for pruritus in human skin. J Neurosci 23: 6176–6180.
14. Reddy VB, Shimada SG, Sikand P (2010) Cathepsin S elicits itch and signals via protease-activated receptors. J Invest Dermatol 130: 1468–1470.
15. Hanifin JM, Rajka G (1980) Diagnostic features of atopic dermatitis. Acta Derm Venereol (Stockh) 92: 44–47.
16. Hanifin JM, Thurston M, Omoto M, Cherill R, Tofte SJ, et al. (2001) The eczema area and severity index (EASI): assessment of reliability in atopic dermatitis. EASI Evaluator Group Exp Dermatol 10: 11–18 (2001).
17. Price DD, Bush FM, Long S, Harkins SW (1994) A comparison of pain measurement characteristics of mechanical visual analogue and simple numerical rating scales. Pain 56: 217–226.
18. Rosier EM, Iadarola MJ, Coghill RC (2002) Reproducibility of pain measurement and pain perception. Pain 98: 205–16.
19. Koyama Y, Koyama T, Kroncke AP, Coghill RC (2004) Effects of stimulus duration on heat induced pain: the relationship between real-time and post-stimulus pain ratings. Pain 107: 256–66.
20. Ishiuji Y, Coghill RC, Patel TS, Dawn A, Fountain J, et al. (2008) Repetitive scratching and noxious heat do not inhibit histamine-induced itch in atopic dermatitis. Br J Dermatol 158: 78–83.
21. Wang H, Papoiu AD, Coghill RC, Patel T, Wang N, et al. (2010) Ethnic differences in pain, itch and thermal detection in response to topical capsaicin: African Americans display a notably limited hyperalgesia and neurogenic inflammation. Br J Dermatol 162: 1023–9.
22. Davidson S, Zhang X, Yoon CH, Khasabov SG, Simone DA, et al. (2007) The itch-producing agents histamine and cowhage activate separate populations of primate spinothalamic tract neurons. J Neurosci 27: 10007–14.
23. Yang HJ, Jeon YH, Pyun BY (2010) Evaluation of patient's subjective severity using various scoring system in Korean children with atopic dermatitis. Asian Pac J Allergy Immunol 28: 130–135.
24. Ikoma A, Rukwied R, Ständer S, Steinhoff M, Miyachi Y, et al. (2003) Neuronal sensitization for histamine-induced itch in lesional skin of patients with atopic dermatitis. Arch Dermatol 139: 1455–1458.
25. Woolf C (2010) Central sensitization: Implications for the diagnosis and treatment of pain. Pain. [Epub ahead of print]; doi:10.1016/j.pain.2010.09.030.

4

Severe Eczema in Infancy Can Predict Asthma Development. A Prospective Study to the Age of 10 Years

Marie Ekbäck[1], Michaela Tedner[2], Irene Devenney[1]*, Göran Oldaeus[3], Gunilla Norrman[4], Leif Strömberg[5], Karin Fälth-Magnusson[1]

1 Division of Pediatrics, Department of Clinical and Experimental Medicine, Faculty of Health Sciences, Linköping University and Department of Pediatrics, County Council of Östergötland, Linköping, Sweden, 2 Pediatric Clinic, Täby, Stockholm, Sweden, 3 Pediatric Clinic, County Hospital Ryhov, Jönköping, Sweden, 4 Pediatric Clinic, Hudiksvall, Sweden, 5 Department of Pediatrics in Norrköping, County Council of Östergötland, Norrköping, Sweden

Abstract

Background: Children with atopic eczema in infancy often develop allergic rhinoconjunctivitis and asthma, but the term "atopic march" has been questioned as the relations between atopic disorders seem more complicated than one condition progressing into another.

Objective: In this prospective multicenter study we followed children with eczema from infancy to the age of 10 years focusing on sensitization to allergens, severity of eczema and development of allergic airway symptoms at 4.5 and 10 years of age.

Methods: On inclusion, 123 children were examined. Hanifin-Rajka criteria and SCORAD index were used to describe the eczema. Episodes of wheezing were registered, skin prick tests and IgE tests were conducted and questionnaires were filled out. Procedures were repeated at 4.5 and 10 years of age with additional examinations for ARC and asthma.

Results: 94 out of 123 completed the entire study. High SCORAD points on inclusion were correlated with the risk of developing ARC, (B = 9.86, P = 0.01) and asthma, (B = 10.17, P = 0.01). For infants with eczema and wheezing at the first visit, the OR for developing asthma was 4.05 (P = 0.01). ARC at 4.5 years of age resulted in an OR of 11.28 (P = 0.00) for asthma development at 10 years.

Conclusion: This study indicates that infant eczema with high SCORAD points is associated with an increased risk of asthma at 10 years of age. Children with eczema and wheezing episodes during infancy are more likely to develop asthma than are infants with eczema alone. Eczema in infancy combined with early onset of ARC seems to indicate a more severe allergic disease, which often leads to asthma development. The progression from eczema in infancy to ARC at an early age and asthma later in childhood shown in this study supports the relevance of the term "atopic march", at least in more severe allergic disease.

Editor: Jacques Zimmer, Centre de Recherche Public de la Santé (CRP-Santé), Luxembourg

Funding: Financial support was given by the Health Research Council in the South-East of Sweden (FORSS), the Swedish Asthma and Allergy Association's Research Foundation, and grants were received from Lion's Club in the South-East of Sweden, GlaxoSmithKline and Konsul Th C Bergh's Foundation for Scientific Research. The funders had no role in study design, data collection and analysis, decision to publish, or preparation of the manuscript.

Competing Interests: GlaxoSmithKline supported the study with a minor grant in 2004 given as a scholarship to one of the junior researchers in the group. There are no competing interests, and the funder has no role in the study design, data collection and analysis, decision to publish, or preparation of the manuscript. No products in development or marketed products from GlaxoSmithKline were part of the study.

* E-mail: irene.devenney@lio.se

Introduction

Background

Children with an atopic constitution are at risk of developing allergic symptoms, such as atopic eczema, food allergy, allergic rhinoconjunctivitis (ARC) and asthma [1–3], with multiple factors influencing these immune responses. Especially in countries with a western life style the prevalence of allergy in childhood has increased remarkably in recent decades [2,4,5]. The "atopic march" is a term that has been used to describe the progression from atopic eczema and food allergy during infancy to ARC and subsequently to asthma later in childhood [6–9]. Previous studies have shown that children with atopic eczema or those sensitized to allergens in early childhood more often develop ARC and asthma [8,10–13]. However, the concept of "atopic march" has been questioned. The relations between the allergic disorders seem to be much more complicated than that of one condition progressing into another [7,8].

Wheezing during infancy is common, but is not necessarily caused by asthma. Epidemiological studies have described different phenotypes of asthma [3,8,14,15], many of which are transient conditions with low risk of asthma and allergy later in life. However, 30–50% of the children involved have been reported to develop persistent asthma, especially if they are sensitized [2,3,16].

Several environmental factors have been associated with asthma in epidemiological studies, for example sensitization to aeroallergens early in life, exposure to pets, maternal diet during pregnancy and lactation, breastfeeding, exposure to tobacco smoke during pregnancy and early in life, viral infections, a disturbed balance of microbes, and psychosocial factors [3,17]. Differences in opinion make it controversial to give advice concerning pets and maternal diet. Breastfeeding has been reported to decrease wheezing associated with respiratory infections in early childhood, but there is not enough evidence as to whether it prevents asthma [3,18].

A better understanding of the process of developing allergic airway symptoms, including early warning signs, would be of great value. This could help to identify children at high risk of developing asthma and thereby enable early intervention and treatment and perhaps even aid prevention.

Aim

The aim of the present study was to follow infants with eczema and suspected food allergy over time, focusing on sensitization to allergens, severity of eczema and the development of allergic airway symptoms at 4.5 and 10 years of age. Furthermore, we wanted to identify any early signs that could be associated with a higher risk of developing allergic airway symptoms.

Methods

Ethics statement

The study was approved by the Human Research Ethics Committees at the Faculty of Health Sciences Linköping University and at the Medical Faculty at Uppsala University. Written informed consent was obtained from the children's parents at all ages and from the children at 10 years of age.

Methods

The study population was 123 children (71 boys and 52 girls) with eczema and suspected food allergy recruited to the study from June 1999 to September 2001. They were all under two years of age (median 6 months, range 1–23) and had been referred from their primary care physician to the pediatric clinics in Linköping, Jönköping, Norrköping and Hudiksvall [19].

Factors studied on inclusion and at follow-up examinations are presented in Table 1. At the first visit, the patients were examined by a pediatrician. Questionnaires regarding other atopic manifestations, family history, environmental factors and nutrition were completed by the parents. The diagnostic criteria proposed by Hanifin and Rajka were used to diagnose atopic dermatitis [20]. The severity of eczema was evaluated by a standardized method, "The Severity Scoring of Atopic Dermatitis" (SCORAD). SCORAD was used to classify eczema as mild (≤25 points), moderate (26–50 points) or severe (>50 points) [21]. Standardized skin prick tests (SPT) were performed in a standardized way [22]; a mean wheal diameter of three mm was used as the lower limit for positivity as recommended in the EAACI position paper [22,23]. The SPTs and the SCORAD were assessed by experienced allergy nurses. All children were recommended treatment with emollients and/or topical steroids. Children with a positive SPT were recommended a temporary elimination diet. For food allergic children, milk and eggs were reintroduced in either open

standardized or double-blind placebo-controlled oral food challenges when SPT was ≤10 mm and SCORAD ≤25points [19]. Six weeks after inclusion, the patients were reexamined by the same nurse using SCORAD and SPT. Venous blood samples were obtained on inclusion, at the six-week follow-up, at 4.5 and 10 years of age. IgE was analyzed with UniCAP, as previously described [24].

The patients were reexamined by a pediatrician at 4.5 years and 10 years of age. Persisting eczema was assessed using Hanifin-Rajka criteria, severity was graded according to SCORAD at both visits, and venous blood samples were obtained. SPTs were performed for foods and aeroallergens (Table 1). Questionnaires enquiring about other allergic manifestations and tolerance to food were completed. At 10 years of age, lung function tests were performed. A standardized spirometric test combined with a standardized exercise test was performed. It included a period of 6 minutes intense running to increase the pulse rate to 160 beats per minute. Heart rate and oxygen saturation were documented. Spirometric values were measured before and immediately after running, after 10 minutes rest, and 15 minutes after inhalation of 1 mg terbutalin, inhaled from a multi-dose powder inhaler. Exhaled nitric oxide was measured with NIOX MINO (Aerocrine, Solna, Sweden) before and directly after the exercise period.

After the final examination at 10 years of age, the patients were divided into three groups. The first group was patients with no persisting allergic airway problems with or without eczema, the second group was patients suffering from ARC, and the third group was patients suffering from asthma. Patients with both ARC and asthma at 10 years were included in the asthma group.

The diagnostic criterion used for asthma in infants and preschool children in this study was any episode of obstructive airway symptoms in combination with IgE-mediated eczema, as recommended by the Swedish National Pediatric Allergy Group [25].

At the final visit for the 10 year-olds, an increase in FEV1 ≥ 10% after inhaling salbutamol or a reduction in FEV1 ≥10% of baseline levels after effort was considered diagnostic for asthma, as were patients previously diagnosed as fulfilling the criteria for asthma [26,27]. ARC was defined as symptoms of rhinitis or conjunctivitis after exposure to allergens, correlating to a positive SPT or a positive test for specific IgE. Sensitization was defined as either a positive SPT or specific IgE values ≥0.35kUA/l [24].

Statistics

Binary logistic regression with ARC and asthma as covariates was used to calculate odds ratios (ORs) with 95% confidence intervals (CIs). Linear regression was used to study the relationship between different dependent scalar variables, ARC and asthma as independent variables. Significance tests of the regression coefficients, here referred to as B, together with estimates and accompanying CIs are presented. T test was used to analyze differences in SCORAD at the first visit between drop-outs and the study population. Differences combined with p values of < 0.05 were considered statistically significant. Descriptive statistics were used to calculate means and confidence intervals for the groups with no airway symptoms, ARC and asthma seen in the Figures 1–4. All calculations were made with SPSS version 20 for Windows.

Results

Participation and summary of symptoms

At the follow-up at 4.5 years of age, 115 out of 123 children participated and several of them displayed more than one

Table 1. An overview of examinations and tests performed on the children with eczema on inclusion, at 4.5 years and at 10 years.

	Inclusion	4,5 years	10 years
Physical examination	X	X	X
SCORAD	X	X	X
Hanifin-Rajka	X	X	X
SPT	X	X	X
IgE	X	X	X
Questionnaries	X	X	X
Wheezing episodes	X		
ARC		X	X
Asthma		X	X
Spirometry			X
Exhaled NO			X

symptom. Of the 115, 60 still suffered from eczema, 26 had ARC, 37 had asthma and 35 had no symptoms of atopic disease at all. Ninety-four out of 123 completed the entire study until 10 years of age, of whom 60 continued to have eczema, 44 had ARC, 27 had asthma and 13 had no symptoms of allergy at all.

Characteristics on inclusion and later risk of disease

At the first visit, the duration of breastfeeding in months, sensitization to cow's milk and egg, having furred pets at home, SCORAD points, eczema fulfilling Hanifin-Rajka criteria, episodes of wheezing and exposure to tobacco smoke were studied.

Higher SCORAD points on inclusion increased the risk of having ARC, B = 9.86 (95%CI 2.18–17.53; P = 0.01) and asthma, B = 10.17 (95%CI 2.82–17.52; P = 0.01) at 10 years of age.

For infants with eczema and wheezing at the first visit, the OR for being diagnosed with asthma at 10 years was 4.05 (95%CI 1.42–11.56; P = 0.01). Sensitization to egg correlated to the risk of an asthma diagnosis at 10 years of age, OR 2.59 (95%CI 1.00–6.67; P = 0.05). On inclusion, no statistically significant differences were found for fulfilled Hanifin-Rajka criteria, sensitization to milk, breastfeeding, having furred pets, or exposure to tobacco smoke.

Characteristics at 4.5 years and later risk of disease

At 4.5 years of age, exposure to tobacco smoke, having furred pets at home, sensitization to milk, egg and aeroallergens, SCORAD points, eczema fulfilling Hanifin- Rajka criteria, ARC and asthma were studied.

For children with remaining sensitization to egg at 4.5 years of age, the OR for ARC at 10 years of age was 10.30 (95%CI 3.28–32.38; P = 0.00). For an asthma diagnosis at 10 years of age, the OR was 3.63 (95%CI 1.25–10.60; P = 0.02). Sensitization to aeroallergens at 4.5 years of age meant an OR of 4.70 (95%CI 1.50–14.75; P = 0.01) for ARC at 10 years of age and an OR of 6.21 (95%CI 1.83–21.06; P = 0.00) for asthma at 10 years of age. ARC at 4.5 years of age gave an OR of 11.28 (95%CI 3.61–35.28; P = 0.00) for asthma development but an OR of 3.05 (95%CI 0.88–10.60; P = 0.08) for only ARC at 10 years of age. For children diagnosed with asthma at 4.5 years of age, the OR for asthma at 10 years of age was 14.44 (95%CI 4.77–43.72; P = 0.00), whereas the OR for only ARC at 10 years of age was 1.08 (95% CI 0.34–3.47; P = 0.89).

No statistically significant differences were found for SCORAD points, having furred pets, remaining sensitization to milk, and fulfilled Hanifin-Rajka criteria at 4.5 years of age.

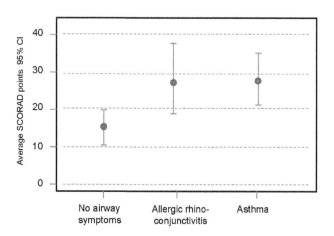

Figure 1. Average SCORAD points on inclusion for children with no airway symptoms, allergic rhinoconjunctivitis or asthma at 10 years.

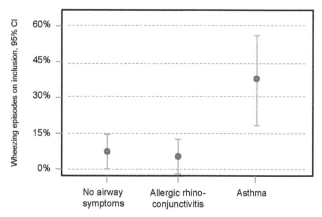

Figure 2. Percentage of children who had had at least one episode of wheezing before inclusion in the groups who had no airway symptoms, allergic rhinoconjunctivitis and asthma at 10 years.

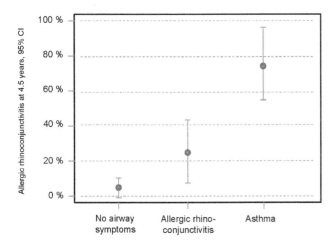

Figure 3. Percentage of children who had allergic rhinoconjunctivitis at 4.5 years among the groups with no airway symptoms, allergic rhinoconjunctivitis and asthma at 10 years.

Figure 4. Percentage of children who were diagnosed with asthma at 4.5 years in the groups with no airway symptoms, allergic rhinoconjunctivitis and asthma at 10 years.

Results at 10 years of age

Heredity, gender, exposure to tobacco smoke during the first 10 years, pets at home, sensitization to foods and aeroallergens, SCORAD, eczema fulfilling Hanifin-Rajka criteria, and values of exhaled NO before and after effort were studied at 10 years of age.

For children with eczema sensitized to aeroallergens at 10 years of age, the OR for ARC was 30.25 (CI 3.69-248.25; P = 0.00) and the OR for asthma was 5.84 (CI 1.65–20.71; P0.01). Higher levels of NO before effort resulted in B = 7.16 (CI 0.26–14.06; P = 0.04) for ARC and B = 13.25 (CI 6.61–19.89; P = 0.00) for asthma. For higher NO values after effort, the B for ARC was 7.76 (CI 0.85–14.66; P = 0.03) and for asthma, 13.26 (CI 6.35–20.16; P = 0.00).

The relation between eczema severity on inclusion and SCORAD points at 10 years of age was also studied. There was no significant difference in SCORAD points at 10 years of age between children with mild, moderate and severe eczema as infants.

Comparing the groups with no airway symptoms, ARC and asthma at ten years displayed no significant difference in positive family history of atopy (defined as at least one first-degree family member suffering from allergic symptoms), gender and fulfilled Hanifin-Rajka criteria.

To compare the representativity of the compliant cases with that of the original cohort, we also studied differences in SCORAD points on inclusion between the patients who had dropped out and those who remained in the study at 10 years of age. The drop-outs had a mean SCORAD point of 22.11, whereas those who remained had a mean SCORAD point of 21.47 on inclusion. The difference was not significant, P = 0.84.

Discussion

In this prospective multicenter study we followed 123 children with eczema from infancy to 10 years of age to study factors that might influence and predict the risk of developing allergic airway symptoms.

Of the 123 patients, 94 completed the entire study. At the age of 10 years, 64% of the children still had problems with eczema, 47% had ARC, 29% had asthma, and only 14% had no symptoms of allergy. Therefore eczema in infancy must be considered a serious warning sign for lasting allergic problems rather than a transient condition, although eczema usually gets less severe with time [28].

Atopic disease during childhood often persists into adulthood [9]. The reported risk for children with atopic eczema of developing asthma varies between different studies. Our results are in line with several other studies [29–32]. Compared with the results from the Swedish birth cohort, BAMSE, which followed 810 children with infantile eczema to 12 years of age, the children in our study more often had persisting symptoms [33,34]. This difference might be explained by the fact that the children in the present study who were diagnosed with eczema and referred to a pediatric clinic are likely to have had more severe symptoms than the children in BAMSE, whose were diagnosed with eczema based on questionnaire data.

We found that the risk of developing ARC and asthma before 10 years of age correlated with high SCORAD points during infancy. The SCORAD system has previously shown adequate validity and reliability to measure the severity of eczema [35,36]. Our findings indicate that high SCORAD points in infancy could also be used to predict the risk of developing asthma and that severe eczema is more associated with allergic airway symptoms is than mild eczema. In contrast, high SCORAD points at the ages of 4.5 and 10 years were not associated with a higher risk of asthma or ARC when the patients were 10 years old. It has previously been shown that the severity of atopic dermatitis predicts the prognosis of eczema and the risk of developing other atopic manifestations [32,37]. This study refutes the notion that severe eczema in infancy, classified according to SCORAD, is a predictor of a poorer prognosis of eczema later in childhood, as we did not find any correlation between high SCORAD points in infancy and high SCORAD points at 10 years of age. Nor did we find any correlation between high SCORAD points in infancy and remaining eczema at 10 years of age that fulfilled the Hanifin-Rajka criteria.

Wheezing in infancy is often transient, and infants tend to outgrow their breathing problems [16]. For our patients with eczema, however, wheezing meant a 4 times greater risk of having an asthma diagnosis at the age of 10 compared with infants affected by eczema only. This is not surprising as other atopic manifestations among wheezing infants are known risk factors for remaining asthma [38]. Children who fulfilled the criteria for asthma at 4.5 years had a 14 times higher risk of suffering from asthma at 10 years of age than had children with only eczema and no wheezing.

The children in our study who had symptoms of ARC at 4.5 years of age had a high risk of developing asthma. At 10 years of age, 67% of them were diagnosed with asthma, and the risk of developing asthma was 11 times higher than for 4.5 year olds without ARC. A strong association between ARC and asthma development was expected as Peroni et al found a strong correlation among 3–5 year olds [39]. Among adults, rhinitis is seen as an independent risk factor for developing asthma [40,41]. Our study confirms the correlation between ARC and asthma for children with eczema. It is likely that eczema in infancy combined with early onset of ARC indicates a more severe allergic disease, which tends to lead to asthma development rather than ARC only.

Concerning food allergy, sensitization to hen's egg in infancy was correlated with a risk of developing asthma. Remaining sensitization to egg at 4.5 years of age was associated with both ARC and asthma development, confirming several other studies [37,42]. In early childhood, sensitization to hen's egg has been associated with sensitization to airborne allergens [43]. At the age of 10 we found no correlation for egg sensitization, ARC and asthma. For our patients, sensitization to aeroallergens at 4.5 and 10 years of age was a strong predictor of allergic airway symptoms, as shown in earlier studies [44,45].

Family history is a well-known risk factor for atopic diseases [46,47]. Almost all patients in our study had a positive family history of atopy, with at least one first-degree family member suffering from allergic symptoms, which probably explains why heredity did not have any impact on the results. Parental smoking, before or immediately after birth, may not increase the risk of allergic sensitization in children, but it is a significant risk factor for recurrent wheezing in the first 1.5 years of life [48,49]. In our study, only six children were exposed to tobacco smoke and almost no parents reported indoor smoking. This might explain why we were unable to find any correlation between tobacco smoke and airway problems in this study population.

To our knowledge, this is the only prospective study that has followed infants with eczema to the age of 10 with standardized methods such as SCORAD index and Hanifin-Rajka criteria to objectively describe the eczema, and with spirometric and NO tests for a reliable asthma diagnosis [50]. One concern was that following children for a long time could increase the number of drop-outs. It is plausible to assume that children who did not have any allergic symptoms would be less enthusiastic to continue the study and more likely to be found among our drop-outs, which could affect the result. This, however, has not been the case in other studies [33,51,52]. To minimize the risk of misinterpreting the results, we compared SCORAD points on inclusion for drop-outs with the rest of the study population and found no significant difference between the groups.

Conclusions

This study indicates that high SCORAD points in infants with eczema are associated with a greater risk of asthma at 10 years of age. Children with eczema and wheezing episodes during infancy are more likely to get asthma later in life compared with infants with eczema only. Eczema in infancy combined with early onset of ARC appears to indicate a more severe allergic disease, which often leads to asthma development. The study shows that the progression from eczema in infancy to ARC at an early age and asthma later in childhood could support the relevance of the term "atopic march", at least for children with a more severe allergic disease.

Acknowledgments

We would like to thank all the children and their parents who participated. We would also like to express our gratitude to the participating nurses. Thanks to Karl Wahlin for invaluable statistical advice. Thanks also to Dr. Lennart Nilsson for valuable advice. The advice on language from Maurice Devenney is gratefully acknowledged.

Author Contributions

Conceived and designed the experiments: MT ID GO GN LS KFM. Performed the experiments: ME MT ID GO GN LS KFM. Analyzed the data: ME ID. Wrote the paper: ME ID KFM.

References

1. Van Bever HP (2009) Determinants in early life for asthma development. Allergy Asthma Clin Immunol 9;5(1):6.
2. Host A, Halken S (2000) The role of allergy in childhood asthma. Allergy 55(7):600–608.
3. Pedersen SE, Hurd SS, Lemanske RF Jr, Becker A, Zar HJ, et al. (2011) Global strategy for the diagnosis and management of asthma in children 5 years and younger. Pediatr Pulmonol 46(1):1–17.
4. Burgess JA, Lowe AJ, Matheson MC, Varigos G, Abramson MJ, et al. (2009) Does eczema lead to asthma? J Asthma 46(5):429–436.
5. Leung DY, Bieber T (2003) Atopic dermatitis. Lancet 11;361(9352):151–160.
6. Ker J, Hartert TV (2009) The atopic march: what's the evidence? Ann Allergy Asthma Immunol 103(4):282–289.
7. Scadding GK (2007) Further marches: allergic and non-allergic. Clin Exp Allergy 37(4):485–487.
8. van der Hulst AE, Klip H, Brand PL (2007) Risk of developing asthma in young children with atopic eczema: a systematic review. J Allergy Clin Immunol 120(3):565–569.
9. Nissen SP, Kjaer HF, Host A, Nielsen J, Halken S (2013) The natural course of sensitization and allergic diseases from childhood to adulthood. Pediatr Allergy Immunol 24(6):549–555.
10. Carlsten C, Dimich-Ward H, Ferguson A, Watson W, Rousseau R, et al. (2013) Atopic dermatitis in a high-risk cohort: natural history, associated allergic outcomes, and risk factors. Ann Allergy Asthma Immunol 110(1):24–28.
11. Dharmage SC, Lowe AJ, Matheson MC, Burgess JA, Allen KJ, et al. (2013) Atopic dermatitis and the atopic march revisited. Allergy 14.
12. Saunes M, Oien T, Dotterud CK, Romundstad PR, Storro O, et al. (2012) Early eczema and the risk of childhood asthma: a prospective, population-based study. BMC Pediatr 24;12:168-2431-12-168.
13. von Kobyletzki LB, Bornehag CG, Hasselgren M, Larsson M, Lindstrom CB, et al. (2012) Eczema in early childhood is strongly associated with the development of asthma and rhinitis in a prospective cohort. BMC Dermatol 27;12:11-5945-12-11.
14. Fitzpatrick AM, Teague WG, Meyers DA, Peters SP, Li X, et al. (2011) Heterogeneity of severe asthma in childhood: confirmation by cluster analysis of children in the National Institutes of Health/National Heart, Lung, and Blood Institute Severe Asthma Research Program. J Allergy Clin Immunol 127(2):382–389.e1–13.
15. Just J, Saint-Pierre P, Gouvis-Echraghi R, Boutin B, Panayotopoulos V, et al. (2013) Wheeze phenotypes in young children have different courses during the preschool period. Ann Allergy Asthma Immunol 111(4):256–261.e1.
16. Martinez FD, Wright AL, Taussig LM, Holberg CJ, Halonen M, et al. (1995) Asthma and wheezing in the first six years of life. The Group Health Medical Associates. N Engl J Med 19;332(3):133–138.
17. Agache I, Ciobanu C (2010) Risk factors and asthma phenotypes in children and adults with seasonal allergic rhinitis. Phys Sportsmed 38(4):81–86.
18. Duncan JM, Sears MR (2008) Breastfeeding and allergies: time for a change in paradigm? Curr Opin Allergy Clin Immunol 8(5):398–405.
19. Devenney I, Norrman G, Oldaeus G, Stromberg L, Falth-Magnusson K (2006) A new model for low-dose food challenge in children with allergy to milk or egg. Acta Paediatr 95(9):1133–1139.
20. Hanifin JM Rajka G (1980) Diagnostic features of atopic dermatitis. Acta Derm Venereol 92:44–47.
21. European Task Force on Atopic Dermatitis (1993) Severity scoring of atopic dermatitis: the SCORAD index. Consensus Report of the European Task Force on Atopic Dermatitis. Dermatology 186(1):23–31.
22. Devenney I, Falth-Magnusson K (2001) Skin prick test in duplicate: is it necessary? Ann Allergy Asthma Immunol 87(5):386–389.
23. The European Academy of Allergology and Clinical Immunology (1993) Position paper: Allergen standardization and skin tests. Allergy 48(14 Suppl):48–82.

24. Tomicic S, Norrman G, Falth-Magnusson K, Jenmalm MC, Devenney I, et al. (2009) High levels of IgG4 antibodies to foods during infancy are associated with tolerance to corresponding foods later in life. Pediatr Allergy Immunol 20(1):35–41.

25. Swedish National Pediatric Allergy Group (nd) 1st Asthma in Toddlers - terminology and diagnoses. Available: http://www.barnallergisektionen.se/stenciler_nya06/b1_astmadefinitioner.html. Accessed 2005.

26. Dalen G, Kjellman B (1979) Assessment of lung function on healthy children using an electronic spirometer and an air-flowmeter before and after inhalation of an adrenergic receptor stimulant. Acta Paediatr Scand 68(1):103–108.

27. Silverman M AS (1972) Standardization of exercise test in asthmatic children. Arch Dis Child 47:882–889.

28. Illi S, von Mutius E, Lau S, Nickel R, Gruber C, et al. (2004) The natural course of atopic dermatitis from birth to age 7 years and the association with asthma. J Allergy Clin Immunol 113(5):925–931.

29. van der Hulst AE, Klip H, Brand PL (2007) Risk of developing asthma in young children with atopic eczema: a systematic review. J Allergy Clin Immunol 120(3):565–569.

30. Spergel JM, Paller AS (2003) Atopic dermatitis and the atopic march. J Allergy Clin Immunol 112(6 Suppl):S118–27.

31. Bergmann RL, Edenharter G, Bergmann KE, Forster J, Bauer CP, et al. (1998) Atopic dermatitis in early infancy predicts allergic airway disease at 5 years. Clin Exp Allergy 28(8):965–970.

32. Gustafsson D, Sjoberg O, Foucard T (2000) Development of allergies and asthma in infants and young children with atopic dermatitis—a prospective follow-up to 7 years of age. Allergy 55(3):240–245.

33. Ballardini N, Kull I, Lind T, Hallner E, Almqvist C, et al. (2012) Development and comorbidity of eczema, asthma and rhinitis to age 12: data from the BAMSE birth cohort. Allergy 67(4):537–544.

34. Ballardini N, Bergström A, Böhme M, van Hage M, Hallner E, et al. Infantile Eczema - prognosis and risk of asthma an rhinitis in pre-adolescence. J.Allergy Clin.Immunol. In press.

35. Schmitt J, Langan S, Williams HC (2007) European Dermato-Epidemiology Network. What are the best outcome measurements for atopic eczema? A systematic review. J Allergy Clin Immunol 120(6):1389–1398.

36. Schram ME, Spuls PI, Leeflang MM, Lindeboom R, Bos JD, et al. (2012) EASI, (objective) SCORAD and POEM for atopic eczema: responsiveness and minimal clinically important difference. Allergy 67(1):99–106.

37. Ricci G, Patrizi A, Baldi E, Menna G, Tabanelli M, et al. (2006) Long-term follow-up of atopic dermatitis: retrospective analysis of related risk factors and association with concomitant allergic diseases. J Am Acad Dermatol 55(5):765–771.

38. Frank PI, Morris JA, Hazell ML, Linehan MF, Frank TL (2008) Long term prognosis in preschool children with wheeze: longitudinal postal questionnaire study 1993–2004. BMJ 21;336(7658):1423–1426.

39. Peroni DG, Piacentini GL, Alfonsi L, Zerman L, Di Blasi P, et al. (2003) Rhinitis in pre-school children: prevalence, association with allergic diseases and risk factors. Clin Exp Allergy 33(10):1349–1354.

40. Shaaban R, Zureik M, Soussan D, Neukirch C, Heinrich J, et al. (2008) Rhinitis and onset of asthma: a longitudinal population-based study. Lancet 20;372(9643):1049–1057.

41. Guerra S, Sherrill DL, Martinez FD, Barbee RA (2002) Rhinitis as an independent risk factor for adult-onset asthma. J Allergy Clin Immunol 109(3):419–425.

42. Gaffin JM, Sheehan WJ, Morrill J, Cinar M, Borras Coughlin IM, et al. (2011) Tree nut allergy, egg allergy, and asthma in children. Clin Pediatr (Phila) 50(2):133–139.

43. Gustafsson D, Sjoberg O, Foucard T (2003) Sensitization to food and airborne allergens in children with atopic dermatitis followed up to 7 years of age. Pediatr Allergy Immunol 14(6):448–452.

44. Govaere E, Van Gysel D, Verhamme KM, Doli E, De Baets F (2009) The association of allergic symptoms with sensitization to inhalant allergens in childhood. Pediatr Allergy Immunol 20(5):448–457.

45. Arshad SH, Tariq SM, Matthews S, Hakim E (2001) Sensitization to common allergens and its association with allergic disorders at age 4 years: a whole population birth cohort study. Pediatrics 108(2):E33.

46. Burke W, Fesinmeyer M, Reed K, Hampson L, Carlsten C (2003) Family history as a predictor of asthma risk. Am J Prev Med 24:160.

47. Litonjua AA, Carey VJ, Burge HA, Weiss ST, Gold DR (1998) Parental history and the risk for childhood asthma. Does mother confer more risk than father? Am J Respir Crit Care Med 158(1):176–181.

48. Strachan DP, Cook DG (1998) Health effects of passive smoking .5. Parental smoking and allergic sensitisation in children. Thorax 53(2):117–123.

49. Halken S (2004) Prevention of allergic disease in childhood: clinical and epidemiological aspects of primary and secondary allergy prevention. Pediatr Allergy Immunol 15 Suppl 16:4–5, 9–32.

50. Jenkins C, Seccombe L, Tomlins R (2012) Investigating asthma symptoms in primary care. BMJ 344:e2734.

51. Savenije OE, Granell R, Caudri D, Koppelman GH, Smit HA, et al. (2011) Comparison of childhood wheezing phenotypes in 2 birth cohorts: ALSPAC and PIAMA. J Allergy Clin Immunol 127(6):1505–12.e14.

52. Ostblom E, Lilja G, Pershagen G, van Hage M, Wickman M (2008) Phenotypes of food hypersensitivity and development of allergic diseases during the first 8 years of life. Clin Exp Allergy 38(8):1325–1332.

5

Prevalence of Childhood Atopic Dermatitis: An Urban and Rural Community-Based Study in Shanghai, China

Feng Xu[1,9], Shuxian Yan[1,9], Fei Li[1,9], Minqiang Cai[2], Weihan Chai[3], Minmin Wu[4], Chaowei Fu[4], Zhuohui Zhao[4], Haidong Kan[4], Kefei Kang[1], Jinhua Xu[1]*

1 Department of Dermatology, Huashan Hospital, Shanghai Medical College, Fudan University, Shanghai, People's Republic of China, 2 Xinjing Community Health Service Center, Shanghai, People's Republic of China, 3 Department of Dermatology, Jiading District Traditional Chinese Medicine Hospital, Shanghai, People's Republic of China, 4 School of Public Health, Key Lab of Public Health Safety of the Ministry of Education, Shanghai Medical College, Fudan University, Shanghai, People's Republic of China

Abstract

Background: Atopic dermatitis (AD) is a common inflammatory and chronically relapsing disorder with increasing prevalence. However, little is known about its prevalence in Shanghai, the top metropolitan of China. This study will estimate and compare the prevalence of AD in urban and rural areas in representative samples of 3 to 6-year-old children in Shanghai.

Methodology/Principal Findings: A descriptive cross-sectional study was performed. Pre-school children were obtained by cluster sampling from 8 communities in different districts in Shanghai. The main instrument was the core questionnaire module for AD used in the U.K. Working Party's study. All the data were statistically analyzed by EpiData 3.1 and SPSS16.0. A total of 10436 children completed the study satisfactorily, with a response rate of 95.8%. The prevalence of AD in 3 to 6-year-old children was 8.3% (Male: 8.5%, Female: 8.2%). The prevalence in urban areas of Shanghai was gradiently and significantly higher than that in rural areas. The highest prevalence was in the core urban area (10.2% in Xuhui Tianping) vs. the lowest far from the urban areas (4.6% in Chongming Baozhen).

Conclusions/Significance: The prevalence of AD was 8.3% (95%CI: 7.6%–9.1%) in children aged 3 to 6 in Shanghai. The prevalence of AD decreased from the center to the rural areas in Shanghai.

Editor: Devendra Amre, University of Montreal, Canada

Funding: This study was supported by Chinese Medical Fund of Shanghai Municipal Health Bureau (2010QL034A), National Natural Science Foundation of China (NSFC no. 30800894) The funders had no role in study design, data collection and analysis, decision to publish, or preparation of the manuscript.

Competing Interests: The authors have declared that no competing interests exist.

* E-mail: xjhhuashan@yahoo.com.cn

9 These authors contributed equally to this work.

Introduction

Atopic dermatitis (AD) is a common inflammatory disease characterized by intense itch and eczematous lesions, which has become an important health problem in children worldwide. There are considerable differences in prevalence between and within countries due to geographic distributions and economical development. A high prevalence of AD is noted in countries such as Sweden, Japan, New Zealand, United Kingdom, Portugal and Thailand, opposed to the countries with lower prevalence rates[1] such as in Iran, Albania, India, Singapore and Spain. In China. A higher prevalence was found in Beijing and Shanghai, reported by Gu Heng in 2002, while a lower prevalence was found in Shenyang[2]. Since then, with the rapid economic development in Shanghai, there has been no follow-up study of the prevalence of AD in children of this city. The objective of this work was to evaluate and compare the prevalence of AD in children aged 3 to 6 year-old in Shanghai with special attention to the difference between urban and rural areas.

Methods

Selection of population

The survey was conducted in eight communities, which are listed in Figure. 1 from March to July, 2010. According to the geographic distribution in Shanghai, eight communities were randomly selected from different areas. The selection of communities was stratified with 2 from urban area, 2 from suburban area and 4 from rural area. All the kindergardens registered in the communities selected were involved in this study by cluster sampling. Children enrolled in the kindergartens in these eight communities were all surveyed in this study. 1-Xuhui Tianping (XT) and 2-Pudong Huamu (PH) are in the center of Shanghai. 3-Changning Xinjing (CX) is at the boundary of the center area, about 10 kilometers from the city center. 4-Jiading Juyuan(JJ)and 5-Baoshan Sitang(BS) are about 30 to 40 kilometers from the center of Shanghai and have experienced significant economic development in the past decade. 6-Nanhui Xinchang(NX), 7-Jinshan Sanyang (JS) and 8-Chongming Baozheng (CB) are typical of the countryside around Shanghai, about 60 to100 kilometers from the center of Shanghai, and much farther away than 4 and 5.

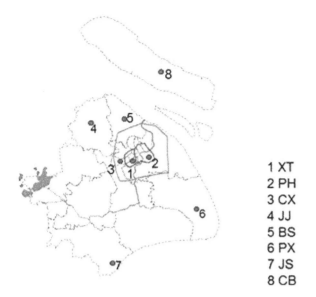

Figure 1. Location of eight communities. The urban area of Shanghai is encircled as the Inner Ring (red) and urbanized suburb of Shanghai is encircled as the Outer Ring (pink).

1 XT
2 PH
3 CX
4 JJ
5 BS
6 PX
7 JS
8 CB

Data collection and diagnostic criteria

One teacher in each kindergarden was responsible for the interview (including communicate with the parents and explain the questions if necessary). All these teachers in charge were undertaken the uniform training by the professional dermatologist to ensure they fully understood the questions in the questionnaire before they helped the children's parents fill out the questionnaire. Personal basic information, such as date of birth, sex, address, telephone number, etc. was recorded and questions based on the U.K. Working Party's diagnostic criteria (UK criteria) for AD were used. In our research, the questionnaire was translated into local language by the teachers in the kindergarten if the parents couldn't understand the written language. The study and the questionnaire were approved by the Ethics Committee of Huashan Hospital, Fudan University, Shanghai, China.

The diagnostic UK criteria [3] require: itchy skin (or parental report of scratching or rubbing in a child) plus 3 or more of the following:

1. History of involvement of the skin creases such as folds of elbows, behind the knees, front of ankles or around the neck (including cheeks in those under 10 years old).
2. A personal history of asthma or hay fever (or history of atopic disease in a first degree relative in those under 4 years old).
3. A history of generally dry skin in the last year.
4. Visible flexural dermatitis (or dermatitis involving the cheeks/forehead and outer aspect of the limbs in children under 4).
5. Onset under the age of 2.

If the child had a history of pruritus and 3 or more minor criteria, he/she would be diagnosed as AD.

We selected inclusion criteria of 3 to 6 years old as the majority of AD patients have early childhood onset, and this also provides many years of life for sequential follow-up studies.

Data analysis

Data were entered on the database (Epidata 3.1). A $\chi 2$ test was used to calculate the difference between groups. OR, 95%

confidence interval (CI), and significance values for the prevalence of AD were calculated using the SPSS statistics analysis package (SPSS for Windows, version 16.0, Chicago, IL, USA). A p-value <0.05 was considered statistically significant. Spearman bivariate analysis was used to evaluate the correlation between the prevalence of AD and GDP (Gross Domestic Product) per capita. Correlation was significant at the 0.01 level.

Results

Of the 10891 subjects, a total of 10436 children were completely surveyed. The responding rate was 95.8%. The reason for no response were sickness or travel of children that their parents could not be informed. But these missing data didn't influence the final results.

A total of 5383 boys and 5053 girls participated in the study and the average age was 5.11 ± 0.90 years old. The prevalence of AD based on the questionnaire was 8.3% (95%CI: 7.6%–9.1%). Boys with AD (8.5% [95%CI: 7.0%–9.9%]) slightly prevailed over girls (8.2% [95%CI:7.3%–9.1%]); this difference was not statistically significant(P value>0.05). The prevalence of AD in boys but not girls decreased from 3 to 5 years old. Table 1 shows the prevalence of AD by ages and gender.

The prevalence of AD according to geographic distribution (Figure. 1 and Figure. 2a) was obviously higher in the core area of the city. The highest prevalence of AD was in 1.XT community, which was located in the center of Shanghai and the lowest prevalence was in 8-CB community, which was typical of the countryside around Shanghai and farthest away from the center of Shanghai (OR = 1.509, 95% CI 1.111–2.050). Figure. 2b shows GDP per capita of different districts in 2008. Table 2 shows the detailed data of the prevalence of AD in eight different communities. The prevalence of AD has significant correlation with GDP per capita in different districts ($r_s = 0.786$, P = 0.001).

Discussion

In this large sample of community-based cross-sectional study, we enrolled 10436 pre-school children aged 3 to 6 in Shanghai using UK criteria. The prevalence of AD was 8.3% (95%CI: 7.6%–9.1%). A high response rate of 95.8% (n = 10436/10891) with statistical results by UK criteria have made this updated data reliable [2]. The symptoms of AD as a rule are expressed within the first two years of life, thus, this data provides a full span of life time for later sequential follow-up studies.

There has been no study reporting the prevalence of AD in Shanghai since 2002. Currently, the prevalence in this study (8.3%) was much higher relative to the 2.78% derived from Gu's study in Shanghai and 4.75% in Beijing in 2002 using the same diagnostic criteria [4]. We then considered the economic

Table 1. Atopic Dermatitis age-grouped by gender.

age	male			female			Total
	population	AD	%	population	AD	%	%
3~	1152	110	9.5%	1042	86	8.3%	8.9%
4~	1729	149	8.6%	1606	122	7.6%	8.1%
5~	1854	140	7.6%	1797	150	8.3%	7.9%
6~	648	56	8.6%	608	57	9.4%	9.0%

The questionnaire was used based on UKWP criteria for AD diagnosis.

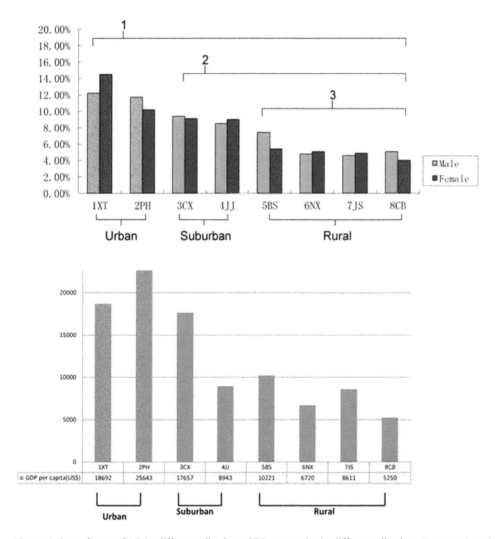

Figure 2. Prevalence of AD in different districts; GDP per capita in different districts. Figure 2a Prevalence of AD in different districts. 1 The prevalence of Urban (#1XT and #2PH) showed statistically significant difference to that of other districts (P<0.05). 2 The prevalence of Suburban (#3CX and #4JJ) showed statistically significant difference to that of the rural areas (P<0.05). 3. Meanwhile the prevalence of different communities in each unit (Urban, Suburban and Rural) showed no statistically significant difference (P>0.05). Figure 2b GDP per capita in different districts. The prevalence of AD has significant correlation with GDP per capita in different districts.(rs = 0.786, P = 0.001)

development in terms of GDP; the data showed that GDP per capita in Shanghai has tremendously grown from US$4900 in 2002 to over US$10,000 in 2010. We found, interestingly, that the AD prevalence in the center of Shanghai was much higher than that of rural area (10.2% in 1XT vs 4.6% in 10CB, P<0.05). The odds ratio was 1.509. The prevalence of AD has significant correlation with GDP per capita in different districts ($r_s = 0.786$, P = 0.001). Some suburban areas, such as 4JJ, have a relatively higher prevalence than that of the other rural areas (5BS). Schram et al [5] had analyzed all twenty-six primary studies comparing the prevalence of eczema between urban and rural populations. Nineteen showed a higher risk for eczema in an urbanized area, of which 11 were significant. Our community-based study now adds more data supporting a higher risk for AD in urban areas. Although China is a developing country, Shanghai is currently a renowned metropolitan city, especially in the core of the city such as the areas located at #1 and #2 shown in Fig. 1. Moreover, in the past 10 years, in addition to the #1 and #2 areas, some areas have also been developing rapidly such as #4JJ and #5BS, and become urbanized with the high-speed development paralleled

with #1 and #2, which may account for the increment of the prevalence of AD in Shanghai. In fact, in recent years, industrial manufacturing has grown rapidly in #4JJ and #5BS, in contrast, #8(CB) still keeps in old production way as some other communities in the countryside. Indeed, there are several variables among rural and urban areas, which might contribute to the differences found in prevalence in Shanghai. Pollution is usually higher in urban areas, as the traffic in urban areas is notably higher than in rural areas. Dotterud et al. [6] found a significant relative risk (3.0, 95%CI 2.5–3.5) for prevalence of eczema in polluted versus nonpolluted areas. Other possible factors that might contribute to the effects are exposure to animals, maternal age, overcrowding in an apartment, differences in food (e.g. processed vs. fresh), socioeconomic factors and time spent indoors[7]. Further studies on environmental circumstances are currently ongoing in our group to reveal the factors associated with a higher prevalence of AD in urban areas.

The result of our study was in agreement with the results of the previous studies performed in other Asian areas and countries nearby. Taiwan found an overall prevalence of 6.7% of AD

Table 2. Atopic Dermatitis in 3 to 6 years old children populated in the different communities.

Community	population	AD	Prevalence			P value*
			Male	Female	Total	
1XT	1214	162	12.2%	14.5%	13.3%	
2PH	1642	180	11.7%	10.2%	11.0%	>0.05
3CX	2309	214	9.4%	9.1%	9.3%	<0.05
4JJ	958	84	8.5%	9.0%	8.8%	<0.05
5BS	1503	96	7.4%	5.4%	6.4%	<0.05
6NX	987	49	4.8%	5.1%	5.0%	<0.05
7JS	990	47	4.6%	4.9%	4.7%	<0.05
8CB	833	38	5.1%	4.0%	4.6%	<0.05

The prevalence of AD ordered by the distance from the core urban to the rural communities surveyed in Shanghai.
*P value refers to the prevalence of each community compared with the prevalence of 1XT.

among the whole population and 9.6% among the people less than 20 years old reported in 2010[8]. In the study of ISAAC (International Study of Asthma and Allergy in Childhood), the overall prevalence of AD in Japan was 11.2% (11.8% among 6–7 years old and 10.5%11–12 years old [9].

According to the latest data reported by Tatyana E. Shaw, prevalence ranged from 8.7 to 18.1% among different areas in the United States with the highest prevalence in many districts of the East Coast states. Metropolitan living style and educational level were found to be associated with prevalence of AD [10].

It is obvious that the economic condition in Shanghai has been rapidly developing and is now similar to that in those areas or countries. The prevalence of AD in Shanghai has become as high as that of other developed areas in Asia. Meanwhile, with comparison of European and American areas, the prevalence of AD is still lower. According to the ISAAC's reports, the prevalence of AD surveyed in several European countries ranged from 13.5% to 21.4% [11–14]. Most likely, differences in diet and lifestyles, environmental and educational levels may add to the different prevalence between eastern and western countries.

Our study gives a strong evidence of the representation and large samples of children from different districts, including urban, urbanized suburb and rural areas and high response rate. Before the survey, kindergarten staffs were trained to explain the questionnaire and to help the parents ascertain flexural dermatitis. AD is usually the first symptom of the "atopic march", so we studied children 3 to 6 years old to allow investigation of the entire march in the following years. While there is still some limitations that this was a questionnaire study without examination of each case by a dermatologist. Misinterpretation could still occur in different populations, and recall bias may exist.

Acknowledgments

We thank Dr. Susan Nedorost for her critical review of this manuscript. We thank Jing Gao, Weiguo Zhou, Yan Wang, Ying Lu, Xiao Chen and Yuxiao Sun for participating or supporting this survey.

Author Contributions

Conceived and designed the experiments: FX SY FL JX. Performed the experiments: FX SY FL MC WC JX. Analyzed the data: FL CF. Contributed reagents/materials/analysis tools: ZZ MW HK. Wrote the paper: FL KK.

References

1. Williams H, Robertson C, Stewart A, Ait-Khaled N, Anabwani G, et al. (1999) Worldwide variations in the prevalence of symptoms of atopic eczema in the International Study of Asthma and Allergies in Childhood. J Allergy Clin Immunol 103: 125–138.
2. Gu H, Chen XS, Chen K, Yan Y, Jing H, et al. (2001) Evaluation of diagnostic criteria for atopic dermatitis: validity of the criteria of Williams et al. in a hospital-based setting. Br J Dermatol 145: 428–433.
3. Williams HC, Burney PG, Hay RJ, Archer CB, Shipley MJ, et al. (1994) The U.K. Working Party's Diagnostic Criteria for Atopic Dermatitis. I. Derivation of a minimum set of discriminators for atopic dermatitis. Br J Dermatol 131: 383–396.
4. Gu H, You LP, Liu YS, Yan Y, Chen K (2004) Survey on the Prevalence of Childhood Atopic Dermatitis in Ten Cities of China. Zhonghua Pifuke Zazhi, 37: 29–31.
5. Schram ME, Tedja AM, Spijker R, Bos JD, Williams HC, et al. (2010) Is there a rural/urban gradient in the prevalence of eczema? A systematic review. Br J Dermatol 162: 964–973.
6. Dotterud LK, Odland JO, Falk ES (2004) Atopic dermatitis and respiratory symptoms in Russian and northern Norwegian school children: a comparison study in two arctic areas and the impact of environmental factors. J Eur Acad Dermatol Venereol 18: 131–136.
7. Braback L, Hjern A, Rasmussen F (2004) Trends in asthma, allergic rhinitis and eczema among Swedish conscripts from farming and non-farming environments. A nationwide study over three decades. Clin Exp Allergy 34: 38–43.
8. Hwang CY, Chen YJ, Lin MW, Chen TJ, Chu SY, et al. (2010) Prevalence of atopic dermatitis, allergic rhinitis and asthma in Taiwan: a national study 2000 to 2007. Acta Derm Venereol 90: 589–594.
9. Saeki H, Iizuka H, Mori Y, Akasaka T, Takagi H, et al. (2005) Prevalence of atopic dermatitis in Japanese elementary schoolchildren. Br J Dermatol 152: 110–114.
10. Shaw TE, Currie GP, Koudelka CW, Simpson EL (2011) Eczema prevalence in the United States: data from the 2003 National Survey of Children's Health. J Invest Dermatol 131: 67–73.
11. van de Ven MO, van den Eijnden RJ, Engels RC (2006) Atopic diseases and related risk factors among Dutch adolescents. Eur J Public Health 16: 549–558.
12. Peters AS, Kellberger J, Vogelberg C, Dressel H, Windstetter D, et al. (2010) Prediction of the incidence, recurrence, and persistence of atopic dermatitis in adolescence: a prospective cohort study. J Allergy Clin Immunol 126: 590-595 e591-593.
13. Hatakka K, Piirainen L, Pohjavuori S, Poussa T, Savilahti E, et al. (2009) Allergy in day care children: prevalence and environmental risk factors. Acta Paediatr 98: 817–822.
14. Guiote-Dominguez MV, Munoz-Hoyos A, Gutierrez-Salmeron MT (2008) Prevalence of atopic dermatitis in schoolchildren in Granada, Spain. Actas Dermosifiliogr 99: 628–638.

6

Interferon and Biologic Signatures in Dermatomyositis Skin: Specificity and Heterogeneity across Diseases

David Wong[1], Bory Kea[1], Rob Pesich[2], Brandon W. Higgs[3], Wei Zhu[3], Patrick Brown[2], Yihong Yao[3], David Fiorentino[1]*

1 Department of Dermatology, Stanford University School of Medicine, Stanford, California, United States of America, 2 Department of Biochemistry, Stanford University School of Medicine, Stanford, California, United States of America, 3 MedImmune, Translational Sciences, One MedImmune Way, Gaithersburg, Maryland, United States of America

Abstract

Background: Dermatomyositis (DM) is an autoimmune disease that mainly affects the skin, muscle, and lung. The pathogenesis of skin inflammation in DM is not well understood.

Methodology and Findings: We analyzed genome-wide expression data in DM skin and compared them to those from healthy controls. We observed a robust upregulation of interferon (IFN)-inducible genes in DM skin, as well as several other gene modules pertaining to inflammation, complement activation, and epidermal activation and differentiation. The interferon (IFN)-inducible genes within the DM signature were present not only in DM and lupus, but also cutaneous herpes simplex-2 infection and to a lesser degree, psoriasis. This IFN signature was absent or weakly present in atopic dermatitis, allergic contact dermatitis, acne vulgaris, systemic sclerosis, and localized scleroderma/morphea. We observed that the IFN signature in DM skin appears to be more closely related to type I than type II IFN based on in vitro IFN stimulation expression signatures. However, quantitation of IFN mRNAs in DM skin shows that the majority of known type I IFNs, as well as IFN g, are overexpressed in DM skin. In addition, both IFN-beta and IFN-gamma (but not other type I IFN) transcript levels were highly correlated with the degree of the *in vivo* IFN transcriptional response in DM skin.

Conclusions and Significance: As in the blood and muscle, DM skin is characterized by an overwhelming presence of an IFN signature, although it is difficult to conclusively define this response as type I or type II. Understanding the significance of the IFN signature in this wide array of inflammatory diseases will be furthered by identification of the nature of the cells that both produce and respond to IFN, as well as which IFN subtype is biologically active in each diseased tissue.

Editor: Serge Nataf, University of Lyon, France

Funding: The authors have no support or funding to report.

Competing Interests: The authors have declared that no competing interests exist.

* E-mail: fiorentino@stanford.edu

Introduction

Dermatomyositis (DM) is a chronic inflammatory disorder that can affect the skin, muscle, and other organs and is associated with significant morbidity and mortality. The prevalence of DM is not well-defined, as it is historically grouped together with polymyositis (PM) and inclusion body myositis (IBM) in most epidemiologic studies. The estimated incidence of DM is approximately 1 per 100,000 per year [1]. There are two forms of DM, juvenile and adult, that have overlapping but some distinct clinical features [1]. DM is considered an autoimmune disease, as it is associated with specific autoantibodies, and its prevalence is associated with particular HLA alleles [2].

Currently classified as an idiopathic inflammatory myopathy (IIM), much of the work in understanding DM has been focused on the muscle pathology that accompanies this disorder. Some authors have suggested that the muscle disease is due to an immune-mediated vasculopathy, with resultant ischemic damage to the muscle fibers resulting in myocyte death and muscle atrophy [3]. However, the precise mechanism of either endothelial cell or myocyte damage is unclear [3]. Inflamed muscle shows infiltration with B lymphocytes, T lymphocytes, and dendritic cells, and the contribution of each to the disease is not well understood [4,5]. Cytokines and chemokines are also postulated to be important in disease pathogenesis [6]. DM muscle expresses large amounts of type I interferon (IFN)-inducible genes [7]. It is possible that these gene products might themselves be causing the vascular and parenchymal cellular damage [7]. In addition, an IFN signature that correlates with overall disease activity is observed in peripheral blood of most DM patients, including patients with juvenile DM [8,9,10]. Thus, much as with other autoimmune diseases such as Systemic Lupus Erythematosus and Sjogren's syndrome, DM is emerging as a potentially type I IFN-driven autoimmune disease.

The pathogenesis of skin inflammation in DM is not well-studied and its pathologic mechanisms may or may not overlap with those causing DM muscle disease. The typical cutaneous histopathologic changes in DM include pathologic apoptosis/necrosis of keratinocytes, perivascular and lichenoid inflammation, increased dermal mucin deposition, endothelial cell damage with loss of capillaries, and vascular dilatation [11,12]. Similarities to muscle disease exist in the skin: first, vasculopathy and vascular deposition of complement components can be detected in cutaneous DM skin [13,14]; second, there is damage to the parenchymal cells (e.g. keratinocytes) [11]; third, DM skin appears to be characterized by increased abundance of several gene products that are known to be upregulated by IFN [15,16] as well as by increased numbers of plasmacytoid dendritic cells [17,18]. It has been proposed that some of these gene products, such as CXCL9/10/11, act as chemoattractants for CXCR3-bearing T lymphocytes which can then perpetuate inflammation and keratinocyte necrosis [16]. In addition, there appears to be a topographical relationship between the site of cell injury, inflammation, and the basement membrane that is shared by both skin and muscle disease in DM [19]. However, there are certain differences between muscle and skin disease in DM patients: clinically, the course of skin and muscle disease is often discordant between patients [20], suggesting different mechanisms of disease pathogenesis; in addition, there are important histopathologic differences between skin and muscle—for example, B lymphocytes are rarely found in the skin disease [21], in contrast to their common perivascular location in DM muscle. Current therapies for DM skin disease include immunosuppressive medications, which are not uniformly efficacious and can be associated with significant morbidity [20]. A better understanding of molecular pathogenesis of DM could potentially unveil better molecular markers for this disease and more effective targets for therapy.

In this study, we performed global gene expression analysis of skin from DM patients and healthy controls. Our results reveal a gene expression signature that is unique to skin inflammation in both DM and lupus, but distinct from other inflammatory skin diseases. Within this signature, we also identify a characteristic IFN-driven expression pattern in DM and lupus that partially overlaps with the pattern seen in other lichenoid dermatoses as well as psoriasis.

Results

Defining expression signature in skin of individuals with DM

In order to understand the molecular characteristics of DM, we hybridized RNA from skin biopsies from patients with active DM (n = 16) and healthy patients (n = 10) (total of 32 independent biopsies, with 12 technical replicates for total of 44 arrays) to HEEBO oligonucleotide arrays. The baseline characteristics of these patients are listed in Table S1. Using significance analysis of microarrays (FDR<0.05), we identified 946 unique genes that were differentially regulated at least 2-fold in DM skin relative to healthy skin: we term this the "DM gene module" (Table S2). Over two-thirds (646 of 946) of the genes identified were up-regulated and 300 were down-regulated in DM skin relative to healthy skin. Two-dimensional hierarchical clustering using these 946 genes segregated all healthy controls and DM patients into 2 distinct clusters (Fig. 1A). The 3 DM patients (4 samples) that segregated with the healthy controls formed a separate sub-cluster unto themselves. There was no apparent clustering with regards to age, gender, or site of biopsy (not shown). When patients with inactive skin disease were included in the cluster analysis, we found that 6 of 7 of the inactive DM patients clustered with the healthy controls (Fig. S1).

We noted that the DM gene module contained groups of genes that are known to function in several distinct biological pathways (Figs. 1A and S2). For example, a group of 13 genes

associated with keratinocyte/epidermal activation (S100A7/8/9, SERPINB3/4, and FABP5) was upregulated in DM (yellow bar, Figs. 1A and S2). In addition, genes involved in epidermal differentiation, including IVL, TGM, SPRR2A/B/E/G, SER-PINB7/8, are induced in DM (red bar, Figs. 1A and S2), which have also been shown to be elevated in other inflammatory skin diseases, such as psoriasis and atopic dermatitis [22,23]. A large cluster of genes upregulated in DM are involved in T cell (IL2RB, CD2, TRAC, CD3D, CTLA4), cytotoxic/NK cell (NKG7), macrophage (CD68), and dendritic cell (CD83) function (green bar, Figs. 1A and Fig. S2), which is consistent with previous observations regarding T cell and macrophage infiltration in DM skin [21]. The overexpression of the cell surface marker CD83 is consistent with previous studies that showed with immunostaining that mature dendritic cells are present in DM skin (either myeloid or plasmacytoid) [16,18]. In addition, skin from patients with DM had induction of markers of endothelial cell activation (VCAM1, SEL-L). A subset of the DM samples showed elevated immunoglobulin expression, indicative of infiltrating mature B lymphocytes and/or plasma cells, the former of which have been shown to be present in low and variable amounts in DM skin (lavender bar, Figs. 1A and S2) [21].

A striking observation in DM skin was the over expression of genes that were induced by IFN (light blue bar, Figs. 1A and S2). In fact, 21 of the top 25 most upregulated genes are known or presumed to be upregulated by IFN [24,25,26] (Table S3). These genes included CXCL10, IFIH1, ISG15/UBE2L6, C1S/R, IRF7, IDO1, MXB and CHN1. Notably this cluster of IFN genes was generally not overexpressed in the skin of DM patients with inactive skin disease (Fig. S1), suggesting that they are induced preferentially in active skin lesions.

Of the downregulated genes in DM, many were involved in either ribosomal synthesis (brown bar, Figs. 1A and S2) or lipid metabolism (dark purple bar, Figs. 1A and S2). The latter group of genes included MVD, MGST1, GCS1, FADS1/2 and GAL. Many of the genes involved in lipid metabolism have been previously reported to be downregulated in other inflammatory skin disorders such as psoriasis and atopic dermatitis [22,27].

To validate our findings from these microarrays, we performed TaqMan quantitative real-time reverse-transcriptase PCR-(QRT-PCR-) based assays on several genes from two of the enriched gene modules, the IFN and lipid gene modules (Fig. 1B). As suggested by the arrays, TaqMan QRT-PCR confirmed that two IFN-induced genes (IFIT3 and OAS2) were upregulated, and two genes involved in lipid metabolism (FADS, HMGCS1) were downregulated in the skin of DM patients. Across patient samples, there was a good correlation between microarray and QRT-PCR values for each of the four genes (Spearman $\rho = 0.76$ to 0.88).

In order to systematically investigate the biological processes that are altered in DM skin, we constructed a gene module map (p<0.05, FDR<0.05) to look for enrichment of gene sets associated with various biologic pathways and/or functions, based on either Gene Ontology (GO) and KEGG pathway annotations and on data derived from publicly available gene expression studies (Figs. 2 and S3). Biologic functions and pathways found to be enriched in the upregulated genes in DM skin included antigen processing, complement activation, MHC I/II receptor activity, T cell function, chemokine activity, antiviral and immune responses and epidermal differentiation (Fig. 2). Besides the IFN signaling pathway, TNF-alpha, IL-1, IL6, IL17 and VEGF pathway activation was also observed in the skin of DM patients (Fig. S3). Downregulated processes in DM skin included fatty acid

A

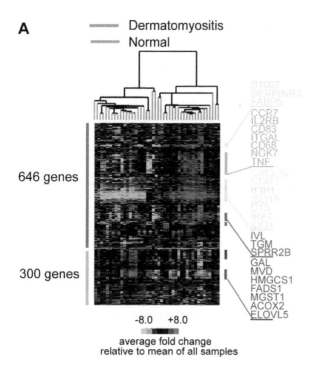

B

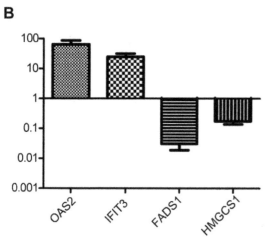

Figure 1. Visualization and validation of DM gene expression on HEEBO oligonucleotide arrays. RNA was prepared from skin biopsies as detailed in Methods, and the same source was used for both gene expression array (**A**) and QRT-PCR experiments (**B**). **A.** Experimental hierarchical clustering dendrogram. Two-dimensional hierarchical clustering was performed on gene expression data from active DM skin lesions and skin from healthy controls. A set of 946 genes whose average expression significantly differed between DM and healthy controls (the "DM module) was used to group sample expression data; 646 genes were upregulated (red bar on left) and 300 genes were downregulated (green bar on left) in DM patients relative to control biopsies. All values are in log$_2$ space and are mean-centered across each gene. Colored bars on right indicate gene clusters evident on dendrogram: yellow bar—epidermal activation; green bar—leukocyte function; light blue bar—IFN signature; red bar—epidermal differentiation; lavender bar—immunoglobulin; brown bar—ribosome; dark purple bar-lipid metabolism. A larger view of the dendrogram and more complete lists of genes in these clusters can be found in **Supplementary Figure S2**. **B.** Validation of array data using TaqMan QRT-PCR of selected transcripts. QRT-PCR was performed (see Methods) on 9 DM skin RNA samples and 8 control skin RNA samples for four selected transcripts that were either found to be upregulated (OAS2, IFIT3) or downregulated (FADS1, HMGCS1) in DM skin. Shown are the mean values (with SEM) for each transcript in DM skin relative to the

mean value in control skin. Relative transcript values for each of the 4 genes across the 9 DM samples showed a high correlation (Pearson's r = 0.71 to 0.86) between the HEEBO array and QRT-PCR.

metabolism, lipid biosynthesis and metabolism, mitochondrial function (electron transport and pyruvate metabolism), peroxisome and ribosomal function.

Mapping the DM gene module across different skin diseases

We next sought to study the specificity of these gene expression changes across various inflammatory skin diseases. With the exception of the cutaneous lupus samples (which were internally collected and processed along with the DM samples), we used publicly available gene expression sets, and all disease data were normalized to internal healthy controls within each study. We examined the expression of genes in the DM gene module across the different diseases (Fig. 3; see also Fig. S4 for a full pairwise correlation matrix). Due to the use of different array platforms in this analysis, only 490 genes of the original 946 genes of the DM module were contained in all of the experimental datasets analyzed and could thus be used for the analysis. Although the data were generated by different investigators on different microarray platforms, diseases for which more than one dataset existed (psoriasis and atopic dermatitis) showed remarkably similar expression patterns between datasets (Spearman ρ = 0.77 to 0.82). A similar correlation analysis between DM samples analyzed using HEEBO arrays and an independent set of DM samples analyzed using Affymetrix arrays demonstrated high correlation (Spearman r = 0.76) (Fig. 3). This suggests that the differences observed between diseases were primarily driven by biological disease-specific characteristics rather than platform or laboratory differences.

The gene expression profiles in DM and lupus skin samples were remarkably similar (Spearman r = 0.87; Fig. 3), suggesting that skin from individuals with DM and lupus, which are both autoimmune interface dermatitis processes, have a common pathophysiology. Interestingly, the upregulated genes in the DM gene module were similarly induced in the muscle of DM patients (Spearman r = 0.56; Fig. 3). DM skin also showed similarity to samples from (herpes simplex-2) HSV-2 infection (Spearman r = 0.64; Fig. 3). The rest of the inflammatory skin diseases appeared to have a small subset of similarly regulated genes as in DM, but overall the pattern was quite different. The epidermal activation genes, such as S100 and SERPIN genes appear to be generally upregulated across most of the skin diseases except for localized and systemic scleroderma (yellow bar, Fig. 3). In addition, many of the inflammatory genes were variably expressed across different diseases, with the highest expression observed in cutaneous lupus and HSV-2, moderately high expression in DM skin and muscle, and modest increase in expression in other diseases (green bar, Fig. 3). Genes involved in the complement cascade (C1S, C1R, C1QB, and C2) were only upregulated in DM skin/muscle, cutaneous lupus, and HSV-2 skin (not shown). IFN-inducible genes were very highly overexpressed in DM skin/muscle, lupus skin, and HSV-2 skin; and to a lesser degree in psoriasis, and the blood of DM and lupus patients (light blue bar, Fig. 3). Genes of lipid metabolism were generally repressed not only in cutaneous DM and lupus but also psoriasis, atopic dermatitis, and morphea, and to a variable extent in other inflammatory skin diseases (dark purple bar, Fig. 3). Of note, this repression of lipid metabolism genes is not found in DM muscle, DM blood, or

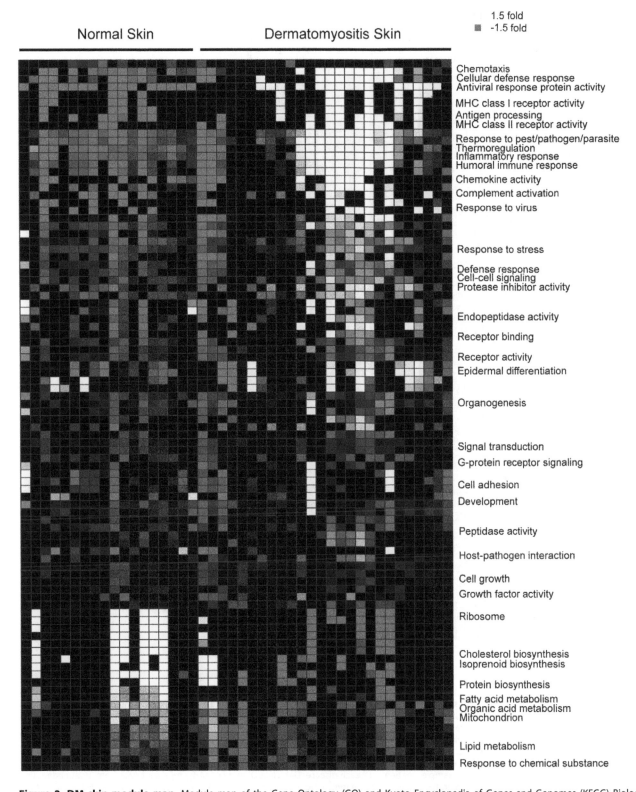

Figure 2. DM skin module map. Module map of the Gene Ontology (GO) and Kyoto Encyclopedia of Genes and Genomes (KEGG) Biological Processes differentially expressed among the active DM samples is shown. Each column represents a single microarray (e.g. patient) and each row represents a single GO or KEGG biological process. Only modules that were significantly enriched (minimum 2-fold change, p = 0.05) on at least 4 microarrays are shown. The average expression of the gene hits from each enriched gene set is displayed here. Only gene sets that show significant differences after multiple hypothesis testing were included. Selected GO or KEGG biological processes are shown. The entire figure with all biological processes can be viewed in Supplementary Figure S3.

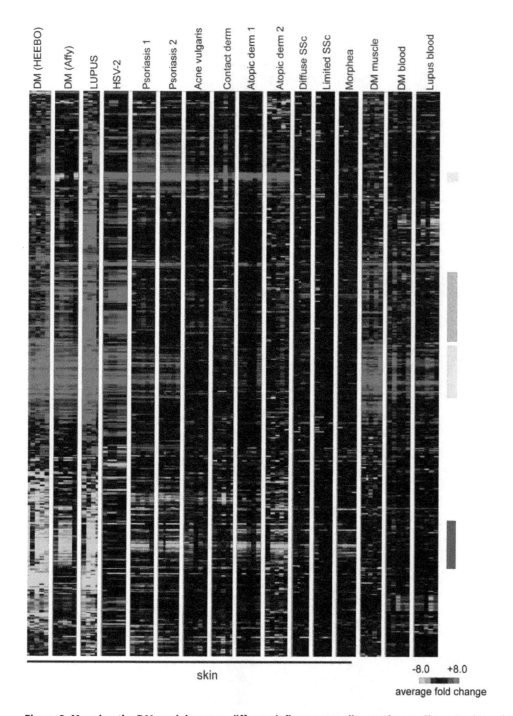

Figure 3. Mapping the DM module across different inflammatory disease tissues. Shown is a hierarchical clustering dendrogram of gene expression data from DM and multiple other diseases. The genes visualized represent all of the genes of the DM module that are common to all of the array platforms used to generate the data shown. The expression pattern of this set of 490 genes across all of the disease states shown was clustered using average linkage clustering, while the columns (samples) were not clustered and grouped by disease and experimental dataset. Expression data for each gene is relative to the mean expression level for all healthy controls (red = upregulated; green = downregulated) within each dataset, with the exception that HSV-2 data is relative to uninvolved skin of *diseased* HSV-2 patients (see Methods). Each disease state is composed of five columns, representing five representative examples (patients) of each disease. DM (HEEBO) and DM (Affy) represent data from independent DM skin biopsies run on either HEEBO or Affymetrix arrays, respectively. The remaining datasets were obtained from publicly available GEO omnibus data (see Methods). All data are derived from skin biopsies with the exception of the three diseases on the right, as indicated. Colored bars on right indicate gene clusters of the DM module that were discussed in the text for Figure 1: yellow bar—epidermal barrier; green bar—leukocyte function; light blue bar—IFN signature; dark purple bar-lipid metabolism.

lupus blood, and may thus be a skin-specific phenomenon. Thus, a cross disease comparison reveals that some gene expression changes may be more commonly seen in inflamma- tory skin diseases, while other (e.g. IFN signature) are more specific, and overall, DM and lupus skin share a highly unique gene expression signature.

Measuring the IFN signature across different skin diseases

Although many IFN-inducible genes were upregulated in our DM module, we wished to determine in more detail how expression of a pre-defined module of IFN-inducible genes was regulated in DM and several other inflammatory skin diseases. A consensus list of 117 IFN-stimulated genes (Table S4) was derived by using publicly available data from in vitro stimulations of various cell types with either type I or II IFNs (see Methods). The expression pattern of these IFN-inducible genes was then surveyed across both the in vitro IFN stimulation data as well as diseased skin expression data. Some variation exists in the in vitro response upon IFN stimulation, depending on the cell type, IFN type, and the independent labs that generated the data (Fig. 4A, left panel). Again it appeared that DM skin and muscle, lupus skin, and HSV-2 skin infection had the most robust overexpression of IFN-inducible genes (Fig. 4B, right panel; also see Fig. S5 for a full pairwise correlation matrix). As was the case for the entire DM module, the expression patterns of IFN-inducible genes in skin of DM and lupus patients appeared almost indistinguishable, and similar to those in DM muscle and HSV-2. DM blood and lupus blood had a weaker induction of IFN genes, which is likely due to the fact that the IFN module was constructed using data from cell types present in skin and not blood. Interestingly, psoriasis demonstrated induction of a subset of IFN-inducible genes. In contrast, most of the skin samples of acne vulgaris, contact dermatitis, atopic dermatitis, allergic contact dermatitis, systemic sclerosis, and morphea did not appear to show significant induction of IFN-driven genes.

We next quantified the strength of the IFN-signature across different disease states. Similar to previous studies, we selected the top 25 most highly IFN-inducible genes from our "core IFN signature", based on the in vitro studies that were used to define this signature (Table S4) [28]. We found that the scores calculated these 25 genes versus the full 117 gene module display a high correlation (Spearman's r = 0.96; not shown). We then calculated the median expression value (relative to healthy controls) of these 25 genes for each sample, which constituted the "IFN score" (Fig. 4B) [28]. DM and lupus skin had the highest average median IFN scores of 20 and 44, respectively. DM muscle and HSV-2 skin had high IFN scores (9.5 and 8.1, respectively), while the two psoriasis datasets yielded mean scores of 2.5 and 2.8. In contrast, all other skin diseases had scores of 1.7 or less.

In addition to the differences in overall IFN score, we were intrigued with the different patterns of IFN-induced genes in the various skin inflammatory diseases (Fig. 4A). These different patterns of IFN signature could be due to multiple factors, including: 1) a difference in cell types responding to IFN stimulation, 2) a difference in IFN subtypes (e.g. type I or II) that are present among the diseases, or 3) the presence of other cytokines that may induce a subset of genes in our "core IFN set". To further investigate the differences in these patterns, we performed principal components analysis of the various disease samples as well as the samples obtained using in vitro IFN stimulations (Fig. 4A) using the in vitro-defined core IFN signature genes (Fig. 5A). We observed that the horizontal component tends to correlate with the strength of IFN signature, specifically in the skin (Figs. 4B and 5). Thus, DM muscle, DM and lupus skin, and HSV-2 are furthest to the right, while psoriasis, DM and lupus blood, and selected systemic sclerosis and atopic dermatitis samples all are modestly displaced to the right from all other skin diseases that are clustered together on the left—this is in general agreement with our IFN scoring data (Fig. 4B). On the other hand, the vertical component (component 2) appears to at least partially

distinguish type I versus type II IFN (see in vitro stimulation data towards the right of Fig. 5). Additionally, the disease samples tend to be more positively positioned along this component, suggesting that DM, lupus and psoriasis all have signatures more consistent with type I IFN than with type II IFN.

IFN gene expression in DM skin

In order to further characterize the IFN response in DM skin, we performed QRT-PCR analysis of the selected IFNs, including IFN-alpha (subtypes 1,2,4,6,8,14 and 21), IFN-beta, IFN-kappa, IFN-omega, and IFN-gamma. Due to unavailability of RNA from samples in our original dataset, these data were derived from skin biopsy samples from an independent cohort of 39 DM patients (see Methods). Importantly, these samples showed similar gene expression patterns to our original dataset (Fig. 4A and S5). We found that expression levels of all IFN transcripts, with the exception of IFN-α4, were elevated in DM skin compared to healthy controls, although there was considerable variation between patients (Fig. 6A). Noting this variation, we next wished to clarify if any of the IFN transcripts were coordinately regulated by performing average linkage hierarchical clustering of the QRT-PCR data for the IFN transcripts across the 39 samples. The IFN-alpha transcripts (with the possible exception of IFN-a21 and IFN-a4) as well as the IFN-omega transcripts were coordinately regulated (Fig. 6B). IFN-beta and IFN-gamma were more closely correlated with one another than any of the other transcripts, while IFN-kappa had the most distinct pattern of expression across the samples.

Our previous data suggested that the IFN signature in DM skin was more similar to the pattern seen with type I rather than type II IFN (Fig. 5). We reasoned that another independent method of identifying the dominant IFN subtype(s) generating the in vivo IFN signature in DM skin was to perform a correlation analysis between the level of each particular IFN family transcript and the IFN score for all of the available samples. Strikingly, IFN-beta transcript level was very highly correlated with IFN signature strength in the skin (Spearman r = 0.82; p<0.0001) (Fig. 6C). Interestingly, IFN-gamma also demonstrated a high correlation with IFN signature score (Spearman r = 0.72; p<0.0001), while none of the IFN-alpha subtypes (as well as IFN-omega) were significantly correlated with the strength of the IFN signature (Fig. 6C; data not shown).

Discussion

This is the first study of global gene expression in the skin of DM patients. We demonstrate an expression signature (the "DM module") in the skin of 16 DM patients relative to skin from 10 normal, unaffected individuals using whole genome HEEBO oligonucleotide arrays. This DM signature was validated in an independent set of DM skin samples on a different microarray platform (Affymetrix). In addition, examination of this signature across multiple different inflammatory skin diseases demonstrated that this signature is unique to DM and lupus, suggesting that cutaneous DM and cutaneous lupus have a similar underlying pathogenetic mechanism. This signature was characterized by up-regulation of genes involved in antigen processing, complement activation, MHC I/II receptor activity, T cell function, chemokine activity, antiviral and immune responses and epidermal differentiation, and down-regulation of genes involved in fatty acid metabolism, lipid biosynthesis and metabolism, mitochondrial function, and ribosomal function.

One might argue that these gene expression changes are simply a function of increased immune cell infiltration in DM skin. Thus,

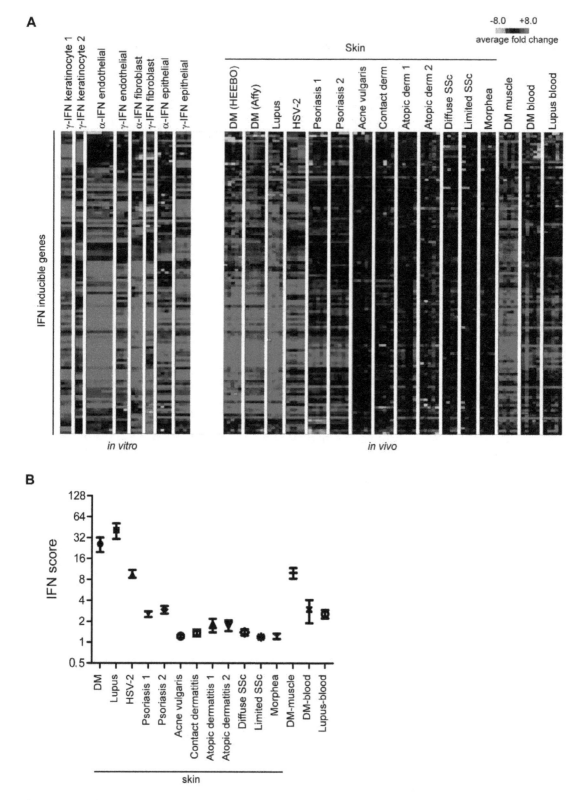

Figure 4. Visualizing the pattern and strength of the IFN signature expression across multiple disease states. A. Heatmaps of gene expression of the IFN inducible genes both *in vitro* and *in vivo* across diseases. The expression of a set of 117 genes comprising the "core IFN signature" (labeled as "IFN inducible genes" in the figure) is shown following one-way hierarchical clustering (genes only) using the entire *in vitro* and *in vivo* dataset. The left panel shows the expression patterns of this IFN signature following various *in vitro* stimulations with IFN-alpha or IFN-gamma on different responding cell types, as indicated. The right panel shows the expression patterns of the IFN signature across multiple disease states. The data from the disease states were derived from publicly available data as described in Figure 3 and Methods. **B.** Comparing the strength of the IFN signature across disease states using an IFN score. The top 25 expressed IFN-inducible genes (a static list) was derived from the same *in vitro* data used to generate the core IFN signature as described in Methods. The median expression value (in linear space) of this set of 25 genes within each

disease sample was defined as the IFN score for that sample. Shown is the mean and SEM for IFN scores calculated for each disease dataset represented in panel A.

we performed a study across multiple inflammatory skin diseases to address the specificity of the altered transcriptional modules seen in DM skin. This cross-disease comparison suggests that, while several gene expression patterns are shared more commonly across inflammatory skin diseases, many of the gene expression patterns are not found uniformly across inflammatory skin diseases. For example, upregulation of genes typically associated with epidermal activation was seen in all skin diseases except scleroderma. In addition, we observed downregulation of a large number of genes involved in lipid metabolism across most of the skin diseases we studied. The only disease in which this was not apparent was HSV-2, and this may actually reflect the fact that this dataset used non-lesional skin from patients (rather than skin from healthy volunteers) as a control—downregulation of lipid genes has been seen in non-lesional skin of psoriasis patients [27] and we have also seen this in the uninvolved skin from DM patients (data not shown). Downregulation of genes involved in lipid metabolism has been previously reported in psoriasis and atopic dermatitis [22,27,29], but our data suggest that it is a more general feature of many inflammatory skin diseases. It is unclear what cell types are being affected to cause these observed changes, although this lipid regulation could indicate the presence of a defective epidermal barrier, as suggested previously [22]. However, we found other signatures, notably the interferon signature as well as others, that appear to be more characteristic of only

selected inflammatory skin diseases, despite the fact that many conditions lacking these signatures (e.g. atopic dermatitis, acne vulgaris) are known to be characterized by inflammatory infiltrates in the skin. Of course, it is still possible that the transcriptional changes seen in DM skin are a direct result of a unique type(s) of infiltrating cell. For the interferon signature, one possible cell type would be the plasmacytoid dendritic cell, and experiments to correlate the strength of various transcriptional responses with infiltrating cell types would be important to perform in the future.

Our data show conclusively that a genuine IFN signature is seen in DM skin, similar to that found in the blood and muscle of DM patients [9,10,30,31]. It is important to look at a complete set of IFN-inducible genes and not simply one gene product, as this can lead to erroneous conclusions of an IFN signature being present. For example, focusing only at MxA, a protein classically characterized as type I IFN-specific, would have led to the conclusion that both atopic dermatitis datasets showed an average of 2.9-fold overexpression relatively to healthy controls (data not shown); this could be misconstrued as evidence of type I IFN activation in the skin of atopic dermatitis, which is clearly not the case. Thus, our results confirm and extend previous reports that demonstrated upregulation of a few selected, IFN-inducible proteins (MxA, CXCL9, CXCL10) in DM skin [15,16]. This signature was found in all patients in which active skin disease was biopsied, but was found at low or absent levels in biopsies from

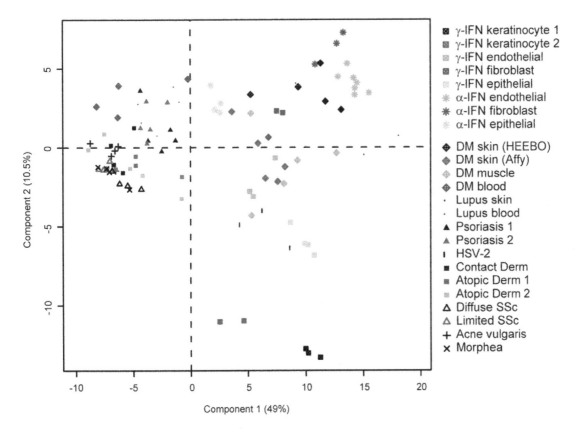

Figure 5. Distinguishing between type I and II IFN expression patterns across disease states. Two-dimensional PCA plot is shown using expression data derived from our data (DM, lupus) and publicly available datasets across the 117 gene "core IFN gene set" as described in Methods. Approximately 60% of the total data variation is summarized in these first two principal components.

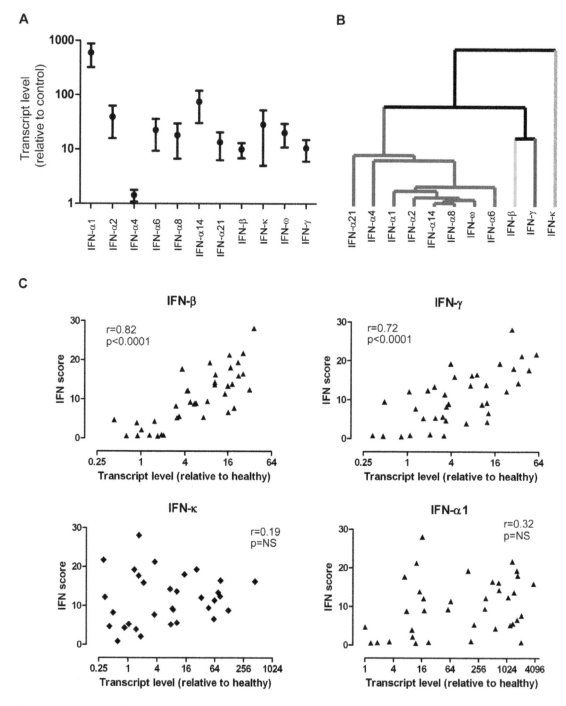

Figure 6. Expression of IFN transcripts in DM skin and correlation with downstream response. A. Upregulation of most IFN transcripts in DM skin. QRT-PCR analysis of different IFN transcripts in DM skin samples. TaqMan PCR was performed (see Methods) on 39 DM skin RNA samples and 4 control skin RNA samples for selected IFN transcripts. Shown are the mean values (with SEM) for each transcript in DM skin relative to the mean value in control skin. **B.** IFN transcripts are not co-regulated across DM skin samples. Hierarchical clustering dendrogram is shown for relative IFN transcript expression levels (using QRT-PCR) across 39 DM samples. Average linkage clustering was performed using correlation (uncentered) similarity metric. Similarity branches (length is inversely correlated with similarity of expression patterns) for IFN-α and IFN-ω are shown in red, IFN-beta in light blue, IFN-gamma in dark purple, and IFN-κ in green. **C.** IFN-beta and IFN-gammacorrelate most closely with the IFN score in DM skin. For each RNA sample made from 39 independent DM skin biopsies, an IFN score was calculated based on transcript levels of downstream IFN-inducible genes from array data (as described in Figure 4B and Methods) as well as a relative transcript level (using QRT-PCR) for several IFN transcripts (see panel A). Shown are correlation plots (for each of the 39 samples) of the IFN score and IFN transcript levels for IFN-a1, IFN-beta, IFN-gamma, and IFN-kappa.

patients with inactive skin disease, despite the presence of active myositis in the latter group. Thus, the IFN signature in the skin might serve as a useful marker for cutaneous disease activity in DM.

This study also provides information regarding the specificity of the IFN signature across many inflammatory skin diseases. We found that DM, lupus, and HSV-2 skin, and to a lesser degree, psoriasis, had moderate-to-robust IFN signatures, whereas atopic dermatitis, contact dermatitis, systemic sclerosis, and acne vulgaris had relatively weak or absent IFN signatures. Psoriasis was characterized by induction of a large subset of the IFN "core" genes whose expression pattern appeared to correlate with a type I IFN response, in agreement with prior observations [32]. The subtle differences between the IFN signatures of DM and lupus compared with psoriasis may be due to a different source of IFN in the two diseases, different population of responding cells, or modulating cytokines. It is curious that psoriasis appears to have an IFN signature, as all other skin diseases that we found to have this signature are characterized by a predominance of keratinocyte injury and/or death. Indeed, it has been suggested that the IFN signature is characteristic of the lichenoid skin reaction [33], but, given the fact that keratinocyte death is not associated with psoriasis, it is clear that the significance of an IFN signature in skin disease may be more complicated. However, it should be noted that the IFN score was much lower in psoriasis skin than in the other lichenoid disorders, and thus may not reach a threshold required to initiate pathways involved in keratinocyte death.

Our data have highlighted the difficulty in assigning an IFN signature as being "type I" or "type II", especially in tissue that contains multiple cell types and cannot be easily modeled *in vitro*. Although a type I IFN signature has been suggested to be present in multiple inflammatory skin diseases, this has yet to be shown conclusively [32,33,34]. Many genes thought to be specifically induced by type I IFN can also be induced by type II IFN, and this relationship is highly dependent on responding cell type and IFN dose. We have employed two methodologies to address this question in DM skin. First, we used various methods of comparing patterns of IFN-inducible gene expression with those obtained from various *in vitro* stimulations using recombinant type I or type II IFN. Although these comparisons suggest that DM skin is more characteristic of Type I IFN rather than type II IFN activity (see Fig. 5), it is difficult to draw firm conclusions from these data. One weakness of this approach is that it is difficult to compare patterns of gene expression obtained under in vitro conditions in cell lines and that which occurs in a dynamic tissue with multiple responding cell types and unknown concentrations of various IFN proteins. Our data certainly could be consistent with activation of either the type I or II IFN pathways in DM skin.

We also performed a correlation analysis between specific IFN transcript levels and a composite measurement of IFN-activity, namely the IFN gene score. We found that IFN-beta and IFN-gamma levels most closely correlate with activation of IFN-induced genes (see Fig. 6C), also suggesting that either type I or II IFNs could be driving the IFN response. Although we did not find a correlation between the IFN-alpha (and other type I) transcripts we measured, this does not rule out a role for these interferons in DM skin disease. It is possible that a threshold level of IFN-alpha is required for the IFN response, which may then be modulated by varying levels of other interferons. The involvement of specific interferons in disease activity will only be conclusively answered by treating patients with specific IFN inhibitors. An alternative interpretation of these data is that IFN-betaand IFN-gamma) are

regulated in the same manner as the other IFN-induced transcripts in DM skin, although this is unlikely given the striking difference in abundance of IFN-beta mRNA versus the other IFN-induced transcripts in DM skin (data not shown). One weakness of this approach is that it assumes that IFN transcript level faithfully reflects the level of active IFN protein in the skin biopsies—however, this assumption would only serve to weaken any positive correlation, and thus the high correlation coefficients we observed are likely of significance.

The fact that many biopsies have high levels of other type I IFN transcripts (which share the same receptor as IFN-beta) in the absence of an IFN signature (Fig. 6C) suggests that other considerations are critical for the strong induction of IFN-induced genes seen in the skin of DM patients—these may include translation of IFN transcripts, localization of IFN production and/ or presence of a responder cell population that is sensitive signaling via the IFN receptor. Thus, our data do not rule out an essential role for other type I or II IFNs in the pathogenesis of DM skin disease. They also point out the important fact that elevation of a particular IFN transcript does not provide proof of its activity *in vivo*.

One limitation of our study is that our data are derived from whole skin biopsies, and thus it is unclear what cell(s) constitute the source of IFN, as well as what cell(s) are responsible for producing such high levels of IFN-induced mRNA transcripts. Previous data suggest that keratinocytes as well as inflammatory cells are included in the latter "responding" population in DM skin [16]. However, it is clear that the pattern of expression of IFN-inducible proteins depends on the protein examined [15,16,33]. In addition, it will be important to detect the source of different IFN transcripts and proteins in DM skin, which can be technically demanding. Without detailed understanding of these issues, the role of IFN in DM skin disease will remain unclear.

Another potential weakness of our study is that many of our analyses compared data generated by different investigators, using different methodologies, across different microarray platforms. We attempted to mitigate this problem by only using datasets in which a control group was included, so that all data could be expressed relative to healthy patient skin. In addition, where possible, we used identical methodologies for normalizing array data. Despite this, we realize that this can always be a concern when analyzing microarray data, and thus we were more interested in the patterns of gene expression rather than absolute levels of selected genes. We believe our methodology had internal validation in that, for a given disease, independent patient samples run by independent investigators across disparate microarray platforms showed astonishingly similar patterns of gene expression over the gene modules that we were interested in studying (see Figure 3).

Our study defines patterns of gene expression that readily distinguish normal from DM skin. Many of these genes may prove to be useful as specific molecular markers that correlate with disease progression and prognosis. Our analysis provides further insight into the underlying pathogenesis of DM, including characterization of a specific IFN response in DM that may provide more effective targets for therapy.

Methods

Ethics Statement

The Stanford Panel on Medical Human Subjects approved human subjects involvement in this research project (last renewal on 04/18/2011). All subjects entered in this study signed an Informed Consent document before donating tissue.

Patients

All patients were seen in the adult Stanford Dermatology Clinics between August 2004 and March 2006 and agreed to sign an Informed Consent before participating in the study. All patients were diagnosed with DM based upon diagnostic cutaneous findings suggested previously [35] and all patients had a skin biopsy consistent with DM. Exclusion criteria included: (1) age less than 18 years old, and/or (2) evidence of medication-induced DM or mixed-connective tissue disease or other overlap syndromes. There were no restrictions on concomitant medications. We analyzed skin biopsies from 23 DM patients (16 active and 7 inactive) and 10 healthy controls (Table S1). All biopsies were taken from an area that was considered to be representative of active disease. In patients considered to have inactive skin disease (but active myositis), biopsies were taken from areas of telangiectasia and/or pigmentary alteration consistent with prior active DM skin disease. Because skin disease localization in DM patients can be variable, many of these biopsies are from different anatomic sites, although the majority of biopsies were from the arm or neck/upper back (Table S1). 23 DM patients provided a total of 25 biopsies, with 9 technical replicates for a total of 34 samples. 10 healthy controls provided a total of 15 biopsies, with 3 technical replicates, for a total of 18 samples. The DM patients were significantly older than the healthy control patients (mean age 53.1 vs 38.2, p = .019) and had a mean disease duration of 6.0 years. Four of the patients (17%) had cancer-associated DM. 8 of the patients (35%) had skin predominant disease–5 of them with a past history of myositis, and 3 never experiencing myositis (amyopathic). We also included skin biopsies from 4 patients with cutaneous lupus erythematosus (2 with acute cutaneous lupus and 2 with discoid lupus lesions).

Skin biopsy Processing and Microarray Analysis

Poly-adenylated RNA was extracted from snap-frozen skin biopsy specimens (DM and lupus) using a two step method. First, total RNA was extracted with phenol-guanidine thiocyaniate extraction (RNAbee, Tel-Test, Friendswood TX). Next, poly-adenylated RNA was purified using RNeasy Kit (Quiagen, Chatsworth, CA) according to the manufacturer's instructions. Sample RNA and reference mRNA (Stratagene) were amplified using an Amino Allyl MessageAmp II aRNA kit (Ambion, Austin, TX). Amplified skin RNA (labeled with Cy5) and amplified Human Universal Reference RNA (labeled with Cy3) (Stratagene, La Jolla, CA) were competitively hybridized to HEEBO (human exon evidence-based oligonucleotide) microarrays as described (http://www.microarray.org/sfgf/heebo.do).

Array data were filtered based on fluorescent hybridization signal $\geq$1.5-fold over local background in either the Cy5 or the Cy3 channel and if the data were technically adequate in $\geq$80% of experiments. Array data underwent LOWESS normalization, and the data were displayed as a $\log_2$ ratio of LOWESS-normalized Cy5/Cy3 ratio (span parameter = 0.4). These array data are publicly available at Gene Expression Omnibus (GEO), accession number GSE32245.

For experiments assessing the platform independence of our DM array findings (Fig. 3) and for quantifying IFN expression in DM skin (Fig. 6), several independent DM (n = 39) and healthy control (n = 18) biopsies were obtained in the exact manner as described above. These biopsies were processed and hybridized to Affymetrix Human Genome U133 Plus 2.0 GeneChip arrays as described [32]. These array data were normalized using Robust Multichip Averaging (RMA) using Genespring (www.agilent.com/chem/genespring).

For all datasets, after filtering and normalization, expression data of each sample for all probes mapping to the same UnigeneID were averaged in linear space before any analysis was performed. Genes which showed significantly different expression between DM and controls were identified using Significance Analysis of Microarrays, with a false discovery rate (FDR)<0.043 and a minimum average expression of 2-fold greater or less than controls.

Average linkage hierarchical clustering was performed using GeneCluster ver3.0 software (http://bonsai.ims.u-tokyo.ac.jp/~mdehoon/software/cluster/software.htm). Clustered trees and gene expression heat maps were viewed using Java TreeView Software (http://jtreeview.sourceforge.net/).

Module Maps

Gene module map was done as described with the program Genomica (http://genomica.weizmann.ac.il/) using gene sets derived from Gene Ontology and KEGG Pathway annotations and the gene expression profiles of skin from patients with dermatomyositis and normal controls.

Briefly, given this collection of precompiled gene sets and this compendium of expression arrays, the method identifies the gene sets that are induced or repressed significantly in the set of arrays (p$\leq$0.05, hypergeometric distribution).

Comparisons with publicly available microarray data

Publicly available gene expression data was obtained for psoriasis (GSE13355, GSE14905), atopic dermatitis (GSE5667, GSE6012), acne vulgaris (GSE6475), allergic contact dermatitis (GSE6281), HSV-2 infection (GSE18527), systemic sclerosis and morphea (GSE9285), DM muscle (GSE1551, GSE5370), DM blood (courtesy S. Greenberg, Brigham and Women's Hospital), and systemic lupus (GSE8650). The following array platforms were used for these studies: Affymetrix U133A (GSE5667, GSE6012, GSE1551, GSE5370, GSE8650) Affymetrix U133A 2.0 (GSE6475, 5667); Affymetrix U133 plus 2.0 (GSE6281, GSE13355, GSE14905); Agilent Whole Human Genome Oligo Microarray G4112A (GSE9285); Illumina humanref-8 v. 2.0 (GSE18527). Only scleroderma samples that classified as "inflammatory subgroup" were used for comparisons [36], given that we wished to enrich these data for samples that might express an IFN signature. For Affymetrix data, all array data was normalized using Robust Multichip Averaging (RMA) using Genespring (www.agilent.com/chem/genespring).

In order to compare data from different experiments, all expression data were first mapped to a common EntrezGene number. A set of 7783 unique EntrezGene IDs that were common to all platforms was used in these comparisons ("comparison matrix"). Probes that matched to multiple genes were not used. For instances in which multiple probes mapped to the same EntrezGene, these data were averaged by calculating the mean value in linear space to give a single value for each EntrezGene ID. Next, data for each gene in a given disease sample were normalized to the mean expression value of all control samples for that gene. Control samples were always skin biopsies from healthy donors, with the exception of the data from the HSV-2 patients (GSE18527), as the only control data available were derived from patient skin from uninvolved sites. Thus, each experiment was normalized to its own internal control samples, in order to facilitate comparison across experiment sets.

RT PCR analysis of individual transcripts

The expression level of several microarray target genes was assessed in patient tissue using Taqman quantitative one-step RT-

PCR (Applied Biosystems, Foster City, California, United States). Fifty nanograms of total RNA was used in each assay. Assay on demand primers for fatty acid desaturase 1 (Assay ID: Hs00203685_m1), IFN-b1 (Assay ID: Hs00277188_s1), 3-hydroxy-3-methylglutaryl-Coenzyme A synthase 1 (Assay ID: Hs00266810_m1), IFN α 2 (Assay ID: Hs02621172_s1), IFN-a1 (Assay ID: Hs00256882_s1), IFN-induced protein with tetratricopeptide repeats 3 (Assay ID: Hs00155468_m1) and IFN-alpha-inducible protein 6 (Assay ID: Hs00242571_m1) were normalized to GAPDH (Assay ID: Hs99999905_m1) levels and relative abundance was calculated using delta-delta threshold analysis. All assays were conducted on a Stratagene MX3000P thermocycler (La Jolla, CA). RT-PCR analysis of IFN mRNA transcripts was performed as described previously [32].

Mapping the DM module across disease states

Due to differences across array platforms, we first determined that 490 of the 946 genes from the DM module were present across all samples in the "comparison matrix" (defined above). One-way hierarchical clustering was performed (genes only) and the data were viewed as described above, with 5 representative examples from each inflammatory disease used for comparison.

Method for defining genes comprising core IFN signature

We reasoned that the skin has keratinocytes, fibroblasts, endothelial cells, and leukocytes, among other cells that could potentially respond differently to IFN. Thus we generated our list of IFN-stimulated genes from all publicly available expression data pertaining to in vitro stimulation with either IFN-gamma, -alpha, -beta, or other IFN preparations—these included data derived from the use of keratinocytes, lung epithelial cells, macrophages, endothelial cells, and fibroblasts as responder cells. These specific datasets used had the following GEO identifiers: GSE1132, GSE7216, GSE5542, GSE3920, GSE1925, GSE1740. The time of stimulation and concentration of IFN varied between studies. For each study, pre- and post-stimulation data were placed in $\log_2$ space and mean-centered for each gene. All data were then combined and evaluated using Statistical Analysis of Microarrays using a two-class analysis (pre vs post-treatment). From this analysis, 749 genes were identified as significantly regulated by IFN. From this set, we selected only genes that were regulated by an average of two-fold or greater, leaving a final set of 161 genes. Of these 161 genes, 117 were contained in the set of 7783 comprised in the "comparison matrix" gene list discussed above, and thus this set was used as the final "core IFN signature" (Table S4).

Correlation matrices and principal components analysis

Spearman's rank correlations were calculated between individual arrays for various disease/specimen sources and various in vitro stimulations with IFN-alpha or IFN-gamma on different responding cell types using the DM module gene set (490 genes) as well as the IFN signature (as described above). The same expression data of the 117 core IFN signature were further utilized to calculate principal components analysis (PCA). Both the correlations and PCA were conducted using the R statistical computing environment (http://r-project.org). The missing values in the data matrix were imputed by the method svdImpute (from the R package "pcaMethods") and the principal components were calculated with the function prcomp.

Supporting Information

Figure S1 Inactive DM skin samples cluster with healthy controls and not active DM skin samples. Shown

is a hierarchical clustering dendrogram using two-dimensional clustering of gene expression data from active DM skin (gold branches), skin from patients with inactive skin disease (green branches), and healthy controls (light blue branches). The 946 gene "DM module" was used to cluster the skin samples. The red bar to the right of the dendrogram indicates the cluster of IFN-induced genes.

Figure S2 Detailed view of heat map of expression of DM module across skin samples. Two-dimensional hierarchical clustering was performed on gene expression data from active DM skin lesions and skin from healthy controls. A set of 946 genes whose average expression significantly differed between DM and healthy controls (the "DM module) was used to group sample expression data and is shown on the thumbnail diagram at the left. Major clusters of genes are shown with the colored bars and labeled with letters A-G. Shown at the panel on the right are enlarged details of expression data for the labeled clusters, with selected groups of genes labeled at the right. Clusters of genes are: A—epidermal activation; B—leukocyte function; C-IFN signature; D-epidermal differentiation; E—immunoglobulin expression; G—lipid metabolism.

Figure S3 DM skin module map (detailed). Module map of the Gene Ontology (GO), Kyoto Encyclopedia of Genes and Genomes (KEGG), and selected other Biological Processes differentially expressed among the active DM samples is shown. Each column represents a single microarray (e.g. patient) and each row represents a single biological process. Only modules that were significantly enriched (minimum 2-fold change, p = 0.05) on at least 4 microarrays are shown. The average expression of the gene hits from each enriched gene set is displayed here. Only gene sets that show significant differences after multiple hypothesis testing were included. Selected GO or KEGG biological processes are shown. The entire figure with all biological processes can be viewed in Supplementary Figure S3.

Figure S4 Spearman's rank coefficient matrix using the DM module across different inflammatory disease tissues. Correlation correlation similarity matrix for 16 cohorts of disease/specimen source groups with 4–5 replicates per each cohort using the 490 genes in the DM module. DM (HEEBO) and DM (Affy) represent data from independent DM skin biopsies run on either HEEBO or Affymetrix arrays, respectively. The remaining datasets were obtained from publicly available GEO omnibus data (see Methods). All data are derived from skin biopsies with the exception of the three diseases on the rightmost region of the x-axis, as indicated. The color legend at the bottom indicates the range of Spearman p values, with general degrees of correlation indicated at each threshold (e.g. low, no (no correlation), mod (moderate), high, or identity). This figure represents the individual array comparisons from the data presented in Figure 3.

Figure S5 Spearman's rank coefficient matrix using 117 IFN inducible genes both in vitro and in vivo across diseases. Correlation correlation similarity matrix for 16 cohorts of disease/specimen source groups as well as various in vitro stimulations with IFN-alpha or IFN-gamma on different responding cell types with 2–7 replicates per each cohort using 117 IFN inducible genes. Similar to the information presented in Figure 4A, the leftmost columns on the x-axis shows the correlation patterns of this IFN signature following various in vitro stimulations with

IFN-alpha or IFN-gamma on different responding cell types, as indicated. The rightmost columns on the x-axis show the expression patterns of the IFN signature across multiple disease states. The data from the disease states were derived from publicly available data as described in Figure 3 and Methods. The color legend at the bottom indicates the range of Spearman p values, with general degrees of correlation indicated at each threshold (e.g. low, no (no correlation), mod (moderate), high, or identity). This figure represents the individual array comparisons from the data presented in Figure 4A.

Table S1 Patients in this study. [1]Limited to immunomodulatory medications. [2]Skin disease graded as active or inactive. Active disease considered based on erythema, induration and/or pruritus. Inactive disease based on absence of erythema with pigmentary alteration and/or telangiectasia. [3]Defined if any of the following were found: proximal muscle weakness, eleveated muscle enzymes (CPK, aldolase), EMG findings consistent with inflammatory myopathy, muscle biopsy consistent with DM. Abbreviations. DM = DM; NT = not tested; Pred = prednisone (daily dose in mg); MTX = methotrexate; AZA = azathioprine; CSA = cyclosporine; MMF = mycophenolate moefitil; HCQ = hydroxychloroquine; Doxy = doxycycline; homo = homogeneous; unk = unknown; Ca = cancer; ILD = interstitial lung disease.

Table S2 List of genes significantly dysregulated in DM skin. Genes significantly dysregulated in DM skin (compared to skin from healthy donors) were determined using SAM analysis as described in Methods. "Average fold change" refers to the ratio of the mean of the average expression in DM samples divided by the mean of the average expression in control (healthy) samples.

Table S3 Top 25 upregulated genes in DM skin. The top 25 upregulated genes from Table S2 are ordered (highest to lowest expression values relative to healthy controls). Genes previously identified to be induced by IFN are bolded.

Table S4 Core IFN gene list. The 117 genes comprising the "core IFN gene list" are listed (highest to lowest expression values relative to unstimulated cells). The list was derived as described in Methods.

Author Contributions

Conceived and designed the experiments: DW BK DF. Performed the experiments: DW BK RP BH WZ DF. Analyzed the data: DW BK BH YY PB DF. Contributed reagents/materials/analysis tools: DW BK WZ YY PB DF. Wrote the paper: DW BK DF.

References

1. Mammen AL (2010) Dermatomyositis and polymyositis: Clinical presentation, autoantibodies, and pathogenesis. Ann N Y Acad Sci 1184: 134–153.
2. O'Hanlon TP, Miller FW (2009) Genetic risk and protective factors for the idiopathic inflammatory myopathies. Curr Rheumatol Rep 11: 287–294.
3. Greenberg SA, Amato AA (2004) Uncertainties in the pathogenesis of adult dermatomyositis. Curr Opin Neurol 17: 359–364.
4. Arahata K, Engel AG (1984) Monoclonal antibody analysis of mononuclear cells in myopathies. I: Quantitation of subsets according to diagnosis and sites of accumulation and demonstration and counts of muscle fibers invaded by T cells. Ann Neurol 16: 193–208.
5. Page G, Chevrel G, Miossec P (2004) Anatomic localization of immature and mature dendritic cell subsets in dermatomyositis and polymyositis: Interaction with chemokines and Th1 cytokine-producing cells. Arthritis Rheum 50: 199–208.
6. De Paepe B, Creus KK, De Bleecker JL (2009) Role of cytokines and chemokines in idiopathic inflammatory myopathies. Curr Opin Rheumatol 21: 610–616.
7. Greenberg SA (2010) Dermatomyositis and type 1 interferons. Curr Rheumatol Rep 12: 198–203.
8. Niewold TB, Kariuki SN, Morgan GA, Shrestha S, Pachman LM (2009) Elevated serum interferon-alpha activity in juvenile dermatomyositis: associations with disease activity at diagnosis and after thirty-six months of therapy. Arthritis Rheum 60: 1815–1824.
9. Baechler EC, Bauer JW, Slattery CA, Ortmann WA, Espe KJ, et al. (2007) An interferon signature in the peripheral blood of dermatomyositis patients is associated with disease activity. Mol Med 13: 59–68.
10. Walsh RJ, Kong SW, Yao Y, Jallal B, Kiener PA, et al. (2007) Type I interferon-inducible gene expression in blood is present and reflects disease activity in dermatomyositis and polymyositis. Arthritis Rheum 56: 3784–3792.
11. Krathen MS, Fiorentino D, Werth VP (2008) Dermatomyositis. Curr Dir Autoimmun 10: 313–332.
12. Crowson AN, Magro CM (1996) The role of microvascular injury in the pathogenesis of cutaneous lesions of dermatomyositis. Hum Pathol 27: 15–19.
13. Mascaro JM, Jr., Hausmann G, Herrero C, Grau JM, Cid MC, et al. (1995) Membrane attack complex deposits in cutaneous lesions of dermatomyositis. Arch Dermatol 131: 1386–1392.
14. Magro CM, Crowson AN (1997) The immunofluorescent profile of dermatomyositis: a comparative study with lupus erythematosus. J Cutan Pathol 24: 543–552.
15. Wenzel J, Scheler M, Bieber T, Tuting T (2005) Evidence for a role of type I interferons in the pathogenesis of dermatomyositis. Br J Dermatol 153: 462–463; author reply 463–464.
16. Wenzel J, Schmidt R, Proelss J, Zahn S, Bieber T, et al. (2006) Type I interferon-associated skin recruitment of CXCR3+ lymphocytes in dermatomyositis. Clin Exp Dermatol 31: 576–582.
17. Shrestha S, Wershil B, Sarwark JF, Niewold TB, Philipp T, et al. (2010) Lesional and nonlesional skin from patients with untreated juvenile dermatomyositis displays increased numbers of mast cells and mature plasmacytoid dendritic cells. Arthritis Rheum 62: 2813–2822.
18. McNiff JM, Kaplan DH (2008) Plasmacytoid dendritic cells are present in cutaneous dermatomyositis lesions in a pattern distinct from lupus erythematosus. J Cutan Pathol 35: 452–456.
19. Greenberg SA, Fiorentino D (2009) Similar topology of injury to keratinocytes and myofibres in dermatomyositis skin and muscle. Br J Dermatol 160: 464–465.
20. Callen JP, Wortmann RL (2006) Dermatomyositis. Clin Dermatol 24: 363–373.
21. Caproni M, Torchia D, Cardinali C, Volpi W, Del Bianco E, et al. (2004) Infiltrating cells, related cytokines and chemokine receptors in lesional skin of patients with dermatomyositis. Br J Dermatol 151: 784–791.
22. Saaf AM, Tengvall-Linder M, Chang HY, Adler AS, Wahlgren CF, et al. (2008) Global expression profiling in atopic eczema reveals reciprocal expression of inflammatory and lipid genes. PLoS One 3: e4017.
23. Gudjonsson JE, Ding J, Johnston A, Tejasvi T, Guzman AM, et al. (2010) Assessment of the psoriatic transcriptome in a large sample: additional regulated genes and comparisons with in vitro models. J Invest Dermatol 130: 1829–1840.
24. Der SD, Zhou A, Williams BR, Silverman RH (1998) Identification of genes differentially regulated by interferon alpha, beta, or gamma using oligonucleotide arrays. Proc Natl Acad Sci U S A 95: 15623–15628.
25. Sanda C, Weitzel P, Tsukahara T, Schaley J, Edenberg HJ, et al. (2006) Differential gene induction by type I and type II interferons and their combination. J Interferon Cytokine Res 26: 462–472.
26. Indraccolo S, Pfeffer U, Minuzzo S, Esposito G, Roni V, et al. (2007) Identification of genes selectively regulated by IFNs in endothelial cells. J Immunol 178: 1122–1135.
27. Gudjonsson JE, Ding J, Li X, Nair RP, Tejasvi T, et al. (2009) Global gene expression analysis reveals evidence for decreased lipid biosynthesis and increased innate immunity in uninvolved psoriatic skin. J Invest Dermatol 129: 2795–2804.
28. Yao Y, Richman L, Higgs BW, Morehouse CA, de los Reyes M, et al. (2009) Neutralization of interferon-alpha/beta-inducible genes and downstream effect in a phase I trial of an anti-interferon-alpha monoclonal antibody in systemic lupus erythematosus. Arthritis Rheum 60: 1785–1796.
29. Plager DA, Leontovich AA, Henke SA, Davis MD, McEvoy MT, et al. (2007) Early cutaneous gene transcription changes in adult atopic dermatitis and potential clinical implications. Exp Dermatol 16: 28–36.
30. Greenberg SA, Pinkus JL, Pinkus GS, Burleson T, Sanoudou D, et al. (2005) Interferon-alpha/beta-mediated innate immune mechanisms in dermatomyositis. Ann Neurol 57: 664–678.
31. Tezak Z, Hoffman EP, Lutz JL, Fedczyna TO, Stephan D, et al. (2002) Gene expression profiling in DQA1*0501+ children with untreated dermatomyositis: a novel model of pathogenesis. J Immunol 168: 4154–4163.
32. Yao Y, Richman L, Morehouse C, de los Reyes M, Higgs BW, et al. (2008) Type I interferon: potential therapeutic target for psoriasis? PLoS One 3: e2737.
33. Wenzel J, Tuting T (2008) An IFN-associated cytotoxic cellular immune response against viral, self-, or tumor antigens is a common pathogenetic feature in "interface dermatitis". J Invest Dermatol 128: 2392–2402.

34. Ghoreishi M, Martinka M, Dutz JP (2010) Type 1 interferon signature in the scalp lesions of alopecia areata. Br J Dermatol 163: 57–62.

35. Sontheimer RD (2002) Dermatomyositis: an overview of recent progress with emphasis on dermatologic aspects. Dermatol Clin 20: 387–408.

36. Milano A, Pendergrass SA, Sargent JL, George LK, McCalmont TH, et al. (2008) Molecular subsets in the gene expression signatures of scleroderma skin. PLoS One 3: e2696.

7

Variants of C-C Motif Chemokine 22 (*CCL22*) Are Associated with Susceptibility to Atopic Dermatitis: Case-Control Studies

Tomomitsu Hirota[1,⑨], Hidehisa Saeki[2,⑨], Kaori Tomita[1,3], Shota Tanaka[1,4], Kouji Ebe[5], Masafumi Sakashita[3], Takechiyo Yamada[3], Shigeharu Fujieda[3], Akihiko Miyatake[6], Satoru Doi[7], Tadao Enomoto[8], Nobuyuki Hizawa[9], Tohru Sakamoto[9], Hironori Masuko[9], Takashi Sasaki[10], Tamotsu Ebihara[10], Masayuki Amagai[10], Hitokazu Esaki[11], Satoshi Takeuchi[11], Masutaka Furue[11], Emiko Noguchi[12], Naoyuki Kamatani[13], Yusuke Nakamura[14], Michiaki Kubo[15], Mayumi Tamari[1]*

1 Laboratory for Respiratory Diseases, Center for Genomic Medicine, The Institute of Physical and Chemical Research (RIKEN), Kanagawa, Japan, 2 Department of Dermatology, The Jikei University School of Medicine, Tokyo, Japan, 3 Division of Otorhinolaryngology Head & Neck Surgery, Department of Sensory and Locomotor Medicine, Faculty of Medical Science, University of Fukui, Matsuoka, Fukui, Japan, 4 Department of Otorhinolaryngology Head and Neck Surgery, University of Yamanashi Faculty of Medicine, Yamanashi, Japan, 5 Takao Hospital, Kyoto, Japan, 6 Miyatake Asthma Clinic, Osaka, Japan, 7 Department of Pediatric Allergy, Osaka Prefectural Medical Center for Respiratory and Allergic Diseases, Osaka, Japan, 8 Nonprofit Organization (NPO) Japan Health Promotion Supporting Network, Wakayama, Japan, 9 Division of Respiratory Medicine, Institute of Clinical Medicine, University of Tsukuba, Ibaraki, Japan, 10 Department of Dermatology, Keio University School of Medicine, Tokyo, Japan, 11 Department of Dermatology, Graduate School of Medical Sciences, Kyushu University, Fukuoka, Japan, 12 Department of Medical Genetics, Majors of Medical Sciences, Graduate School of Comprehensive Human Sciences, University of Tsukuba, Ibaraki, Japan, 13 Laboratory for International Alliance, Center for Genomic Medicine, The Institute of Physical and Chemical Research (RIKEN), Kanagawa, Japan, 14 Laboratory of Molecular Medicine, The Institute of Medical Science, The University of Tokyo, Tokyo, Japan, 15 Laboratory for Genotyping Development, Center for Genomic Medicine, The Institute of Physical and Chemical Research (RIKEN), Kanagawa, Japan

Abstract

Atopic dermatitis (AD) is a common inflammatory skin disease caused by multiple genetic and environmental factors. AD is characterized by the local infiltration of T helper type 2 (Th2) cells. Recent clinical studies have shown important roles of the Th2 chemokines, CCL22 and CCL17 in the pathogenesis of AD. To investigate whether polymorphisms of the *CCL22* gene affect the susceptibility to AD, we conducted association studies and functional studies of the related variants. We first resequenced the *CCL22* gene and found a total of 39 SNPs. We selected seven tag SNPs in the *CCL22* gene, and conducted association studies using two independent Japanese populations (1st population, 916 cases and 1,032 controls; 2nd population 1,034 cases and 1,004 controls). After the association results were combined by inverse variance method, we observed a significant association at rs4359426 (meta-analysis, combined $P = 9.6 \times 10^{-6}$; OR, 0.74; 95% CI, 0.65–0.85). Functional analysis revealed that the risk allele of rs4359426 contributed to higher expression levels of *CCL22* mRNA. We further examined the allelic differences in the binding of nuclear proteins by electrophoretic mobility shift assay. The signal intensity of the DNA-protein complex derived from the G allele of rs223821, which was in absolute LD with rs4359426, was higher than that from the A allele. Although further functional analyses are needed, it is likely that related variants play a role in susceptibility to AD in a gain-of-function manner. Our findings provide a new insight into the etiology and pathogenesis of AD.

Editor: Jacques Zimmer, Centre de Recherche Public de la Santé (CRP-Santé), Luxembourg

Funding: This work was supported by grants from the Ministry of Education, Culture, Sports, Science and Technology and from the Ministry of Health, Labour and Welfare, Japan. This work was conducted as part of the BioBank Japan Project. The funders had no role in study design, data collection and analysis, decision to publish or preparation of the manuscript.

Competing Interests: The authors have declared that no competing interests exist.

* E-mail: tamari@src.riken.jp

⑨ These authors contributed equally to this work.

Introduction

Atopic dermatitis (AD) is a pruritic and chronically relapsing inflammatory skin disease involving disturbed skin barrier functions, cutaneous inflammatory hypersensitivity and defects in the antimicrobial immune defense with a strong genetic background [1]. Predominant infiltration of Th2 cells is a hallmark of acute atopic AD skin lesions [2]. Most patients with AD have peripheral blood eosinophilia and increased serum IgE levels, which are reflected in an increased frequency of peripheral blood skin-homing Th2 cells producing IL-4, IL-5 and IL-13 [1]. C-C motif chemokine 22 (CCL22) and CCL17 are high-affinity ligands for CC-chemokine receptor 4 (CCR4) and induce selective migration of Th2 cells [3]. CCL22 plays a crucial role in controlling the trafficking of Th2 cells into sites of allergic inflammation and is considered to be involved in the pathology of

AD [4]. Keratinocytes from patients with AD highly express thymic stromal lymphopoietin (TSLP), and CCL22 is produced by TSLP-treated dendritic cells [5]. CCL22 is upregulated in lesional atopic dermatitis skin compared with healthy skin [6], and keratinocytes in the epidermal layer of AD skin express CCL17 and CCL22 [7]. Serum levels of CCL22 in AD patients are significantly higher than those found in normal controls [8], and the levels correlate positively with disease severity in AD patients [9]. Strong positive correlations between the levels of CCL17, CCL22, and total IgE in serum of patients with AD and SCORing Atopic Dermatitis (SCORAD) have also been reported [10]. Another study reported that overproduction of IgE induced CCL22 secretion from basophils, which are essential for IgE-mediated chronic allergic dermatitis [11]. These findings prompt-

Table 1. Frequencies of polymorphisms of the *CCL22* gene.

	SNP*	Location	Amino acid	MAF‡	NCBI†	
1	-3075G/A	5'-flanking region	-	0.125	rs223884	
2	-2938G/A	5'-flanking region	-	0.208	rs223885	
3	-2903T/A	5'-flanking region	-	0.333	rs223886	
4	-2668G/T	5'-flanking region	-	0.458	rs34569362	
5	-2550G/C	5'-flanking region	-	0.458	rs76295899	
6	-2511G/T	5'-flanking region	-	0.458	rs4784799	
7	-2191G/C	5'-flanking region	-	0.042	rs76720124	
8	-1795G/A	5'-flanking region	-	0.458	rs34885482	
9	-1775G/T	5'-flanking region	-	0.083	rs72784894	
10	-1618C/T	5'-flanking region	-	0.458	rs77239447	
11	-1515G/T	5'-flanking region	-	0.333	rs223887	
12	-1338A/G	5'-flanking region	-	0.208	rs182668	
13	-961G/A	5'-flanking region	-	0.208	rs223888	
14	-740A/G	5'-flanking region	-	0.083	rs3760071	
15	-488T/C	5'-flanking region	-	0.333	rs223889	§
16	-215WT/DelG	5'-flanking region	-	0.333	rs3214179	
17	5C/A	exon 1	Ala2Asp	0.125	rs4359426	§
18	88C/A	intron 1	-	0.458	rs2074543	§
19	493T/C	intron 1	-	0.458	rs72784897	
20	559G/A	intron 1	-	0.333	rs223816	
21	902C/T	intron 1	-	0.333	rs223817	
22	2030G/C	intron 2	-	0.208	rs223818	§
23	2134T/C	intron 2	-	0.208	rs223819	
24	2198T/C	intron 2	-	0.208	rs223820	
25	2314G/A	intron 2	-	0.292	rs598366	
26	2936A/G	intron 2	-	0.125	rs170359	
27	3062A/G	intron 2	-	0.458	rs73557194	
28	3766T/A	intron 2	-	0.042		
29	3970G/A	intron 2	-	0.125	rs223821	
30	4064WT/InsAAAAC	intron 2	-	0.125	rs72030112	
31	5222T/C	3' UTR	-	0.125	rs170360	
32	5978WT/DelT	3' UTR	-	0.125	rs57450696	
33	5979C/G	3' UTR	-	0.375	rs57186204	
34	6089T/C	3' UTR	-	0.125	rs223823	
35	6621A/G	3' UTR	-	0.458	rs121565	§
36	6910G/A	3' UTR	-	0.417	rs658559	§
37	7858C/T	3'-flanking region	-	0.458	rs3859048	§
38	7883G/A	3'-flanking region	-	0.458	rs72301	
39	8021G/A	3'-flanking region	-	0.042	rs11865093	

*Numbering according to the genomic sequence of *CCL22* (AC003665). Position 1 is the A of the initiation codon.
‡Minor allele frequencies (MAF) in the screening population (N = 12).
†NCBI, number from the dbSNP of NCBI (http://www.ncbi.nlm.nih.gov/SNP/).
§SNPs were genotyped in this study.

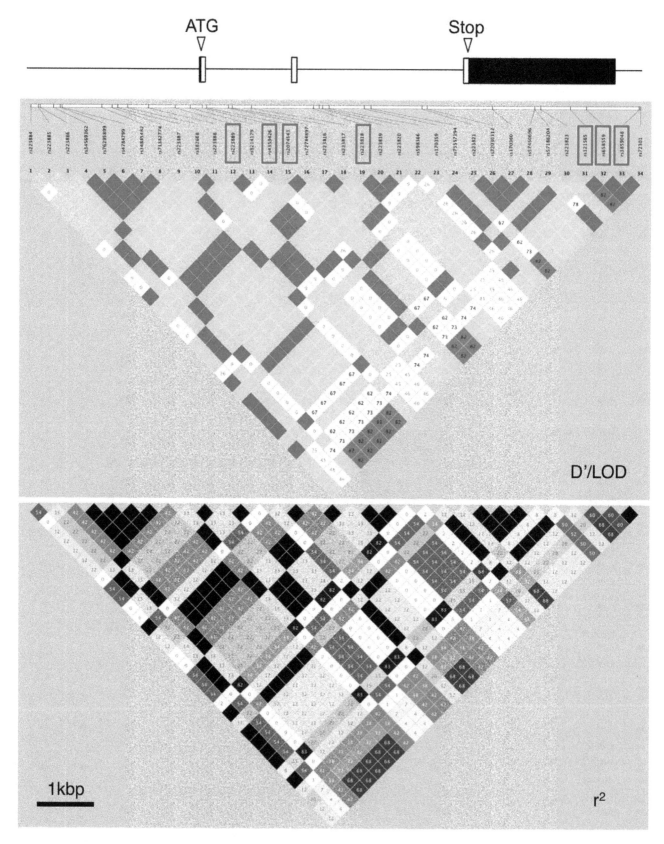

Figure 1. Pairwise linkage disequilibrium between 34 SNPs. LD was measured by D'/LOD (upper) and r[2] (lower) estimated using the Haploview 4.2 program (http://www.broad.mit.edu/mpg/haploview/). Boxed variants were genotyped in this study.

Table 2. Clinical characteristics of the subjects.

	Case	Control
1st population		
Source	The University of Tokyo Keio University Kyushu University Takao Hospital	Control volunteers
Number of samples	916	1,032
Ethnicity	Japanese	Japanese
Female	43.6%	33.0%
Age (mean ± sd)	30.1±9.5	48.5±13.7
2nd population		
Source	BioBank Japan	University of Tsukuba
Number of samples	1,034	1,004
Ethnicity	Japanese	Japanese
Female	43.8%	54.4%
Age (mean ± sd)	30.8±12.7	50.0±9.2

ed us to conduct an association and functional study to test whether genetic variations of *CCL22* contribute to AD susceptibility.

Several association studies using genetic variants of genes *CCL17* and *CCR4* in the CCR4 pathway have been conducted to discover genetic components in the pathogenesis of atopic dermatitis [12,13]. A promoter polymorphism of *CCL17*, -431C>T, increases the promoter activity and the 431T allele influences higher serum levels of CCL17 [12], but genetic variants in the *CCL17* gene are not associated with susceptibility to AD. A recent study also reported that C1014T polymorphism in the *CCR4* gene was not associated with AD [13]. However, those studies were performed with small sample sizes and without replication studies. Genetic study of the *CCL22* gene has not been conducted.

In this study, we focused on the *CCL22* gene, resequenced the gene regions including all exons and introns, and carried out linkage disequilibrium mapping. We performed an association study using two independent populations and functional analyses of the related variants.

Results

Polymorphisms of the *CCL22* gene and LD mapping

We identified a total of 39 polymorphisms (Table 1). We next performed linkage disequilibrium (LD) mapping and calculated

Table 3. Genotype counts and case-control association test results of seven tag SNPs.

db SNP ID	Allele 1/2	Case 1/1	1/2	2/2	N	Control 1/1	1/2	2/2	N	Frequency of allele 2 Case	Control	P value	OR (95%CI)
1st population													
rs223889	T/C	321	435	151	907	360	502	161	1023	0.406	0.403	0.82	-
rs4359426	C/A	706	191	12	909	736	269	16	1021	0.118	0.147	0.0072	0.77(0.64–0.93)
rs2074543	G/C	386	404	113	903	447	469	110	1026	0.349	0.336	0.39	-
rs223818	A/G	563	311	39	913	596	369	56	1021	0.213	0.236	0.093	-
rs121565	A/G	294	439	173	906	325	509	195	1029	0.433	0.437	0.82	-
rs658559	G/A	333	434	134	901	374	491	162	1027	0.390	0.397	0.65	-
rs3859048	C/T	399	410	103	912	466	448	108	1022	0.338	0.325	0.40	-
2nd population													
rs223889	T/C	369	497	163	1029	364	485	150	999	0.400	0.393	0.65	-
rs4359426	C/A	815	202	12	1029	722	249	22	993	0.110	0.148	0.00037	0.71(0.59–0.86)
rs2074543	G/C	404	484	133	1021	418	459	120	997	0.367	0.351	0.26	-
rs223818	A/G	647	331	42	1020	585	351	57	993	0.203	0.234	0.019	0.84(0.72–0.97)
rs121565	A/G	317	530	179	1026	317	500	180	997	0.433	0.431	0.92	-
rs658559	G/A	389	486	154	1029	363	479	148	990	0.386	0.391	0.71	-
rs3859048	C/T	425	484	117	1026	441	446	113	1000	0.350	0.336	0.35	-
Combined													
rs223889	T/C	690	932	314	1936	724	987	311	2022	0.403	0.398	0.63	-
rs4359426	C/A	1521	393	24	1938	1458	518	38	2014	0.114	0.147	0.0000096	0.74(0.65–0.85)
rs2074543	G/C	790	888	246	1924	865	928	230	2023	0.359	0.343	0.16	-
rs223818	A/G	1210	642	81	1933	1181	720	113	2014	0.208	0.235	0.0044	0.86(0.77–0.95)
rs121565	A/G	611	969	352	1932	642	1009	375	2026	0.433	0.434	0.93	-
rs658559	G/A	722	920	288	1930	737	970	310	2017	0.388	0.394	0.56	-
rs3859048	C/T	824	894	220	1938	907	894	221	2022	0.344	0.330	0.21	-

P values of the two populations were calculated by logistic regression analysis under an additive model. The combined P values were calculated using the inverse variance method. OR, odds ratio; CI, confidence interval; -, not significant.

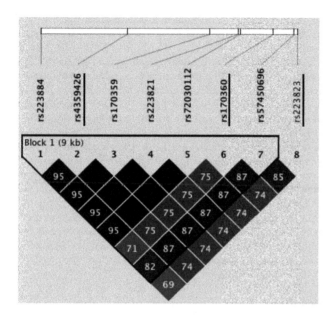

Figure 2. Pairwise linkage disequilibrium (r²) among eight SNPs in strong LD with rs4359426 in 94 control subjects. Two tag SNPs, rs170360 and rs223823, were selected for further association study. Underlined SNPs were examined.

pairwise LD coefficients D′ and r² among the 34 polymorphisms with MAF>10% using the Haploview 4.2 program (Figure 1). Seven tag SNPs were selected for association studies using tagger in Haploview 4.2, and these polymorphisms captured 34 of the 34 alleles with a mean r² of 0.990 (r²>0.82). The HapMap JPT database contains genotype data for six SNPs with MAF>10% in the region (data not shown). The SNPs examined in this study covered all six SNPs shown in the HapMap JPT database.

Association of *CCL22* SNPs with susceptibility to atopic dermatitis

We recruited 916 cases and 1,032 control subjects for the 1st population and 1,034 cases and 1,004 control subjects for the 2nd population, respectively (Table 2). We genotyped seven tag SNPs and all genotype frequencies are shown in Table 3. The rs4359426 (A2D) SNP was associated with AD under an additive genotype model by logistic regression analysis in the first population (*P*= 0.0072; OR, 0.77; 95% CI, 0.64–0.93) (Table 3). In a replication study, rs4359426 was also associated with AD in the second population (*P*= 0.00037; OR, 0.71; 95% CI, 0.59–0.86) (Table 3). The direction of association of the SNP was similar in both of the populations. We combined the results using inverse variance method, and observed a significant association at rs4359426 (meta-analysis, *P*= 0.0000096; OR, 0.74; 95% CI, 0.65–0.85) (Table 3). We next performed further mapping analyses using two genetic variants, rs170360 and rs223823. The two SNPs were selected from among SNPs that were in strong LD (r²>0.87) with rs4359426 (Figure 2). Among the three variants, the strongest association was observed at rs4359426 (Table 4).

Contribution of 5′UTR rs4359426 SNP to mRNA expression levels of *CCL22*

Next, using allele-specific transcript quantification (ASTQ), we evaluated whether the related variants could affect the mRNA expression level in EBV-transformed lymphoblastoid cells. As rs4359426 was located at the 16th nucleotide from the 5′ end of the *CCL22* gene (NM_002990.3), we were not able to design primers of the SNP for ASTQ analysis. We therefore designed PCR primers to encompass a SNP in the 3′-UTR of *CCL22* (rs170360) that was in strong LD with rs4359426 (Figure 3A). We isolated total RNA from 24 cell lines that were heterozygous with rs170360, and genomic DNA was used as a control for equal biallelic representation. Predicted haplotype frequencies are shown in Figure 3B. The ratio of PCR products was approximately 1.6 for cDNAs and 1.0 for genomic DNA from 21 subjects who were heterozygous for rs4359426 (Figure 3C, left panel); however, such

Table 4. Genotype counts and case-control association test results for SNPs rs4359426, rs170360 and rs223823.

db SNP ID	Allele 1/2	Case 1/1	1/2	2/2	N	Control 1/1	1/2	2/2	N	Frequency of allele 2 Case	Control	P value	OR (95%CI)
1st population													
rs4359426	C/A	706	191	12	909	736	269	16	1021	0.118	0.147	0.0072	0.77(0.64–0.93)
rs170360	T/C	695	199	12	906	734	269	20	1023	0.123	0.151	0.011	0.78(0.65–0.95)
rs223823	T/C	728	170	11	909	765	252	10	1027	0.106	0.132	0.0093	0.77(0.63–0.94)
2nd population													
rs4359426	C/A	815	202	12	1029	722	249	22	993	0.110	0.148	0.00037	0.71(0.59–0.86)
rs170360	T/C	792	220	19	1031	728	238	26	992	0.125	0.146	0.055	0.84(0.70–1.00)
rs223823	T/C	823	189	8	1020	780	193	19	992	0.100	0.116	0.11	0.85(0.70–1.04)
Combined													
rs4359426	C/A	1521	393	24	1938	1458	518	38	2014	0.118	0.147	0.0000096	0.74(0.65–0.85)
rs170360	T/C	1487	419	31	1937	1462	507	46	2015	0.123	0.151	0.0017	0.81(0.72–0.93)
rs223823	T/C	1551	359	19	1929	1545	445	29	2019	0.106	0.132	0.0030	0.81(0.70–0.93)

P values of the two populations were calculated by logistic regression analysis under an additive model.
The combined *P* values were calculated using the inverse variance method. OR, odds ratio; CI, confidence interval.

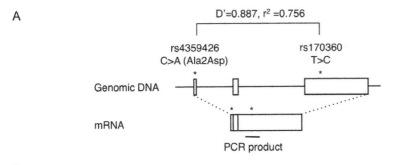

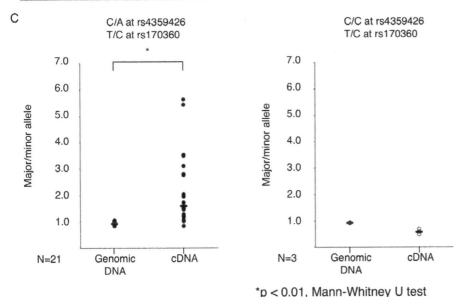

Haplotype	rs4359426 C>A	rs170360 T>C	Frequency
I	C	T	0.849
II	A	C	0.120
III	C	C	0.018
IV	A	T	0.013

*p < 0.01, Mann-Whitney U test

Figure 3. Allelic imbalance of gene expression of *CCL22* in EBV-transformed cells with heterozygous genotypes. (A) Genomic structures, locations and LD of the two SNPs. **(B)** Haplotypes for the two SNPs in the 1st population. **(C)** The allelic ratio of PCR products from individuals. Heterozygous (left) and homozygous (right) at rs4359426. *Two-tailed $P = 0.0000006$ by the Mann-Whitney U test.

differences were not observed in cells from three subjects who were homozygous for the C allele at rs4359426 (Figure 3C, right panel). These results implied an effect of rs4359426 and/or variants in strong LD with rs4359426 on mRNA expression levels of *CCL22*. rs4359426 and rs170360 are in absolute LD in the HapMap Caucasian populations. We further examined the expression patterns of rs4359426 and rs170360 using Genevar 3.0.2 dataset, and confirmed that the expression patterns were similar to our findings (data not shown).

Transcription factor binding to the rs223821 SNP

As rs4359426 was in absolute LD with rs170359, rs223821 and rs72030112 (n = 94) (Figure 2), we further examined the allelic differences of these three SNPs in the binding of nuclear proteins by electrophoretic mobility shift assay (EMSA). We could not find any specific binding of nuclear factor(s) to oligonucleotides containing rs170359 and rs72030112. However, we observed that

the signal intensity of the DNA-protein complex derived from the G allele of rs223821 was higher than that from the A allele in the presence of THP-1 nuclear extract stimulated with LPS (1 µg/ml) (Figure 4). We confirmed that the complex was diminished by an excess amount of a non-labeled allele-specific competitor probe (Figure 4). This result suggested that an unidentified nuclear factor(s) interacted with the genomic region at intron 2 of *CCL22* and the SNP might have an allele-specific effect on expression through varying affinity for a transcription factor.

Discussion

CCL22 plays an important role in the recruitment of Th2 cells into the inflammatory lesions of Th2-related diseases such as AD [14]. A recent study reported upregulation of *CCL17*, *CCL18* and *CCL22* expression in patients with AD, and suggested that the disease-specific chemokines might recruit specific memory T-cell subsets into the skin [15]. The plasma levels of CCL22 are

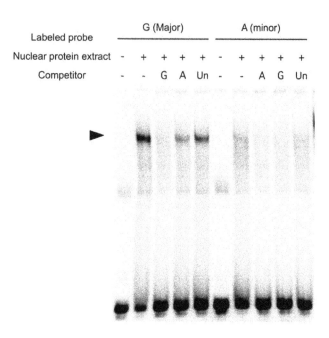

Figure 4. Electrophoretic mobility shift assays of rs223821. EMSA was performed using nuclear extracts from THP-1 cells stimulated with LPS (1.0 µg/ml) for 1 hour. DIG-labeled oligonucleotides corresponding to the G allele (lanes 1–5) and A allele (lanes 6–10) were used as probes. Three independent experiments were performed with similar results.

significantly elevated in AD patients, and the values strongly correlate with disease severity [7,10]. We identified and replicated the rs4359426 (A2D) variant of *CCL22*, which was significantly associated with AD. rs4359426 is a non-synonymous SNP and causes an amino acid substitution in the signal peptide-encoding region. We examined the influence of the amino acid substitution on the structure using SIFT (Sorting Intolerant From Tolerant) software, and the substitution at position 2 from Ala to Asp was predicted to be tolerated. In addition, no possible impacts of the amino acid substitution on the structure and function of CCL22 were predicted by PolyPhen-2 (polymorphism phenotyping v2).

Functional analyses of the related variants of *CCL22* polymorphisms showed that the susceptible allele of rs4359426 might be involved in higher mRNA expression in ASTQ analysis. We confirmed that the expression patterns from Genevar 3.0.2 dataset were similar to our findings. We also demonstrated that the genomic fragment including the risk allele of rs223821 had much higher binding affinity to the nuclear factor(s). Although it is unclear whether higher mRNA expression is influenced by altering expression enhancer activity or mRNA stability, polymorphisms in the *CCL22* gene appear to be a genetic component of the pathologic mechanisms leading to atopic dermatitis, putatively via increased *CCL22* mRNA expression.

Genetic studies reveal underlying cellular pathways, and in some cases, point to new therapeutic approaches. A recent study using a humanized model of asthma showed a critical role for DC-derived CCL17 and CCL22 in attracting Th2 cells and inducing airway inflammation [16]. In the study, administration of a CCR4-blocking antibody abolished airway eosinophilia, goblet cell hyperplasia, IgE synthesis and bronchial hyperreactivity [16]. IL-13 is an important mediator of Th2 immune responses, and there many IL-13-positive cells in AD skin lesions [17]. A recent study has shown that IL-13 induces a significant increase in the expression of CCL22 in human keratinocytes, and blocking of

CCL22 in IL-13-stimulated cells results in 70–90% inhibition in migration of CD4+CCR4+ T cells [18]. These findings suggest that targeting the CCL22/CCR4 pathway might be therapeutically efficacious as a new treatment for atopic dermatitis.

The involvement of CCL22 has been reported in several immune-mediated diseases. A recent study has shown by immunohistochemistry that CCL22 is not expressed in normal skin and is markedly expressed in the lesions of atopic dermatitis, allergic contact dermatitis, and psoriasis vulgaris [19]. Another report has shown that CCL22 is present within the synovial membrane in rheumatoid arthritis and osteoarthritis patients and in high amounts in the synovial fluid of patients with rheumatoid arthritis and psoriatic arthritis [20]. To examine whether the functional SNPs found in this study are associated with those diseases will be needed for understanding of the interconnectivity of the molecular mechanisms underlying distinct diseases.

In summary, we found a significant association between susceptibility to AD and polymorphisms affecting *CCL22* expression in Japanese populations. Our findings strongly support the important role of CCL22 in AD. Although the effect of the non-synonymous SNP on protein function remains unclear, it is likely that related variants play a role in susceptibility to AD in a gain-of-function manner. Further functional analyses and replication studies in other populations are needed; however, our findings provide insights into the pathophysiology of AD.

Materials and Methods

Subjects

A total of 1,950 case subjects with AD were recruited from several hospitals as described [21]. Case subjects in a second population were obtained from the BioBank Japan [22]. All case subjects were diagnosed according to the criteria of Hanifin and Rajka [23]. A total of 1,032 control volunteers in the first set who had no history of AD were recruited by detailed physicians' interviews. For the second set, a total of 1,004 controls who had never been diagnosed with AD were recruited during their annual health checkup in the University of Tsukuba (Table 2). All individuals were Japanese and gave written informed consent to participate in the study. This research project was approved by the ethics committees at the Institute of Medical Science, the University of Tokyo and the RIKEN Yokohama Institute.

Resequencing of the *CCL22* gene and genotyping

We first resequenced the *CCL22* region to identify genetic variations using DNA from 12 subjects with AD. We surveyed the gene from 3 kb of the 5′ flanking region to a 1 kb continuous 3′ flanking region of the last exon on the basis of genomic sequences from the NCBI database (NC_000016.9). The PCR product was reacted with BigDye Terminator v3.1 (Applied Biosystems), and sequences were assembled and polymorphisms identified using the SEQUENCHER program (Gene Codes Corporation, Ann Arbor, MI).

Genotyping of the seven SNPs in *CCL22* was performed by the TaqMan^{TM} allele-specific amplification (TaqMan-ASA) method (Applied Biosystems) and multiplex-PCR based Invader assay (Third Wave Technologies).

Allele-specific transcript quantification (ASTQ)

We conducted allelic expression analyses by TaqMan assay using SNP genotyping probes as described [24]. EBV-transformed lymphoblastoid cells were obtained from the Health Science Research Resources Bank of Japan. Genomic DNA was used as a control for equal biallelic representation. The allelic ratio for each cDNA and genomic DNA was measured.

Electrophoresis Mobility Shift Assay

EMSA was performed using nuclear extracts from THP-1 cells stimulated with LPS (1.0 µg/ml) for 1 hour. DIG-labeled oligonucleotides corresponding to the G allele (lanes 1–5) and A allele (lanes 6–10) were used as probes. The oligonucleotide sequences were 5′-ATCGCCTGAACCCGGGGAGTTGGAG-GTT for the G allele and 5′-ATCGCCTGAACCCAG-GAGTTGGAGGTT for the A allele. For competition, a 100-fold excess of unlabeled G or A allele oligonucleotides or unrelated oligonucleotides (Un) (TFIID) was used.

Statistical analysis

We calculated allele frequencies and tested agreement with Hardy-Weinberg equilibrium using a chi-square goodness-of-fit test. We then compared differences in the allele frequencies between case and control subjects by logistic regression analysis under an additive model and calculated odds ratios (ORs) with 95% confidence intervals (CIs). Results for the 1st and 2nd populations were combined by fixed effect inverse-variance method using Genome-Wide Association Meta Analysis (GWAMA, http://www.well.ox.ac.uk/gwama/tutorial.shtml) [25]. We applied Bonferroni correc-

tions, the multiplication of P values by the number of variants investigated. Corrected P values of less than 0.05 were judged to be significant. The expression patterns of SNPs were obtained from Genevar (GENe Expression VARiation) 3.0.2 (Wellcome Trust Sanger Institute). We examined the influence of amino acid substitution on the structure using SIFT software (http://sift.jcvi.org/) and PolyPhen-2 (polymorphism phenotyping v2) (http://genetics.bwh.harvard.edu/pph2/).

Acknowledgments

We thank all the patients for participating in the study as well as the collaborating physicians for collecting samples. We also thank the members of BioBank Japan and the Rotary Club of Osaka-Midosuji District 2660 Rotary International in Japan for supporting our study and M. T. Shimizu, H. Sekiguchi, A. I. Jodo, N. Kawaraichi and the technical staff of the Center for Genomic Medicine for providing technical assistance. We thank K. Barrymore for proof reading this document.

Author Contributions

Conceived and designed the experiments: TH MT. Performed the experiments: TH KT STanaka HM TSasaki STakeuchi. Analyzed the data: TH. Contributed reagents/materials/analysis tools: HS KE MS TY SF AM SD TE NH TSakamoto HM TSasaki TE MA HE STakeuchi MF EN YN MK. Wrote the paper: MT. Supervised the study: NK YN.

References

1. Fonacier LS, Dreskin SC, Leung DY (2010) Allergic skin diseases. J Allergy Clin Immunol 125: S138–149.
2. Fiset PO, Leung DY, Hamid Q (2006) Immunopathology of atopic dermatitis. J Allergy Clin Immunol 118: 287–290.
3. Andrew DP, Chang MS, McNinch J, Wathen ST, Rihanek M, et al. (1998) STCP-1 (MDC) CC chemokine acts specifically on chronically activated Th2 lymphocytes and is produced by monocytes on stimulation with Th2 cytokines IL-4 and IL-13. J Immunol 161: 5027–5038.
4. Guttman-Yassky E, Lowes MA, Fuentes-Duculan J, Whynot J, Novitskaya I, et al. (2007) Major differences in inflammatory dendritic cells and their products distinguish atopic dermatitis from psoriasis. J Allergy Clin Immunol 119: 1210–1217.
5. Soumelis V, Reche PA, Kanzler H, Yuan W, Edward G, et al. (2002) Human epithelial cells trigger dendritic cell-mediated allergic inflammation by producing TSLP. Nat Immunol 3: 673–680.
6. Guttman-Yassky E, Suárez-Fariñas M, Chiricozzi A, Nograles KE, Shemer A, et al. (2009) Broad defects in epidermal cornification in atopic dermatitis identified through genomic analysis. J Allergy Clin Immunol 124: 1235–1244.
7. Horikawa T, Nakayama T, Hikita I, Yamada H, Fujisawa R, et al. (2002) IFN-gamma-inducible expression of thymus and activation-regulated chemokine/CCL17 and macrophage-derived chemokine/CCL22 in epidermal keratinocytes and their roles in atopic dermatitis. Int Immunol 14: 767–773.
8. Shimada Y, Takehara K, Sato S (2004) Both Th2 and Th1 chemokines (TARC/CCL17, MDC/CCL22, and Mig/CXCL9) are elevated in sera from patients with atopic dermatitis. J Dermatol Sci 34: 201–208.
9. Hashimoto S, Nakamura K, Oyama N, Kaneko F, Tsunemi Y, et al. (2006) Macrophage-derived chemokine (MDC)/CCL22 produced by monocyte derived dendritic cells reflects the disease activity in patients with atopic dermatitis. J Dermatol Sci 44: 93–99.
10. Jahnz-Rozyk K, Targowski T, Paluchowska E, Owczarek W, Kucharczyk A (2005) Serum thymus and activation-regulated chemokine, macrophage-derived chemokine and eotaxin as markers of severity of atopic dermatitis. Allergy 60: 685–688.
11. Watanabe M, Satoh T, Yamamoto Y, Kanai Y, Karasuyama H, et al. (2008) Overproduction of IgE induces macrophage-derived chemokine (CCL22) secretion from basophils. J Immunol 181: 5653–5659.
12. Sekiya T, Tsunemi Y, Miyamasu M, Ohta K, Morita A, et al. (2003) Variations in the human Th2-specific chemokine TARC gene. Immunogenetics 54: 742–745.
13. Tsunemi Y, Sekiya T, Saeki H, Hirai K, Ohta K, et al. (2004) Lack of association of CCR4 single nucleotide polymorphism with atopic dermatitis in Japanese patients. Acta Derm Venereol 84: 187–190.
14. Yamashita U, Kuroda E (2002) Regulation of macrophage-derived chemokine (MDC, CCL22) production. Crit Rev Immunol 22: 105–114.
15. Fujita H, Shemer A, Suárez-Fariñas M, Johnson-Huang LM, Tintle S, et al. (2011) Lesional dendritic cells in patients with chronic atopic dermatitis and psoriasis exhibit parallel ability to activate T-cell subsets. J Allergy Clin Immunol. In press.
16. Perros F, Hoogsteden HC, Coyle AJ, Lambrecht BN, Hammad H (2009) Blockade of CCR4 in a humanized model of asthma reveals a critical role for DC-derived CCL17 and CCL22 in attracting Th2 cells and inducing airway inflammation. Allergy 64: 995–1002.
17. Hamid Q, Naseer T, Minshall EM, Song YL, Boguniewicz M, et al. (1996) In vivo expression of IL-12 and IL-13 in atopic dermatitis. J Allergy Clin Immunol 98: 225–231.
18. Purwar R, Werfel T, Wittmann M (2006) IL-13-stimulated human keratinocytes preferentially attract CD4+CCR4+ T cells: possible role in atopic dermatitis. J Invest Dermatol 126: 1043–1051.
19. Vulcano M, Albanesi C, Stoppacciaro A, Bagnati R, D'Amico G, et al. (2001) Dendritic cells as a major source of macrophage-derived chemokine/CCL22 in vitro and in vivo. Eur J Immunol 31: 812–822.
20. Flytlie HA, Hvid M, Lindgreen E, Kofod-Olsen E, Petersen EL, et al. (2010) Expression of MDC/CCL22 and its receptor CCR4 in rheumatoid arthritis, psoriatic arthritis and osteoarthritis. Cytokine 49: 24–29.
21. Shimizu M, Matsuda A, Yanagisawa K, Hirota T, Akahoshi M, et al. (2005) Functional SNPs in the distal promoter of the ST2 gene are associated with atopic dermatitis. Hum Mol Genet 14: 2919–2927.
22. Nakamura Y (2007) The BioBank Japan Project. Clin Adv Hematol Oncol 5: 696–697.
23. Hanifin JM, Rajka G (1980) Diagnostic features of atopic dermatitis. Acta Derm Venereol 92: 44–47.
24. Onouchi Y, Ozaki K, Buns JC, Shimizu C, Hamada H, et al. (2010) Common variants in CASP3 confer susceptibility to Kawasaki disease. Hum Mol Genet 19: 2898–2906.
25. Mägi R, Morris AP (2010) GWAMA: software for genome-wide association meta-analysis. BMC Bioinformatics 11: 288.

8

Eosinophils Increase Neuron Branching in Human and Murine Skin and *In Vitro*

Erin L. Foster[1], Eric L. Simpson[2], Lorna J. Fredrikson[3], James J. Lee[3], Nancy A. Lee[3], Allison D. Fryer[4], David B. Jacoby[4]*

1 Department of Molecular Microbiology and Immunology, Oregon Health & Science University, Portland, Oregon, United States of America, 2 Department of Dermatology, Oregon Health & Science University, Portland, Oregon, United States of America, 3 Department of Biochemistry, Mayo Clinic, Scottsdale, Arizona, United States of America, 4 Division of Pulmonary and Critical Care, Department of Medicine, Oregon Health & Science University, Portland, Oregon, United States of America

Abstract

Cutaneous nerves are increased in atopic dermatitis, and itch is a prominent symptom. We studied the functional interactions between eosinophils and nerves in human and mouse skin and in culture. We demonstrated that human atopic dermatitis skin has eosinophil granule proteins present in the same region as increased nerves. Transgenic mice in which interleukin-5 (IL-5) expression is driven by a keratin-14 (K14) promoter had many eosinophils in the epidermis, and the number of nerves was also significantly increased in the epidermis. In co-cultures, eosinophils dramatically increased branching of sensory neurons isolated from the dorsal root ganglia (DRG) of mice. This effect did not occur in DRG neurons co-cultured with mast cells or with dead eosinophils. Physical contact of the eosinophils with the neurons was not required, and the effect was not blocked by an antibody to nerve growth factor. DRG neurons express eotaxin-1, ICAM-1 and VCAM-1, which may be important in the recruitment, binding, and activation of eosinophils in the region of cutaneous nerves. These data indicate a pathophysiological role for eosinophils in cutaneous nerve growth in atopic dermatitis, and suggest they may present a therapeutic target in atopic dermatitis and other eosinophilic skin conditions with neuronal symptoms such as itch.

Editor: George C. Tsokos, Beth Israel Deaconess Medical Center, United States of America

Funding: This work was supported by NIH T32AI007472 (DBJ) and an OHSU Tartar Fellowship to E.F., and the Mayo Foundation for Medical Education and Research, as well as NIH HL61013 (DBJ), HL71795 (DBJ), AI75064 (DBJ), HL55543 (ADF), ES14601 (ADF), HL065228 (JJL), RR109709 (JJL), and HL058723 (NAL). The funders had no role in study design, data collection and analysis, decision to publish, or preparation of the manuscript.

Competing Interests: The authors have declared that no competing interests exist.

* E-mail: jacobyd@ohsu.edu

Introduction

Atopic dermatitis is characterized by itch, which greatly affects the quality of life of patients [Jacquet, 1904 and [1]]. The itch often begins before any lesions appear, and marks on the skin can be limited to excoriations, or scratches, made by the patient. Patients with atopic dermatitis experience itch instead of pain when tested with mechanical, electrical, low pH, or heat stimuli [2]. The sensory neurons that transmit itch are primary afferents whose cell bodies are in the dorsal root ganglia (DRG). These free nerve endings in the epidermis and upper dermis can be activated by a variety of stimuli, including proteases, neurotrophins, cytokines and other small molecules (reviewed in [3]).

The mechanisms for enhanced itch sensations in atopic dermatitis are unclear. One potential mechanism is an increase in nerve endings in atopic dermatitis skin [4]. Specifically, there are more nerve fibers in the papillary and upper dermis as disease progresses from clinically normal-appearing, or *non-lesional*, skin to active disease, or *lesional*, skin [5].

Eosinophils have been linked to atopic dermatitis for well over forty years, due to high numbers circulating in the blood of atopic dermatitis patients [6]. Serum concentrations of eosinophil granule proteins correlate with the severity of atopic dermatitis [7,8], and peripheral blood eosinophils from patients have more neurotrophin receptors and more functional activity in response to

neurotrophins than eosinophils from healthy controls [9]. Intact eosinophils are not found in high numbers in atopic dermatitis biopsies, leading some to question whether these cells have a role in the pathogenesis of this disease. However, the presence of eosinophil granule proteins in lesional skin suggests that activated eosinophil are present, but not identifiable, having degranulated [10,11].

Previously, we showed that eosinophils interact with nerves in the airways of patients with asthma, in animal models of asthma, and in culture. Eosinophils are found adjacent to nerves in airway biopsies of humans who died from asthma attacks, a histological finding that is recapitulated in antigen-challenged guinea pigs and rats [12]. Primary cultures of parasympathetic neurons from guinea pig and human airways express eotaxin-1, as well as ICAM-1 and VCAM-1, and these participate in binding of eosinophils to neurons [13,14]. The association of eosinophils with airway nerves is important in the pathophysiological changes that lead to airway hyperreactivity [12,15].

Eosinophils communicate with other cell types through a variety of specific signals. They can act as antigen-presenting cells, release cytokines and chemokines after activation, or release granule proteins, such as major basic protein (MBP) and eosinophil peroxidase (EPO) [16,17]. They also constitutively synthesize specific neurotrophins, including nerve growth factor (NGF), brain-derived neurotrophic factor (BDNF), and neurotrophin-3

(NT-3), and they can be triggered to release these factors upon stimulation [9,18].

In this study, we investigated the physical and functional relationship between eosinophils and sensory nerves in the skin of humans with atopic dermatitis, in a mouse model of atopic dermatitis, and in co-cultures of eosinophils with primary sensory neurons. We report here that eosinophil granules are located near neurons in the upper, or papillary, dermis of human skin, the region in which nerves are also increased. In a transgenic mouse in which IL-5 is driven by a K14 promoter, eosinophils localize to the epidermis and lead to increased nerves in this region. In culture, eosinophils directly cause branching of sensory neurons, through a mechanism that does not involve NGF. These data indicate a potential mechanism and therapeutic target for the increase in nerves seen in human atopic dermatitis.

Results

Human skin biopsies are representative of healthy skin and different stages of atopic dermatitis

Skin biopsies were gathered from five healthy volunteers and six subjects with atopic dermatitis. Patients with atopic dermatitis had not used topical corticosteroids for a minimum of a week before the biopsies were taken. Each subject was examined by a dermatologist and confirmed to have atopic dermatitis, both by clinical exam and patient and family history. All atopic dermatitis subjects were previously diagnosed with the Hanifin and Rajka criteria [1]. One biopsy was taken from each healthy control, and two were taken from each atopic dermatitis subject, for paired lesional (L) and non-lesional (NL) skin. Non-lesional skin throughout this report refers to normal appearing skin from an atopic dermatitis patient. Subject characteristics and biopsy sites are shown in Table 1. All patients had positive family and personal history for atopic dermatitis, including allergies and asthma. Hematoxylin and eosin (H&E) staining of the human skin biopsies confirmed the clinical diagnoses of healthy control, non-lesional atopic dermatitis or lesional atopic dermatitis (Figure 1A).

Atopic dermatitis lesional skin biopsies have more nerves than non-lesional skin from the same subjects

Biopsy sections were stained with an antibody to the pan-neuronal marker PGP9.5. Photographs were taken along the

length of the skin section, and nerves staining positively for PGP9.5 were counted in the papillary dermis and basement membrane zone of the skin. Representative photomicrographs of normal, non-lesional and lesional skin are shown with quantification (Figure 1 B, C). Nerves were increased, both in number and in length, in lesional atopic dermatitis skin, compared to each non-lesional skin sample from the same patient. Overall, nerves were also increased compared to healthy control skin, except for one healthy control with many more cutaneous nerves. It may be significant that this outlier subject had high numbers of eosinophils in the blood and also had increased eosinophil granule proteins in the skin.

Atopic dermatitis skin biopsies have more eosinophil granule proteins, which are located around nerves in the papillary dermis

In order to determine if eosinophil localization to nerves in the skin occurs in atopic dermatitis biopsies, we first performed single immunohistochemistry with an antibody to eosinophil peroxidase (EPO), a protein present in eosinophil granules. EPO was present in lesional atopic dermatitis skin at higher quantities than normal or non-lesional skin, and it was often located in the papillary dermis (Figure 2 A,B and Table 2). This localization correlated with both the location and stage of disease in which nerves are increased. Intact eosinophils were present in some lesional skin sections, more often in blood vessels (data not shown), suggesting that eosinophils that have migrated into tissues tended to degranulate. In addition, double immunohistochemistry for eosinophil peroxidase and PGP9.5 determined that eosinophil peroxidase could be found around nerves in the papillary dermis, especially in lesional skin samples (Figure 2C).

Mast cells are increased in non-lesional atopic dermatitis skin and are not increased in lesional skin

Because mast cells are found in the skin in association with nerves, under both normal and pathological conditions [19,20], and previous reports have shown mast cells are increased in lesional skin compared to healthy controls [21,22], we stained biopsies with toluidine blue. A non-significant trend toward more mast cells was seen in non-lesional atopic dermatitis skin, but not in lesional skin (Figure 3).

Nerves are increased in the epidermis of a transgenic mouse that expresses IL-5 in basal keratinocytes

NJ.692 mice were generated to constitutively express IL-5 under the control of keratin 14 regulatory elements in basal keratinocytes. The mice have mild peripheral blood eosinophilia with greater than 30-fold increased numbers of eosinophils in the skin. Some mice develop spontaneous skin lesions and clinically apparent inflammation. These animals also have deposition of eosinophil granule proteins in the skin, predominantly in the epidermis, which can be detected using anti-MBP antibodies (figure 4C).

We examined skin sections from these mice for the number of nerves and found that they have more nerves in the epidermis and basement membrane zone than wild-type controls, but similar numbers of nerves in the dermis (Figure 4). Thus the increase in nerves was seen in the same regions where IL-5 was expressed and where eosinophils were located.

Eosinophils increase sensory neuron branching *in vitro*

The cell bodies of the sensory neurons that innervate the skin are located in the dorsal root ganglia (DRG), and these were dissected

Table 1. Human skin biopsies.

Subject	Skin type	Samples taken	Region
001	Atopic Dermatitis	Lesional/Non-lesional	Flexor knee
002	Healthy Control	Normal	Interior arm
003	Healthy Control	Normal	Interior arm
004	Atopic Dermatitis	Lesional/Non-lesional	Flexor knee
005	Atopic Dermatitis	Lesional/Non-lesional	Flexor elbow
006	Atopic Dermatitis	Lesional/Non-lesional	Exterior arm
007	Healthy Control	Normal	Interior arm
008	Healthy Control	Normal	Interior arm
009	Healthy Control	Normal	Interior arm
010	Atopic Dermatitis	Lesional/Non-lesional	Interior arm
011	Atopic Dermatitis	Lesional/Non-lesional	Extensor elbow

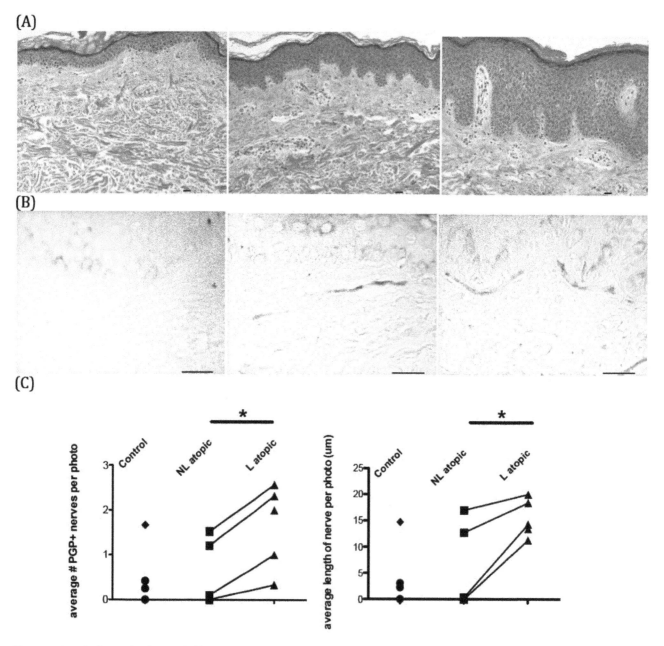

Figure 1. Atopic dermatitis lesional skin has more nerves than paired non-lesional skin. (A) Human skin biopsies are typical of healthy control skin (left), non-lesional atopic dermatitis (center), and lesional atopic dermatitis (right). (B) Nerves were stained (in gray), and representative sections are shown of healthy control (left), non-lesional (center) and lesional atopic dermatitis (right). (C) Quantification of number and length of nerves in healthy control or atopic dermatitis skin. Paired t-test was performed between lesional and non-lesional skin biopsies from the same subject. Outlier control subject with high blood eosinophils and increased nerves is represented by diamond. * denotes significantly different from control. Scale bar in photographs = 50 um.

from wild-type mice, enzymatically dissociated and plated on Matrigel. Blood was taken from NJ1638 mice, in which the IL-5 gene is expressed under the control of the CD3δ promoter, leading to high levels of circulating eosinophils [23]. Eosinophils were isolated using density centrifugation and fluorescence-activated cell sorting (FACS) of unstained cells based on size and granularity. Eosinophils were added to DRG cell cultures for twenty-four hours. The cultures were then fixed, stained with PGP9.5, and the number of cell bodies, length of neurites, number of neurites per cell body, and number of branchpoints per neurite were quantified by an observer who was blinded to the experimental condition. Neurons

grown with eosinophils had dramatically increased neurite branching, compared to neurons grown alone (Figure 5 A, B). The number of cell bodies, number of neurites per cell body and the length of the longest neurite were not significantly different between neurons alone or neurons with eosinophils (data not shown). There was also no difference in DRG cell survival with or without eosinophils (data not shown).

Mast cells do not increase neuron branching *in vitro*

Since mast cells were localized around nerves in human skin biopsies, we isolated mast cells from the peritonea of wild-type

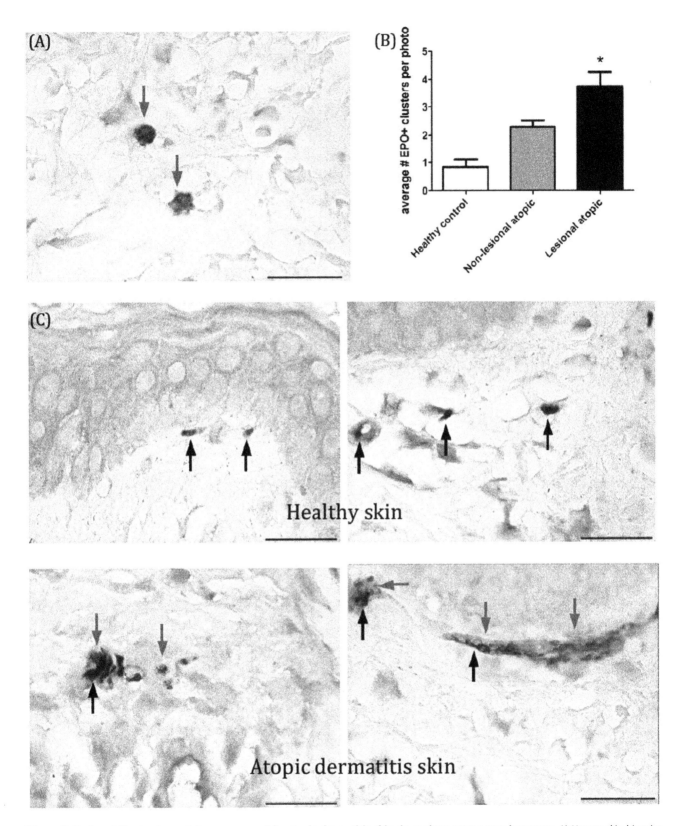

Figure 2. Eosinophil granule proteins are present in atopic dermatitis skin, in regions near nerve increases. A) Human skin biopsies were stained with anti-EPO antibody (dark red-brown). A representative photomicrograph is shown of lesional skin. B) Quantification of EPO-positive clusters in skin. C) Representative photomicrographs of double immunohistochemistry using anti-PGP9.5 (black) for nerves and anti-EPO (red-brown). Top panels are two samples of healthy control skin. Bottom panels are two lesional atopic dermatitis samples. Bottom left shows a nerve with EPO+ cells nearby, while bottom right shows a nerve overlaid with EPO. * denotes significantly different from control. Scale bar = 50 um.

Table 2. Eosinophil peroxidase (EPO) staining in human skin biopsies.

Name of sample	avg # EPO+ clusters	EPO+ regions of skin
NORMAL:		
002 normal	1.5	papillary dermis
003 normal	0.6	basement membrane zone
008 normal	0.25	papillary dermis
009 normal	1	reticular dermis
NON-LESIONAL		
001 non-lesional	1.8	papillary dermis
004 non-lesional	2.43	papillary dermis
005 non-lesional	2.36	papillary dermis
006 non-lesional	3	papillary+reticular dermis
011 non-lesional	1.833	papillary dermis
LESIONAL		
001 lesional	2.5	papillary+reticular dermis
004 lesional	5.08	papillary+reticular dermis
005 lesional	2.3	papillary+reticular dermis
006 lesional	3.125	papillary+reticular dermis
010 lesional (unpaired)	4.36	papillary dermis
011 lesional	2.75	papillary dermis

mice and added them, in the same numbers as eosinophils, to the neuron cultures for twenty-four hours. Mast cells did not increase neurite branching (Figure 5C).

Eosinophils must be alive to increase neuron branching, but physical contact is not required

In order to determine whether the eosinophils needed to be alive to have this effect on neurite branching, we freeze-fractured eosinophils and added them to neuronal cultures for twenty-four

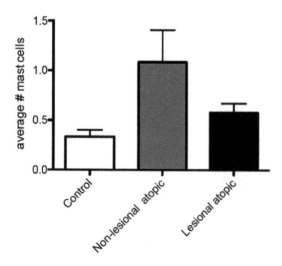

Figure 3. Mast cells in controls and atopic dermatitis patients. A non-significant increase in mast cells was seen in biopsies of non-lesional skin in atopic patients. There was no increase in mast cells in lesional skin.

hours. Eosinophils killed in this way did not increase neurite branching (Figure 5D). Adding culture medium from eosinophils plated on Matrigel for twenty-four hours to DRG cultures increased neuron branching, indicating that the morphological changes do not require cell contact, and adding culture medium from co-cultures of DRG neurons with eosinophils to fresh DRG cultures further increased the amount of neurite branching (Figure 5E).

Blocking nerve growth factor (NGF) does not inhibit eosinophil-induced neurite branching

Adding exogenous murine NGF (40 ng/ml) to DRG cultures increased neurite branching, and this effect was blocked by an antibody to NGF (20 ug/ml) (Figure 5F). However, adding the same concentration of anti-NGF to DRG cultures co-cultured with eosinophils (Figure 5F) or treated with eosinophil culture medium (data not shown) did not prevent the increase in neurite branching. Thus NGF production by eosinophils was not responsible for the effect on nerve branching.

Neurons from dorsal root ganglia produce eotaxin-1, ICAM-1 and VCAM-1

DRG neurons were cultured alone for twenty-four hours and stained for eotaxin-1, a chemokine that acts through the CCR3 chemokine receptor on eosinophils [24,25]. Neurons synthesized eotaxin-1, both in the presence and absence of exogenous NGF (Figure 6A). In addition, neurons also produced the adhesion molecules ICAM-1 and VCAM-1, but only when exogenous NGF was added to the cultures (Figure 6B, C). This indicates a regulated expression of adhesion molecules that could be affected by the presence of eosinophils or other cells that express NGF [9,26].

Discussion

Our data demonstrate for the first time that eosinophils can dramatically increase sensory neuron branching, and that this effect is important in eosinophilic skin diseases, such as atopic dermatitis. We found that there were more nerves in lesional versus non-lesional atopic dermatitis, which correlated with the amount and location of eosinophil granule proteins. In transgenic mice that express IL-5 driven by a K14 promoter, both eosinophils and increased innervation were localized to the epidermis. Finally, eosinophils dramatically increased neurite branching in cultured dorsal root ganglion sensory neurons. The ability of eosinophils to promote neurite branching in sensory neurons in culture supports the role of eosinophils in the neural changes in atopic dermatitis. Sensory neuron expression of ICAM-1 and VCAM-1, as well as eotaxin-1, suggests active recruitment of eosinophils to the nerves, as we have previously demonstrated for parasympathetic neurons in the airways [13].

Our biopsies were taken from several places anatomically, and the control patients' biopsies were all taken from the inner arm (Table 1). While this might have affected the number of nerves, the regional variation in cutaneous nerve density would favor more nerves in the arm than in the leg [27], and we found the opposite when comparing atopic dermatitis biopsies to control biopsies. Although there was a general increase in cutaneous mast cells in our human skin biopsies, unlike the eosinophils cutaneous mast cells were not increased in the lesional skin, where nerves were increased. This finding, along with the failure of mast cells to promote nerve branching in vitro, suggests that eosinophils are more likely responsible.

In human and mouse skin, we did not identify which types of nerves were increased in number, although the locations of these

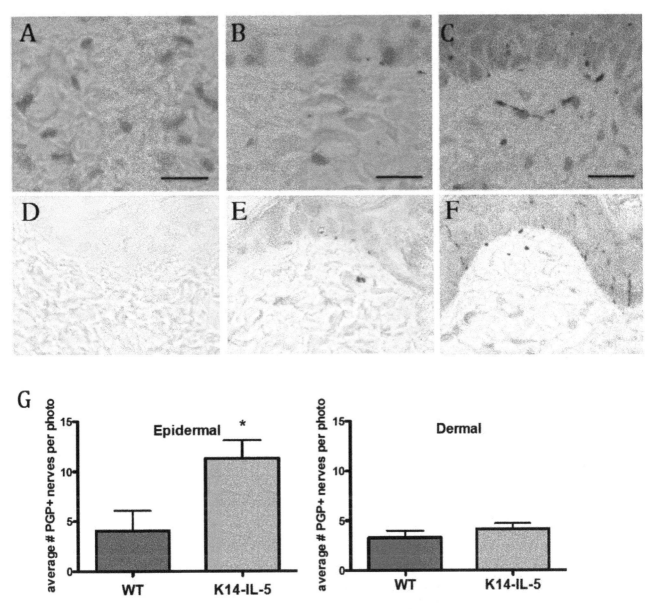

Figure 4. Keratin 14-Interleukin 5 mice have eosinophil major basic protein (MBP) primarily in the epidermis, and have more nerves in epidermis and basement membrane zone than wild-type controls, but similar numbers in the dermis. 5 um skin sections on slides were stained using anti-MBP (red, in top three sections) and anti-PGP9.5 to visualize nerves (brown, in bottom three sections). Photographs of each entire section were taken, and random numbers assigned to each for quantification of nerves by an observer blinded to the genotype. (A and D) IgG negative control, (B) anti-MBP staining of wild type mouse,(C) anti-MBP staining of K14-IL-5 skin section. MBP staining is largely seen in the epidermis, which is where the IL-5 is expressed. (E) PGP9.5 stained wild type mouse, (F) PGP9.5 stained K14-IL-5 skin section. Note the extensive linear nerves from the basement membrane zone through many layers of the epidermis. (G) Quantification of nerves shows an increase in the epidermis (where IL-5 is expressed and eosinophil major basic protein is seen) but not in the dermis. Scale bars = 50 μM.

nerves in the papillary dermis and along the basement membrane zone would suggest sensory origins. However, our culture experiments specifically examined the branching of sensory neurons with cell bodies in the dorsal root ganglia, which include the itch-specific C-type neurons [2,28,29].

Itch-specific C-type neurons are reported to have more highly branching terminals, enabling them to innervate exceptionally large regions of tissue [29]. It is possible that eosinophils are not simply stimulating neurite growth but are causing a shift in the phenotype of the affected neurons. A precedent for this type of shift lies in *hyperalgesia* and *allodynia*, in which changes in neurotransmitter release, ion channel regulation and threshold for stimulation lead to perception of non-painful stimuli as pain [30,31].

We showed that NGF was not the necessary factor for eosinophil-induced neurite branching using a blocking antibody that has less than 1% cross-reactivity for BDNF and neurotrophins 3 and 4 (NT-3, NT-4). However, eosinophils synthesize other neurotrophins, including BDNF and NT-3 [18,32], as well as interleukins and other mediators that could be responsible for nerve growth. Thus there may be considerable redundancy in this system, as well as the possibility that other, non-neurotrophin eosinophil products, are involved. For example, major basic protein, the principal constitutent of the eosinophil granule,

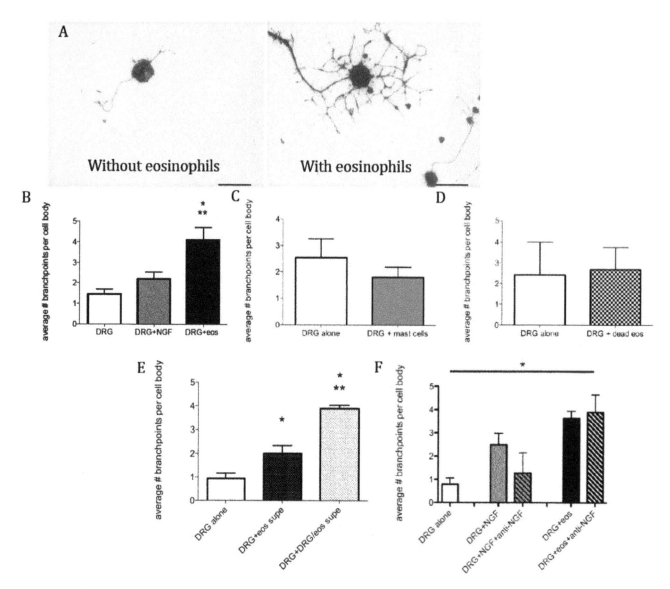

Figure 5. Eosinophils increase branching of dorsal root ganglion (DRG) neurites. (A) Mouse DRG neurons were isolated and co-cultured with eosinophils for 24 hours. Cells were fixed and stained with anti-PGP9.5 to visualize neurons. DRG neurons cultured with eosinophils (right) showed dramatic increases in neurite branching, compared to DRG neurons cultured alone (left). (B) Quantification of number of branchpoints per cell body, n = 7. * denotes significantly different from DRG alone, ** denotes significantly different from DRG+NGF. (C) Mast cells were isolated from the peritonea of wild-type mice and added to DRG neuron cultures for 24 hours. Slides were stained and quantified as above. n = 4. (D) Eosinophils were resuspended in sterile deionized water and freeze-thawed twice, resuspended in culture medium and added to DRG neuron cultures for 24 hours. n = 2. (E) Culture medium from eosinophils cultured alone or with DRG for 24 hours was applied to new DRG cultures for 24 hours. n = 4. (F) DRG neurons were plated and incubated alone (white bar), with 40 ng/ml NGF (gray solid bar), with NGF and 20 ug/ml anti-NGF (gray hatched bar), with eosinophils (black bar), or with eosinophils and 20 ug/ml anti-NGF (black hatched bar) for 24 hours. n = 2. * denotes significant one-way ANOVA across all groups.

interacts with neurons on several levels, including blocking M2 muscarinic receptors on the nerves [15], increasing sensory nerve excitability [33], and activating p38 MAP kinase [34]. The effects of major basic protein, as well as other eosinophil granule proteins and non-granule products, is not known.

Our findings are also important for other eosinophilic skin diseases, several of which induce itch as a predominant symptom. Itchy papular eruptions have been described in the hypereosinophilic syndrome (HES) and can be successfully treated with ultraviolet (UV) therapy [35]. In prurigo nodularis, a disease defined solely by its itchiness, large deposits of eosinophil cationic protein (ECP) and EDN were detected by immunofluorescence.

Intact eosinophils were often located near nerves, and there was an increase in the number of nerves in areas with many eosinophils [36]. Finally, a disease called equine sweet itch results from sensitization to the bite of the midge and subsequent "challenge" or further bites. Eosinophils are recruited by eotaxin and MCP-1, which are expressed in the skin of sensitized horses, and horses scratch, rub and bite the lesions, which results in skin thickening and hair loss [37].

Our report demonstrates the role of eosinophils in nerve branching *in vivo* and *in vitro*, and strongly suggests that this is relevant to human skin diseases, including atopic dermatitis, in which eosinophils and nerves are found together. The ability of

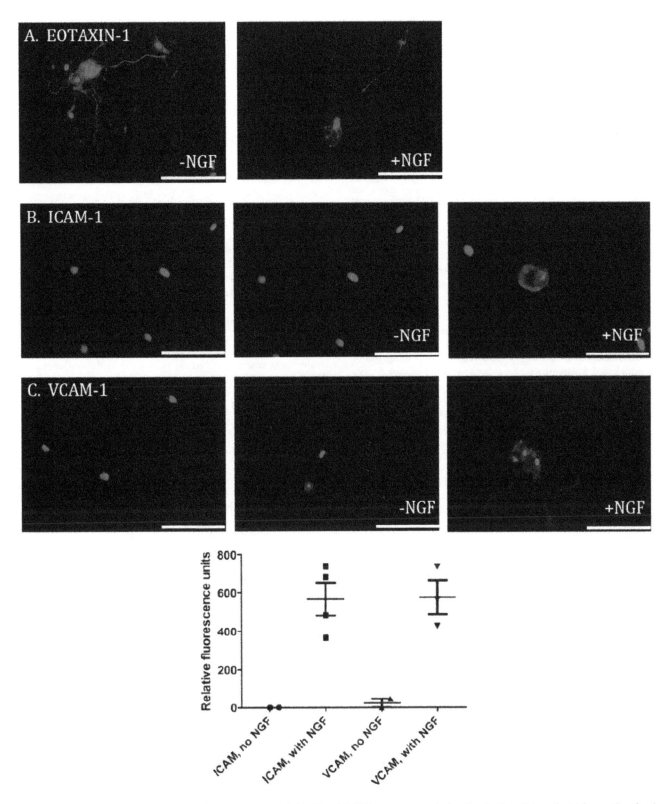

Figure 6. DRG neurons produce eotaxin-1, ICAM-1, and VCAM-1. (A) DRG neurons were isolated and cultured alone for 24 hours, then fixed and stained with anti-eotaxin-1 (red). Cell nuclei were counterstained using DAPI (blue). Two representative photomicrographs are shown. Scale bars = 50 um. (B–C) DRG neurons were cultured alone or with 40 ng/ml NGF for 24 hours, then fixed and stained with anti-ICAM-1 (B) or anti-VCAM-1 (C). Left, no primary with secondary negative control; center, DRG stained with antibody in cultures without exogenous NGF; right, DRG stained with antibody in cultures with NGF added. GRAPH: Quantification of relative fluorescence units, compared to background and to negative controls, was performed using Metamorph.

sensory neurons to express adhesion molecules and chemokines that interact with eosinophils suggests potential drug targets in eosinophil-related skin diseases.

Methods

Human Skin Biopsies

Human studies were approved by the Institutional Review Board of Oregon Health & Science University (IRB approval #2568), and all patients gave written informed consent. Healthy subjects and atopic dermatitis patients were interviewed for their personal and family history of atopy and then examined by a dermatologist to determine extent of disease. A self-reported history of atopy was required for inclusion as an atopic dermatitis patient, and all patients had a previous diagnosis of atopic dermatitis by dermatologists at OHSU. Four millimeter punch biopsies were removed from areas of normal-appearing (non-lesional) or active (lesional) disease. Biopsies of normal skin from healthy subjects were taken from the inner arm or behind the knee. All biopsies were fixed in 10% neutral buffered formalin and embedded in paraffin.

Human Skin Immunocytochemistry

5 um paraffin sections were cut onto slides, and these were rehydrated through xylenes and sequential ethanol dilutions. Antigen unmasking solution was used according to the protocol, [Vector], and 3% hydrogen peroxide in methanol was applied for ten minutes, to quench endogenous peroxidase activity. Sections were blocked with 10% normal goat serum, and mouse anti-human protein gene product 9.5 (PGP9.5) [Serotec] was applied overnight at 4°C. Slides were rinsed in PBS and biotinylated goat anti-mouse IgG was applied for 30 minutes at room temperature. The Vectastain ABC kit and chromogenic substrates were used to visualize positive antibody staining. Slides were rinsed in tap water, then dehydrated through ethanol dilutions and xylenes. Slides were mounted using Cytoseal CrystalMount and dried overnight. Likewise, human skin biopsies stained for eosinophil peroxidase (EPO) were blocked and incubated with antibody at 4°C overnight, then treated identically as PGP9.5-stained slides. Sections stained for both EPO and PGP9.5 were treated with the avidin-biotin blocking kit from Vector to prevent non-specific signal. Sections used for H&E or mast cell identification were deparaffinized and rehydrated as above and then stained using hematoxylin and eosin or toluidine blue.

Semi-quantitative Analysis of Immunostaining of Human Skin

40× or 60× photomicrographs were taken of the entire region of each skin biopsy. Measurements were taken of papillary dermis, reticular dermis, hypodermis, and epidermal-dermal zone; however, only measurements of papillary dermis and epidermis/basement membrane are reported. Nerve length was calculated by calibrating each photograph to the objective with which it was taken and then drawing a straight line between the two furthest points of a PGP 9.5-positive nerve, using Metamorph software. Nerve number was counted manually. Data were reported as average number of nerves per photo, and average length of nerve per photo. Mast cells were counted in double-stained 60× photographs, and proximity to nerves measured using Metamorph software. Fifteen microns, or approximately half a mast cell's diameter, was determined to be the limit of "association" between a mast cell and nerve.

Animals

Female wild-type C57BL/6 mice, 6–8 weeks of age, were purchased from Jackson Laboratories. NJ.1638 IL-5 transgenic mice, in which the full murine IL-5 sequence, with every intron and 1.2 kb of 3′-flanking sequences, but none of the upstream known regulatory elements, is regulated by the promoter and tissue-specific enhancer for CD3δ, overexpresses IL-5 in T cells. These mice were generated, bred and genotyped as previously described (67). NJ.692 mice (K14/IL5 transgenic mice) were generated by creating a plasmid construct containing the 1.9 kb K14 promoter (provided by Dr. Elaine Fuchs [38] fused to the IL-5 gene. The plasmid insert was injected into mouse embryos following excision from the plasmid vector. Mice were bred with C57Bl/6J mice (Jackson Laboratories) and maintained using either Southern analysis of BamHI digested tail DNA blotted to radioactively labelled IL-5 cDNA or PCR reactions using primers specific for the IL-5 injected DNA. PCR primers were (K14) 5′ TTG GCG CTA GCC TGT GGG 3′ and (IL5 beta 2) 5′ CAG CCT ACC CTA CAT AGC AAG TTT G 3′. All animal experiments were approved by the Institutional Animal Care and Use Committee of Oregon Health & Science University (approval # B11249), and were performed in accordance with National Institutes of Health and Mayo Foundation institutional guidelines.

Mouse skin immunocytochemistry

Skin sections from mice were fixed in 4% formaldehyde and embedded in paraffin. Five micron sections were immunostained in the same manner as human skin, using rabbit anti-mammal PGP9.5 and biotinylated goat anti-rabbit IgG. Sequential samples were double-stained with PGP9.5 and major basic protein (MBP) antibodies generated in the Lee Laboratory. Rat anti-mouse MBP was applied overnight at 4°C, and secondary antibody, conjugated to the fluorophore Alexa Fluor-555, was applied for 2 hours at 37°C. Slides were rinsed in PBS, and mounted using Vectastain with DAPI, to stain cell nuclei.

Semi-quantitative analysis of mouse skin immunohistochemistry

60× photographs of entire mouse skin biopsies were taken. Slides were de-identified using an algorithm assigning random numbers to each photograph, and measurements were taken of PGP-positive spots in the papillary dermis, reticular dermis, and epidermal-dermal zone of each blinded photograph by an investigator blinded to the condition of the biopsy. Nerve length was calculated by calibrating each photograph to the 60× objective and then drawing a straight line between the two furthest points of a PGP 9.5-positive nerve, using Metamorph software. Nerve number was counted manually. Data from each photograph were averaged to determine the mean number of nerves per photo, sum of nerve lengths per photo, and average length of nerve per photo. Each photograph was de-coded after all measurements and calculations were completed. Quantification of nerves per area or nerves per length of basement membrane did not give different results from number of nerves per photo.

Isolation of Dorsal Root Ganglia (DRG)

Dorsal root ganglia were isolated according to modifications of previous published protocols [39,40]. Cervical, thoracic and lumbar DRG were dissected from the spines of wild-type C57BL/6 mice and incubated in 0.05% collagenase at 37°C for four hours, centrifuged at 300×g for 10 minutes at room temperature, and resuspended in 3 ml 1.25% Trypsin-EDTA for 15 minutes at 37°C. Cells were centrifuged again and resuspended in DMEM, 10% FBS, penicillin-streptomycin, and pre-plated. The next day, non-adherent cells were centrifuged and resuspended in C2 nerve growth medium that contained penicillin-streptomycin, at a concentration of 5×10^5 cells/ml. Nerves were plated on Matrigel-coated chamber slides. Murine NGF was added to some cultures at a concentration of 40 ng/ml. Sheep anti-NGF was added for a final concentration of 20 ug/ml. At the end of each experiment, cells were fixed in 4% paraformaldehyde for 5 minutes.

Isolation of murine blood eosinophils

Diluted blood from NJ.1638 (IL-5 transgenic) mice was layered over 15 mL sterile Percoll (density 1.084 g/mL) and centrifuged at $2000 \times g$ for 45 minutes. The white layer at the interface, which contained the granulocytes, was collected, washed and centrifuged at $300 \times g$ for 15 minutes at $4°C$. Red cells were lysed and the eosinophils were isolated by size and granularity using fluorescence-activated cell sorting (FACS). Trypan blue exclusion was used to determine viability. Percent purity was determined by Hemacolor assay on cytospin slides. After FACS staining, percent purity of eosinophils was determined by Hemacolor staining and differential cell counts under the $20 \times$ objective of a bright field microscope. The purity of eosinophils after sorting was 91%. Cells were resuspended in C2 nerve medium at the indicated concentrations and added to cultures of DRG neurons for 24 hours.

Isolation of murine peritoneal mast cells

Peritoneal mast cells were isolated according to the method of Jensen et al. [Jensen B, Swindle E, Iwaki S, Gilfillan A, Current Protocols in Immunology, 2006, Wiley Interscience]. A single mouse was killed and the peritoneum was lavaged with HBSS. Lavage fluid was centrifuged at $400 \times g$ for 5 minutes, red blood cells were lysed, and the cells were washed twice with HBSS. The pellet was resuspended in 70% isotonic Percoll solution, and cells were layered over filter-sterilized peritoneal mast cell (PMC) medium (DMEM, 5% FBS, 2 mM L-glutamine, 50 ug/ml gentamicin, 20 mM HEPES) and centrifuged at $580 \times g$ for 15 minutes at room temperature. The mast cell pellet was resuspended in PMC medium. Aliquots of cells were counted and stained with trypan blue to determine viability or toluidine blue to determine purity of mast cells. Finally, cells were adjusted to indicated concentrations, added to slides or wells and incubated at $35.5°C$ with 5% CO_2.

Dorsal Root Ganglion Immunocytochemistry

Slides with DRG were fixed in 4% paraformaldehyde for 5 minutes, rinsed with HBSS with calcium and magnesium, and stored in PBS until stained. Slides were blocked with 10% serum and stained with antibodies to PGP 9.5, ICAM-1, VCAM-1, or eotaxin-1 overnight at $4°C$. After rinsing in PBS, a secondary antibody conjugated to Alexa Fluor-555, or biotin, was applied.

Slides were rinsed and either mounted in Vector Mounting Medium with DAPI, to stain cell nuclei, or completed, using Vector Vectastain Avidin-Biotin Complex immunohistochemistry kit and mounted.

Dorsal Root Ganglion Imaging and Quantification

Thirty $40 \times$ photographs were taken of each chamber after each treatment, stained with anti-PGP 9.5 antibody. Photographs were always taken beginning in the center of each well of a 4-well chamber slide, and then every subsequent field of view was photographed, in the same defined pattern for all slides. Using Metamorph, numbers of cell bodies, neurites, and branchpoints per cell body were counted manually. Each cell body in each photograph was quantified. In addition, neurite length was measured with the segmented line function, which allowed the neurite to be traced from end to end and measured according to the pixel per micron ratio for the $40 \times$ objective. The mean of each measurement (number of cell bodies, neurites, branchpoints and neurite length) for all cell bodies in thirty pictures was determined. Verification of this method was provided two ways: first, one group of photographs each from two experiments was quantified by a blinded observer, who knew neither the treatment groups nor the predicted outcome, and second, photographs were taken at random places in each well for one experiment, and a blinded observer then performed the measurements. Blinded observations were found to match unblinded observations.

Statistical Analysis of Data

All data are expressed as mean +/− SEM. Comparisons between two groups were made using t-tests for unpaired data, while comparisons of nerves in lesional and non-lesional skin from the same human were made using paired t-tests. Multiple comparisons used one-way ANOVA, with a Tukey's post-test to evaluate differences between groups. A p value of less than 0.05 was considered statistically significant.

Acknowledgments

Many thanks to Elizabeth Bivins-Smith, Zhenying Nie, and Jesse Lorton for technical assistance during the project, as well as to Kalmia Buels and Jon Hanifin for advice and productive discussions, and to Gregory Scott, who provided the software coding for assigning random numbers to photos, used in the blinded quantifications.

Author Contributions

Conceived and designed the experiments: EF LF NL JL AF DJ. Performed the experiments: EF ES LF NL. Analyzed the data: EF AF DJ. Contributed reagents/materials/analysis tools: ES LF NL JL. Wrote the paper: ES NL DJ.

References

1. Hanifin J, Rajka G (1980) Diagnostic features of atopic dermatitis. Acta Derm Venereol 92: 44–47.
2. Ikoma A, Fartasch M, Heyer G, Miyachi Y, Handwerker H, et al. (2004) Painful stimuli evoke itch in patients with chronic pruritus: central sensitization for itch. Neurology 62: 212–217.
3. Paus R, Schmelz M, Biro T, Steinhoff M (2006) Frontiers in pruritus research: scratching the brain for more effective itch therapy. J Clin Invest 116: 1174–1186.
4. Tobin D, Nabarro G, Baart de la Faille H, van Vloten WA, van der Putte SC, et al. (1992) Increased number of immunoreactive nerve fibers in atopic dermatitis. J Allergy Clin Immunol 90: 613–622.
5. Sugiura H, Omoto M, Hirota Y, Danno K, Uehara M (1997) Density and fine structure of peripheral nerves in various skin lesions of atopic dermatitis. Arch Dermatol Res 289: 125–131.
6. Byrom NA, Timlin DM (1979) Immune status in atopic eczema: a survey. Br J Dermatol 100: 491–498.
7. Kagi MK, Joller-Jemelka H, Wuthrich B (1992) Correlation of eosinophils, eosinophil cationic protein and soluble interleukin-2 receptor with the clinical activity of atopic dermatitis. Dermatology 185: 88–92.
8. Taniuchi S, Chihara J, Kojima T, Yamamoto A, Sasai M, et al. (2001) Serum eosinophil derived neurotoxin may reflect more strongly disease severity in childhood atopic dermatitis than eosinophil cationic protein. J Dermatol Sci 26: 79–82.
9. Kobayashi H, Gleich GJ, Butterfield JH, Kita H (2002) Human eosinophils produce neurotrophins and secrete nerve growth factor on immunologic stimuli. Blood 99: 2214–2220.
10. Leiferman KM, Ackerman SJ, Sampson HA, Haugen HS, Venencie PY, et al. (1985) Dermal deposition of eosinophil-granule major basic protein in atopic dermatitis. Comparison with onchocerciasis. N Engl J Med 313: 282–285.
11. Kiehl P, Falkenberg K, Vogelbruch M, Kapp A (2001) Tissue eosinophilia in acute and chronic atopic dermatitis: a morphometric approach using quantitative image analysis of immunostaining. Br J Dermatol 145: 720–729.

12. Costello RW, Schofield BH, Kephart GM, Gleich GJ, Jacoby DB, et al. (1997) Localization of eosinophils to airway nerves and effect on neuronal M2 muscarinic receptor function. Am J Physiol 273: L93–103.

13. Sawatzky DA, Kingham PJ, Court E, Kumaravel B, Fryer AD, et al. (2002) Eosinophil adhesion to cholinergic nerves via ICAM-1 and VCAM-1 and associated eosinophil degranulation. Am J Physiol Lung Cell Mol Physiol 282: L1279–1288.

14. Fryer AD, Stein LH, Nie Z, Curtis DE, Evans CM, et al. (2006) Neuronal eotaxin and the effects of CCR3 antagonist on airway hyperreactivity and M2 receptor dysfunction. J Clin Invest 116: 228–236.

15. Evans CM, Fryer AD, Jacoby DB, Gleich GJ, Costello RW (1997) Pretreatment with antibody to eosinophil major basic protein prevents hyperresponsiveness by protecting neuronal M2 muscarinic receptors in antigen-challenged guinea pigs. J Clin Invest 100: 2254–2262.

16. Weller PF, Rand TH, Barrett T, Elovic A, Wong DT, et al. (1993) Accessory cell function of human eosinophils. HLA-DR-dependent, MHC-restricted antigen-presentation and IL-1 alpha expression. J Immunol 150: 2554–2562.

17. Costa JJ, Matossian K, Resnick MB, Beil WJ, Wong DT, et al. (1993) Human eosinophils can express the cytokines tumor necrosis factor-alpha and macrophage inflammatory protein-1 alpha. J Clin Invest 91: 2673–2684.

18. Noga O, Englmann C, Hanf G, Grutzkau A, Seybold J, et al. (2003) The production, storage and release of the neurotrophins nerve growth factor, brain-derived neurotrophic factor and neurotrophin-3 by human peripheral eosinophils in allergics and non-allergics. Clin Exp Allergy 33: 649–654.

19. Arizono N, Matsuda S, Hattori T, Kojima Y, Maeda T, et al. (1990) Anatomical variation in mast cell nerve associations in the rat small intestine, heart, lung, and skin. Similarities of distances between neural processes and mast cells, eosinophils, or plasma cells in the jejunal lamina propria. Lab Invest 62: 626–634.

20. Undem BJ, Hubbard WC, Christian EP, Weinreich D (1990) Mast cells in the guinea pig superior cervical ganglion: a functional and histological assessment. J Auton Nerv Syst 30: 75–87.

21. Jarvikallio A, Naukkarinen A, Harvima IT, Aalto ML, Horsmanheimo M (1997) Quantitative analysis of tryptase- and chymase-containing mast cells in atopic dermatitis and nummular eczema. Br J Dermatol 136: 871–877.

22. Damsgaard TE, Olesen AB, Sorensen FB, Thestrup-Pedersen K, Schiotz PO (1997) Mast cells and atopic dermatitis. Stereological quantification of mast cells in atopic dermatitis and normal human skin. Arch Dermatol Res 289: 256–260.

23. Lee NA, McGarry MP, Larson KA, Horton MA, Kristensen AB, et al. (1997) Expression of IL-5 in thymocytes/T cells leads to the development of a massive eosinophilia, extramedullary eosinophilopoiesis, and unique histopathologies. J Immunol 158: 1332–1344.

24. Kitaura M, Nakajima T, Imai T, Harada S, Combadiere C, et al. (1996) Molecular cloning of human eotaxin, an eosinophil-selective CC chemokine, and identification of a specific eosinophil eotaxin receptor, CC chemokine receptor 3. J Biol Chem 271: 7725–7730.

25. Ponath PD, Qin S, Ringler DJ, Clark-Lewis I, Wang J, et al. (1996) Cloning of the human eosinophil chemoattractant, eotaxin. Expression, receptor binding, and functional properties suggest a mechanism for the selective recruitment of eosinophils. J Clin Invest 97: 604–612.

26. Pincelli C, Sevignani C, Manfredini R, Grande A, Fantini F, et al. (1994) Expression and function of nerve growth factor and nerve growth factor receptor on cultured keratinocytes. J Invest Dermatol 103: 13–18.

27. Lauria G, Holland N, Hauer P, Cornblath DR, Griffin JW, et al. (1999) Epidermal innervation: changes with aging, topographic location, and in sensory neuropathy. J Neurol Sci 164: 172–178.

28. Namer B, Carr R, Johanek LM, Schmelz M, Handwerker HO, et al. (2008) Separate peripheral pathways for pruritus in man. J Neurophysiol 100: 2062–2069.

29. Schmelz M, Schmidt R, Bickel A, Handwerker HO, Torebjork HE (1997) Specific C-receptors for itch in human skin. J Neurosci 17: 8003–8008.

30. Andrew D, Greenspan JD (1999) Mechanical and heat sensitization of cutaneous nociceptors after peripheral inflammation in the rat. J Neurophysiol 82: 2649–2656.

31. Sandkuhler J (2009) Models and mechanisms of hyperalgesia and allodynia. Physiol Rev 89: 707–758.

32. Noga O, Hanf G, Gorges D, Dinh QT, Groneberg DA, et al. (2005) Regulation of NGF and BDNF by dexamethasone and theophylline in human peripheral eosinophils in allergics and non-allergics. Regul Pept 132: 74–79.

33. Gu Q, Lim ME, Gleich GJ, Lee LY (2009) Mechanisms of eosinophil major basic protein-induced hyperexcitability of vagal pulmonary chemosensitive neurons. Am J Physiol Lung Cell Mol Physiol 296: L453–461.

34. Kingham PJ, McLean WG, Walsh MT, Fryer AD, Gleich GJ, et al. (2003) Effects of eosinophils on nerve cell morphology and development: the role of reactive oxygen species and p38 MAP kinase. Am J Physiol Lung Cell Mol Physiol 285: L915–924.

35. van den Hoogenband HM, van den Berg WH, van Diggelen MW (1985) PUVA therapy in the treatment of skin lesions of the hypereosinophilic syndrome. Arch Dermatol 121: 450.

36. Johansson O, Liang Y, Marcusson JA, Reimert CM (2000) Eosinophil cationic protein- and eosinophil-derived neurotoxin/eosinophil protein X-immunoreactive eosinophils in prurigo nodularis. Arch Dermatol Res 292: 371–378.

37. Benarafa C, Collins ME, Hamblin AS, Cunningham FM (2002) Role of the chemokine eotaxin in the pathogenesis of equine sweet itch. Vet Rec 151: 691–693.

38. Vassar R, Rosenberg M, Ross S, Tyner A, Fuchs E (1989) Tissue-specific and differentiation-specific expression of a human K14 keratin gene in transgenic mice. Proc Natl Acad Sci U S A 86: 1563–1567.

39. Sotelo JR, Horie H, Ito S, Benech C, Sango K, et al. (1991) An in vitro model to study diabetic neuropathy. Neurosci Lett 129: 91–94.

40. Delree P, Leprince P, Schoenen J, Moonen G (1989) Purification and culture of adult rat dorsal root ganglia neurons. J Neurosci Res 23: 198–206.

9

Anti-Apoptotic Bfl-1 Is the Major Effector in Activation-Induced Human Mast Cell Survival

Maria Ekoff[1]*, Katarina Lyberg[1], Maryla Krajewska[2], Monica Arvidsson[3], Sabina Rak[3], John C. Reed[2], Ilkka Harvima[4], Gunnar Nilsson[1]

1 Department of Medicine, Centre for Allergy Research, Karolinska Institutet, Stockholm, Sweden, **2** Sanford-Burnham Medical Research Institute, La Jolla, California, United States of America, **3** Department of Respiratory Medicine and Allergology, Sahlgrenska University Hospital, Goteborg, Sweden, **4** Department of Dermatology, Kuopio University Hospital and University of Eastern Finland, Kuopio, Finland

Abstract

Mast cells are best known for their role in allergic reactions, where aggregation of FcεRI leads to the release of mast cell mediators causing allergic symptoms. The activation also induces a survival program in the cells, i.e., activation-induced mast cell survival. The aim of the present study was to investigate how the activation-induced survival is mediated. Cord blood-derived mast cells and the mast cell line LAD-2 were activated through FcεRI crosslinking, with or without addition of chemicals that inhibit the activity or expression of selected Bcl-2 family members (ABT-737; roscovitine). Cell viability was assessed using staining and flow cytometry. The expression and function of Bcl-2 family members *BFL-1* and *MCL-1* were investigated using real-time quantitative PCR and siRNA treatment. The mast cell expression of Bfl-1 was investigated in skin biopsies. FcεRI crosslinking promotes activation-induced survival of human mast cells and this is associated with an upregulation of the anti-apoptotic Bcl-2 family member Bfl-1. ABT-737 alone or in combination with roscovitine decreases viability of human mast cells although activation-induced survival is sustained, indicating a minor role for Bcl-X$_L$, Bcl-2, Bcl-w and Mcl-1. Reducing *BFL-1* but not *MCL-1* levels by siRNA inhibited activation-induced mast cell survival. We also demonstrate that mast cell expression of Bfl-1 is elevated in birch-pollen-provoked skin and in lesions of atopic dermatitis and psoriasis patients. Taken together, our results highlight Bfl-1 as a major effector in activation-induced human mast cell survival.

Editor: Ana Claudia Zenclussen, Otto-von-Guericke University Magdeburg, Germany

Funding: This study was supported by grants from the Swedish Research Council-Medicine, the Centre for Allergy Research at Karolinska Institutet, the Swedish Heart Lung Foundation, the Swedish Cancer Society, Ellen, Walter and Lennart Hesselmans foundation for scientific research, Ollie and Elof Ericsson's foundation, King Gustav V's 80-years foundation, Sweden, Kuopio University Hospital and Abbot, Finland. The authors also acknowledge support from the COST Action BM1007 (Mast cells and basophils – targets for innovative therapies). The funders had no role in study design, data collection and analysis, decision to publish, or preparation of the manuscript.

Competing Interests: The authors have declared that no competing interests exist.

* E-mail: maria.ekoff@ki.se

Introduction

Mast cells are known to be central effectors and regulators in allergic diseases. When a multivalent antigen binds to IgE occupying the high affinity receptor for IgE (FcεRI), receptor aggregation and subsequent mast cell activation occurs. This result in mast cell degranulation, changes in gene expression, and the release of inflammatory mediators causing the symptoms associated with allergic reactions [1,2,3]. In addition, the mast cell has the ability to survive the degranulation process, regranulate, and be activated again, which perpetuates the allergic reaction [4,5]. One important question in mast cell biology is how mast cells survive during this degranulation – regranulation process.

It has previously been demonstrated that the aggregation of FcεRI can result in increased survival of mast cells (activation-induced survival) [6,7,8,9]. Upon crosslinking of FcεRI (IgECL) murine mast cells upregulate anti-apoptotic Bcl-2 family member *A1* and *bcl-XL* and also to a lesser extent *bcl-2* at the mRNA level [8,10,11]. We have previously shown that mouse mast cells deficient in *A1* do not exhibit activation-induced survival upon IgECL [8], suggesting that *A1* is essential for this process in mouse.

Similarly, the human homologue of *A1*, *BFL-1*, is upregulated in human mast cells upon IgECL [12] together with anti-apoptotic Bcl-2 family member *MCL-1* [12,13]. These observations provide a possible explanation for IgE-mediated activation-induced mast cell survival. Furthermore, FcγRI crosslinking also induces *BFL-1* upregulation and activation-induced human mast cell survival [14], further suggesting that activation through these Fc-receptors contributes to mast cell survival.

Here we describe that Bfl-1 is a mediator of activation-induced human mast cell survival as demonstrated by siRNA experiments. We also demonstrate that activation-induced mast cell survival is sustained when the anti-apoptotic proteins Bcl-X$_L$, Bcl-2, Bcl-W and Mcl-1 are targeted using inhibitors, indicating a minor role for the targeted anti-apoptotic Bcl-2 family members. Furthermore, Bfl-1 is upregulated in mast cells in various skin inflammatory models. Therefore, the observations highlight Bfl-1 as a potential target for treatment of allergic and inflammatory diseases.

Results

IgECL promotes activation-induced survival in cytokine deprived human mast cells

IgECL has been shown to promote survival of mast cells cultured in the absence of their required growth factors [7,8,9]. We therefore investigated the survival capacity of human cytokine-deprived cord blood-derived mast cells (CBMCs) and the human mast cell line LAD-2 following IgECL using a fixed concentration of human IgE (1 μg/ml) and 0.2, 2 or 20 μg/ml of anti-human IgE. The results show that IgECL resulted in prolonged survival of cytokine-deprived CBMCs for all anti-human IgE concentrations tested (Fig. 1A). Also LAD-2 cells responded with an increased survival after activation with 2 μg/ml of anti-human IgE (Fig. 1B). For further studies the concentration of 2 μg/ml of anti-human IgE was chosen since the results indicated that this concentration is superior (P = 0.039 and 0.031 respectively) as compared to 0.2 and 20 μg/ml for achieving activation-induced survival of CBMCs and LAD-2 cells.

Activation-induced mast cell survival is not dependent on Bcl-2, Bcl-X$_L$, Bcl-w or Mcl-1

The family of pro-survival Bcl-2 proteins in humans consists of Bcl-2, Bcl-X$_L$, Bcl-W, A1/Bfl-1, Bcl-B and Mcl-1. The activation-induced survival following IgECL is a complex process where Bcl-X$_L$, Bfl-1 and Mcl-1 has been demonstrated to be induced in human mast cells, and hence have a possible role in activation-induced mast cell survival [8,13]. To evaluate the role of Bcl-2, Bcl-X$_L$, Bcl-W and Mcl-1 we used the BH3-only mimetic ABT-737 alone or in combination with roscovitine. ABT-737 is a small molecular inhibitor mimicking the binding of the BH3 domain of the pro-apoptotic protein Bad [15]. It binds with high affinity to the anti-apoptotic proteins Bcl-X$_L$, Bcl-2 and Bcl-W but not Mcl-1, Bcl-B or A1/Bfl-1. The cyclin-dependent kinase (CDK) inhibitor roscovitine has been reported to down-regulate the anti-apoptotic protein Mcl-1 [16,17,18,19]. The concentrations of ABT-737 and roscovitine used were chosen based on dose-response data (not shown) and with the purpose of inducing a degree of apoptosis similar to cytokine deprivation in our system.

Upon treating CBMCs with 0.5 μM ABT-737, mast cell viability decreased by approximately 10% and combination of 0.5 μM ABT-737 and 5 μM roscovitine decreased this viability even further by another 20% (Fig. 2A). Decreased viability could also be observed for LAD-2 cells where the viability was decreased by approximately 25% in response to ABT-737 or ABT-737 in

combination with roscovitine (Fig. 2B). The results show that IgECL resulted in prolonged survival of both ABT-737 and ABT-737/Roscovitine-treated CBMCs and LAD-2 cells (Fig. 2A–B). These results demonstrate that the ability to induce survival is sustained in an experimental setting where Bcl-2, Bcl-X$_L$, Bcl-W and Mcl-1 are inhibited, and suggest that one of the remaining pro-survival Bcl-2 family members (i.e. Bfl-1 and Bcl-B) was responsible for the activation-induced survival response. Since mice lack an obvious ortholog of Bcl-B, we focused on Bfl-1, the human ortholog of A1 which was shown to be essential for murine activation-induced mast cell survival [8].

siRNA targeting BFL-1 inhibits activation-induced survival of human mast cells

Having demonstrated a minor role of Bcl-X$_L$, Bcl-2, Bcl-W and possibly also Mcl-1 we next examined how inhibition of *BFL-1* affects activation-induced survival of CBMC and LAD-2 cells. To inhibit gene expression, cells were electroporated using siRNA oligonucleotides targeting *BFL-1*, *MCL-1* or non-targeting siRNA. Activation-induced upregulation of both *BFL-1* and *MCL-1* at the mRNA level following IgECL were abolished by siRNA treatment, as demonstrated by quantative PCR (Fig. 3A and C). The expression of *BCL-2*, *BCL-XL*, or *C-KIT* was not affected (data not shown). In contrast, activation-induced survival was diminished by *BFL-1* targeting siRNA but not by *MCL-1* targeting siRNA (Fig. 3B and D). We could also demonstrate, by immunohistochemical staining, Bfl-1 to be down-regulated on the protein level in CBMC and LAD-2 cells by *BFL-1* siRNA treatment as compared to non-targeting siRNA (fig. 3E). Taken together our results demonstrate the critical role of Bfl-1 in prolonging the survival of cytokine-deprived human mast cells after IgECL and support our hypothesis that Bfl-1 is a major survival factor promoting activation-induced survival. Mcl-1 by comparison, seems to play a minor role in activation-induced mast cell survival, even though IgECL induces Mcl-1 expression.

Bfl-1 is expressed in skin tissue mast cells and is increased under inflammatory conditions

CBMCs as well as LAD-2 cells express tryptase and chymase (data not shown) [20,21,22] exhibiting a human MC$_{TC}$ phenotype, which is the dominating phenotype in connective tissues, e.g. the skin [23]. To examine if Bfl-1 is regulated in tissue mast cells, we therefore used a doublestaining technique on skin biopsies as previously described [24]. An enzymatical staining followed by an

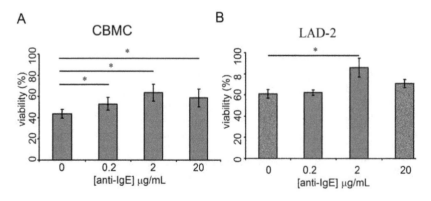

Figure 1. IgECL-induced survival of human mast cells. (A). CBMC upon IgECL. (B) LAD-2 cells upon IgECL. Cells were sensitized with 1 μg/mL of IgE overnight before cytokine-deprived and challenged with anti-IgE. After 24 hrs the cell viability was enumerated using trypan blue exclusion. N = 3–4.

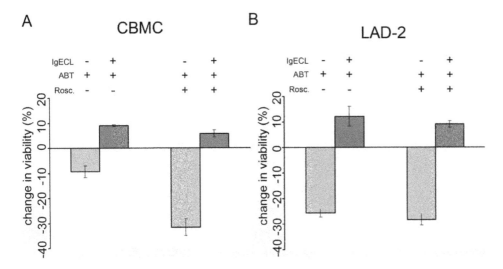

Figure 2. Activation-induced mast cell survival following IgECL in presence of ABT-737 and roscovitine. (A) CBMC treated with 0.5 μM ABT-737 alone or in combination with 5 μM roscovitine following IgECL. N = 6–3. (B) LAD-2 treated with 0.5 μM ABT-737 alone or in combination with 5 μM roscovitine following IgECL. N = 3 Viability was assessed after 24 hrs using propidium iodide plus FITC-conjugated Annexin V. Change in viability is expressed as percentage viable cells after treatment deducted from untreated cells. ABT-737 = ABT, roscovitine = rosc.

immunohistochemical staining of the same tissue section demonstrated that Bfl-1 is expressed in skin tissue mast cells (Fig. 4).

To examine if Bfl-1 is regulated in skin mast cells *in vivo* we performed allergen challenge on birch-pollen allergic patients. Skin biopsies were obtained 24 h following challenge with pollen allergen or diluent. A significant increase in mast cell Bfl-1 expression in the biopsies from allergen provoked skin compared with control was observed (Fig. 5a). We could not observe any significant changes in mast cell number (data not shown). Thus, IgE-receptor activated human mast cells upregulate Bfl-1 upon allergic provocation *in vivo*.

Although mast cells are perhaps best known for their involvement in allergic diseases, growing evidence also suggest that mast cells are involved in inflammatory mechanisms of chronic skin diseases. Atopic dermatitis (AD), psoriasis (PSO), and basal cell carcinoma (BCC) are chronic cutaneous inflammatory diseases where the number of mast cells is higher to varying extents in lesional compared with nonlesional skin [24,25]. We therefore investigated if expression of the pro-survival protein Bfl-1 was increased concomitant to increased mast cell numbers in the lesional skin. A significant increase in mast cell Bfl-1 expression in the lesional skin of AD and PSO patients compared with nonlesional skin from the same patients was observed (Fig. 5b). In addition, Bfl-1 was increased in the lesional BCC skin in every case, though statistical significance was not reached (p = 0.078).

Discussion

In the present study we provide strong evidence that activation-induced human mast cell survival is dependent on the expression of Bfl-1 and that Bfl-1 is induced in skin mast cells *in vivo*.

We have previously demonstrated that, in the mouse, mRNA levels for the anti-apoptotic Bcl-2 family member *A1* are increased following IgECL and that mast cells lacking *A1* do not gain a survival advantage from IgECL [8]. Similarly, our results using quantative PCR confirm that *BFL-1* is upregulated at mRNA level following IgECL in human mast cells ([12] and this study). However, activation-induced mast cell survival following IgECL is a complex process where also other anti-apoptotic Bcl-2 family members apart from A1/Bfl-1 are regulated. In the murine

system, anti-apoptotic Bcl-X_L is increased following IgECL [8,26] and in human mast cells Mcl-1 [12,13] is upregulated. Our results using the BH3 mimetic compound ABT-737 suggests a minor role of anti-apoptotic Bcl-X_L, Bcl-2 and Bcl-W in human mast cell survival following IgECL. Furthermore, the use of ABT-737 combined with roscovitine also implicates a minor role for Mcl-1 in activation-induced survival following IgECL. In contrast, mast cell survival was impaired by *BFL-1* (but not *MCL-1*) knockdown using siRNA. Altogether, our results establish the importance of *BFL-1* for activation-induced survival of human mast cells *in vitro*.

To examine if Bfl-1 is regulated in activated mast cells *in vivo* we used human skin biopsies from birch-pollen allergic patients. We found a significant increase in mast cell Bfl-1 expression in allergen provocated skin. Although we could not detect a statistically significant change in mast cell numbers after 24 hours following allergen challenge it seems plausible that an increased mast cell Bfl-1 expression over time would lead to an increase in mast cell numbers. Thus, both our *in vivo* and *in vitro* findings suggest that activated mast cells upregulate Bfl-1 upon allergic provocation, highlighting Bfl-1 as a potential target for treatment of allergic diseases.

In addition, we also found a significant increase in mast cell Bfl-1 expression in lesional skin of AD and PSO patients compared with nonlesional skin from the same patients. FcεRI-dependent activation of mast cells is not commonly associated with these diseases, but it has been reported that in IFN-γ-rich psoriatic skin [27] mast cells express FcγRI [28]. Interestingly, we have previously shown that also FcγRI crosslinking of *in vitro*-generated human mast cells induce *BFL-1* upregulation and activation-induced mast cell survival [14]. Thus, we believe that activation-induced mast cell survival is an Fc-mediated mechanism, as we have not been able to observe this *BFL-1* upregulation and activation-induced survival for other types of mast cell stimuli, e.g. through adenosine receptors [11] or compound 48/80 [8]. Since our findings suggest that activation-induced mast cell survival is dependent on the upregulation of *BFL-1* and that there is an increase of mast cell Bfl-1 expression in lesional skin of AD and PSO patients, this could be an important explanation to increased mast cell numbers seen in AD, PSO and BCC. Still, the role of

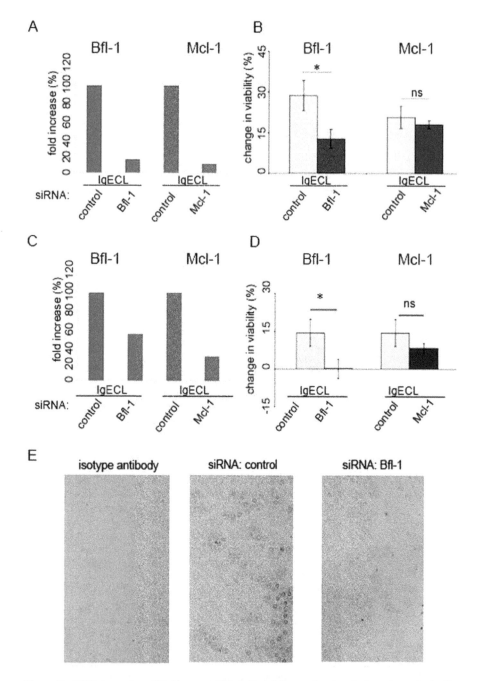

Figure 3. siRNA targeting *BFL-1* but not *MCL-1* diminishes activation-induced survival of human mast cells. (A) The upregulation of *BFL-1* and *MCL-1* following IgECL in CBMCs is abolished following targeted siRNA treatment as verified 30 hours post-transfection by quantative PCR. Cells were transfected with 100 nM siRNA, sensitized with 1 µg/mL of IgE and challenged with 2 µg/mL anti-IgE before expression was determined. Data correspond to one representative experiment using one donor. Similar result was obtained for another donor. (B) *BFL-1* but not *MCL-1* siRNA treated CBMCs show decreased survival upon IgECL compared to control siRNA treated cells. Cells were transfected, sensitized with 1 µg/mL of IgE and 24 hours post-transfection cytokine-deprived and challenged with 2 µg/mL anti-IgE before being enumerated 24 hours later using the vital dye trypan blue. N = 6. (C) The upregulation of *BFL-1* and *MCL-1* following IgECL in LAD-2 cells is abolished following targeted siRNA treatment as described above. (D) *BFL-1* but not *MCL-1* siRNA treated LAD-2 cells show decreased survival upon IgECL compared to control siRNA treated cells. N = 4. Change in viability is percentage viable cytokine-deprived cells deducted from viable cytokine-deprived cells following IgECL. (E) Bfl-1 is down-regulated in LAD-2 cells following siRNA treatment targeting *BFL-1* as compared to control siRNA in immunohistochemical stainings for Bfl-1 expression.

mast cells and the implications elevated Bfl-1 expression might have in mast cell survival in AD, PSO and BCC remains to be determined.

Altogether, the results reported here suggest that Bfl-1 is among the contributors to survival of mast cells, raising the possibility that agents neutralizing this Bcl-2 family member could find a role in the treatment of a wide variety of allergic and chronic inflammatory diseases.

Atopic dermatitis (AD) lesional skin

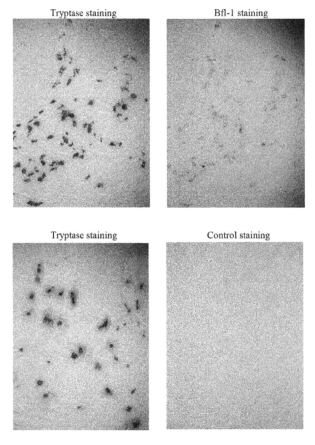

Figure 4. Bfl-1 is expressed in skin tissue mast cells. An enzymatical staining for tryptase followed by an immunohistochemical staining of Bfl-1 (upper panel) and was performed on atopic dermatitis (AD) lesional skin. Isotype control staining following tryptase staining (lower panel).

Materials and Methods

Ethics statement

All patients provided written informed consent. The regional ethics review board for medical research in Gothenburg, Sweden and the etical committee of Kuopio University Hospital, Kuopio, Finland approved the studies.

Cell cultures

Cord blood-derived mast cells (CBMCs) were derived in supplemented StemPro-34 SFM medium (Invitrogen Corp., Carlsbad, CA, USA) including 100 ng/mL recombinant human SCF (hSCF, Peprotech EC Ltd, London, UK) and 10 ng/mL human IL-6 (Peprotech EC Ltd) as previously described [12]. The human mast cell line LAD-2 (kindly provided by Drs. A. Kirshenbaum and D. Metcalfe, NIH, Bethesda, MD, USA) [22] was maintained in supplemented StemPro-34 SFM medium with 100 ng/mL hSCF.

Mast cell activation

Cells (10^6 cells/mL) were incubated with 1 µg/mL IgE (AG30P, Millipore, Billerica, MA, USA) overnight, washed with PBS, and activated with 0.2, 2 or 20 µg/mL anti-human IgE (Sigma, St. Louis, MO, USA) for 24 hours in medium deprived of cytokines. For inhibition studies, 0.5 µM ABT-737 (provided by Abbott laboratories) was added at the time of activation, whereas 5 µM roscovitine (Sigma) was added two hours prior activation.

Cell survival assays

Enumeration of viable cells was performed by trypan blue exclusion or propidium iodide (PI, 2 µg/mL) and FITC-conjugated annexin V (0.3 µg/mL) analyzed by FACScan (Becton Dickinson, Franklin Lakes, NJ, USA).

RNA preparation and real-time quantitative PCR

RNA was extracted using TriPure isolation reagent (Roche Diagnostics) according to the manufacturer's protocol. cDNA was synthesised using a First Strand cDNA Synthesis Kit (Roche Diagnosticss) and amplified using 1xSYBR Green PCR master mix (Applied Biosystems, Foster City, CA, USA) and 700 nM of

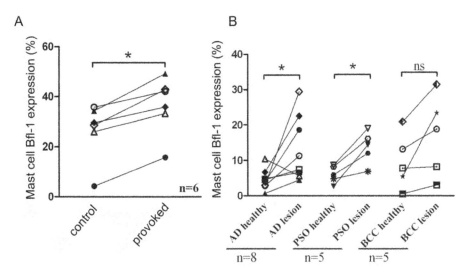

Figure 5. Elevated Bfl-1 expression upon allergen provocation in birch-pollen allergic patients (A) and in lesions of atopic dermatitis (AD) and psoriasis patients (PSO) (B). An enzymatical staining for tryptase followed by an immunohistochemical staining of Bfl-1 was performed. The results are presented as the percentage of mast cells expressing Bfl-1.

primer. Relative changes in gene expression were calculated by the comparative ΔCt method in which human gyceraldehyde-3-phosphate dehydrogenase (*GAPDH*) was used for normalization. Listed 5′ to 3′, primer sequences were as follows: *BFL-1* forward, AAATGTTGCGTTCTCAGTCC; *BFL-1* reverse, AGCCTCCGTTTTGCCTTATC; *MCL-1* forward, TTACCGCGTTTCTTTTGAGG; *MCL-1* reverse CACTTCT-CACTTCCGCTTCC; *GAPDH* forward, TCGGAGTCAACG-GAT; *GAPDH* reverse, CTCCGACGCCTGCTT.

siRNA-mediated inhibition of *BFL-1* and *MCL-1* gene expression

CBMC and LAD-2 cells were transfected using Human MCL1 SMARTpool siRNA Reagent, BCL2A1 SMARTpool siRNA Reagent or human ON-TARGETplus Non-targeting siRNA (Dharmacon Inc., Lafayette, CO, USA). 100 nM siRNA was introduced using a Nucleoporator (nucleofector kit VPI-1002; program X-001 (Amaxa AG, Cologne, Germany)). 24 hours post-transfection, the dead cell removal kit MACS (Miltenyi Biotec, Bergisch Gladbach, Germany) was used before anti-human IgE was added as described previously. Inhibition of *BFL-1* and *MCL-1* expression was verified by real-time quantitative PCR 30 hours post-transfection.

Antibody generation and characterization

The anti-Bfl-1 serum (SB-50) was generated in rabbits using recombinant Bfl-1 protein. Bfl1 was produced as GST fusion protein from pGEX vectors using Escherichia coli BL21 (DE3) as the host strain. The protein purification method has been described previously [29]. New Zealand white female rabbits were injected subcutaneously with a mixture of recombinant protein (0.1 to 0.25 μg protein/immunization) and 0.5 ml Freund's complete adjuvant (dose divided over 10 injection sites), boosted three times at weekly intervals, followed by another 3 to 20 boostings at monthly intervals with recombinant protein in Freund's incomplete adjuvant, collecting blood at 1 to 3 weeks after each boosting to obtain serum.

Detection of mast cell Bfl-1 expression

Bfl-1 expression in IgECL-activated CBMC and LAD-2 cells following siRNA treatment was investigated using an immunohistochemical staining of Bfl-1. Slides were immunohistochemically stained with an anti-Bfl-1 polyclonal rabbit antibody and the EnVision system and the 3-amino-9-etyhlcarbazole (AEC) method (Sigma) were performed according to the manufacturer's instructions (Dakocytomation, Carpinteria, CA, USA).

Bfl-1 expression in mast cells in skin inflammatory conditions was investigated in a blinded fashion using a sequential double-staining, combining an enzymatical staining for tryptase with the immunohistochemical staining of Bfl-1 [24,30]. Tryptase containing cells were visualized using 1 mM Z-Gly-Pro-Arg-4-methoxy-2-naphthylamide (MNA) (Bachem, Bubendorf, Switzerland) and Fast Garnet GBC (Sigma) and the sections were immunohistochemically stained for Bfl-1 as described above. The mast cells were counted in a total area of 0.2–0.4 mm^2 just beneath the epidermis.

Six birch-allergic patients with a clinical history of birch pollen-induced rhinoconjunctivitis were included in the study. The birch allergy was confirmed by positive skin prick test: 3 mm and serum-specific IgE antibodies to birch: class 2 (CAP system, Phadia, Uppsala, Sweden). Allergen challenge was performed and biopsies were collected outside birch pollen season. 50 SQ-U birch pollen allergen extracts (Aquagen® SQ *Betula verrucosa*; ALK-Abello, Hørsholm, Denmark) was injected intracutaneously in the forearm. Albumin diluent (Aquagen® SQ) was injected in the opposite forearm as a negative control. Skin biopsies were taken 24 h following challenge using a 3 mm disposable punch, under local anaesthesia with Xylocain® (Astra AB, Södertälje, Sweden). Samples were snap frozen, embedded immediately in TissueTek (Zoeterwoude, Netherlands) OCT medium and stored at −70°C. For staining, 6 μm thick sections were cut by cryostat (Leica CM1800, Nusstoch bei Heidelberg, Germany).

We also included three skin biopsy series from patients with atopic dermatitis, psoriasis, and basal cell carcinoma. The patients had not received any effective internal or UV-light treatment before biopsing. Punch biopsies (4 mm) were taken from untreated lesional skin and from healthy-looking skin at least 2 cm apart from the lesions. The biopsies were immediately embedded in OCT compound (Miles Scientific, Naperville, IL, USA) and frozen for preparation of 5-μm-thick cryosections [24,30].

Statistics

All data, unless otherwise stated, are presented as the mean ± SEM. The differences among different groups were determined by the Student's t test. $P<0.05$ was considered significant.

Acknowledgments

We wish to thank Agnetha Beinhoff and Anne Koivisto for expert technical assistance.

Author Contributions

Conceived and designed the experiments: ME GN MA SR IH. Performed the experiments: ME KL IH. Analyzed the data: ME KL IH. Contributed reagents/materials/analysis tools: MK MA SR JR IH. Wrote the paper: ME GN IH.

References

1. Metcalfe DD, Baram D, Mekori YA (1997) Mast cells. Physiol Rev 77: 1033–1079.
2. Galli SJ (2000) Allergy. Curr Biol 10: R93–95.
3. Ishizaka T, Ishizaka K (1984) Activation of mast cells for mediator release through IgE receptors. In: Ishizaka K, editor. Mast Cell Activation and Mediator Release. Basel: Karger. 188–235.
4. Kobayasi T, Asboe-Hansen G (1969) Degranulation and regranulation of human mast cells. An electron microscopic study of the whealing reaction in urticaria pigmentosa. Acta Derm Venereol 49: 369–381.
5. Dvorak AM, Schleimer RP, Lichtenstein LM (1987) Morphologic mast cell cycles. Cell Immunol 105: 199–204.
6. Kawakami T, Galli SJ (2002) Regulation of mast-cell and basophil function and survival by IgE. Nat Rev Immunol 2: 773–786.
7. Kitaura J, Xiao W, Maeda-Yamamoto M, Kawakami Y, Lowell CA, et al. (2004) Early divergence of Fc epsilon receptor I signals for receptor up-regulation and internalization from degranulation, cytokine production, and survival. J Immunol 173: 4317–4323.
8. Xiang Z, Ahmed AA, Moller C, Nakayama K, Hatakeyama S, et al. (2001) Essential role of the prosurvival bcl-2 homologue A1 in mast cell survival after allergic activation. J Exp Med 194: 1561–1569.
9. Yoshikawa H, Nakajima Y, Tasaka K (1999) Glucocorticoid suppresses autocrine survival of mast cells by inhibiting IL-4 production and ICAM-1 expression. J Immunol 162: 6162–6170.
10. Alfredsson J, Puthalakath H, Martin H, Strasser A, Nilsson G (2005) Proapoptotic Bcl-2 family member Bim is involved in the control of mast cell survival and is induced together with Bcl-X(L) upon IgE-receptor activation. Cell Death Differ 12: 136–144.
11. Möller C, Xiang Z, Nilsson G (2003) Activation of mast cells by immunoglobulin E-receptor cross-linkage, but not through adenosine receptors, induces A1 expression and promotes survival. Clin Exp Allergy 33: 1135–1140.
12. Xiang Z, Moller C, Nilsson G (2006) IgE-receptor activation induces survival and Bfl-1 expression in human mast cells but not basophils. Allergy 61: 1040–1046.

13. Berent-Maoz B, Salemi S, Mankuta D, Simon HU, Levi-Schaffer F (2008) TRAIL mediated signaling in human mast cells: the influence of IgE-dependent activation. Allergy 63: 333–340.

14. Karlberg M, Xiang Z, Nilsson G (2008) Fc gamma RI-mediated activation of human mast cells promotes survival and induction of the pro-survival gene Bfl-1. J Clin Immunol 28: 250–255.

15. Oltersdorf T, Elmore SW, Shoemaker AR, Armstrong RC, Augeri DJ, et al. (2005) An inhibitor of Bcl-2 family proteins induces regression of solid tumours. Nature 435: 677–681.

16. MacCallum DE, Melville J, Frame S, Watt K, Anderson S, et al. (2005) Seliciclib (CYC202, R-Roscovitine) induces cell death in multiple myeloma cells by inhibition of RNA polymerase II-dependent transcription and down-regulation of Mcl-1. Cancer Res 65: 5399–5407.

17. Raje N, Kumar S, Hideshima T, Roccaro A, Ishitsuka K, et al. (2005) Seliciclib (CYC202 or R-roscovitine), a small-molecule cyclin-dependent kinase inhibitor, mediates activity via down-regulation of Mcl-1 in multiple myeloma. Blood 106: 1042–1047.

18. van Delft MF, Wei AH, Mason KD, Vandenberg CJ, Chen L, et al. (2006) The BH3 mimetic ABT-737 targets selective Bcl-2 proteins and efficiently induces apoptosis via Bak/Bax if Mcl-1 is neutralized. Cancer Cell 10: 389–399.

19. Ortiz-Ferron G, Yerbes R, Eramo A, Lopez-Perez AI, De Maria R, et al. (2008) Roscovitine sensitizes breast cancer cells to TRAIL-induced apoptosis through a pleiotropic mechanism. Cell Res 18: 664–676.

20. Nilsson G, Blom T, Harvima I, Kusche-Gullberg M, Nilsson K, et al. (1996) Stem cell factor-dependent human cord blood derived mast cells express alpha- and beta-tryptase, heparin and chondroitin sulphate. Immunology 88: 308–314.

21. Saito H, Ebisawa M, Sakaguchi N, Onda T, Iikura Y, et al. (1995) Characterization of cord-blood-derived human mast cells cultured in the presence of Steel factor and interleukin-6. Int Arch Allergy Immunol 107: 63–65.

22. Kirshenbaum AS, Akin C, Wu Y, Rottem M, Goff JP, et al. (2003) Characterization of novel stem cell factor responsive human mast cell lines LAD 1 and 2 established from a patient with mast cell sarcoma/leukemia; activation following aggregation of FcepsilonRI or FcgammaRI. Leuk Res 27: 677–682.

23. Nilsson G, Costa JJ, Metcalfe DD (1999) Mast Cells and Basophils. In: Gallin JI, Snyderman R, editors. Inflammation: Basic Principles and Clinical Correlates. 3rd ed. ed. Philadelphia: Lippincott Williams & Wilkins. 97–117.

24. Diaconu NC, Kaminska R, Naukkarinen A, Harvima RJ, Nilsson G, et al. (2007) Increase in CD30 ligand/CD153 and TNF-alpha expressing mast cells in basal cell carcinoma. Cancer Immunol Immunother 56: 1407–1415.

25. Ackermann L, Harvima IT (1998) Mast cells of psoriatic and atopic dermatitis skin are positive for TNF-alpha and their degranulation is associated with expression of ICAM-1 in the epidermis. Arch Dermatol Res 290: 353–359.

26. Alfredsson J, Moller C, Nilsson G (2006) IgE-receptor activation of mast cells regulates phosphorylation and expression of forkhead and Bcl-2 family members. Scand J Immunol 63: 1–6.

27. Barker JN (1991) The pathophysiology of psoriasis. Lancet 338: 227–230.

28. Tkaczyk C, Okayama Y, Woolhiser MR, Hagaman DD, Gilfillan AM, et al. (2002) Activation of human mast cells through the high affinity IgG receptor. Mol Immunol 38: 1289–1293.

29. Schendel SL, Azimov R, Pawlowski K, Godzik A, Kagan BL, et al. (1999) Ion channel activity of the BH3 only Bcl-2 family member, BID. J Biol Chem 274: 21932–21936.

30. Fischer M, Harvima IT, Carvalho RF, Moller C, Naukkarinen A, et al. (2006) Mast cell CD30 ligand is upregulated in cutaneous inflammation and mediates degranulation-independent chemokine secretion. J Clin Invest 116: 2748–2756.

10

ORAI1 Genetic Polymorphisms Associated with the Susceptibility of Atopic Dermatitis in Japanese and Taiwanese Populations

Wei-Chiao Chang[10,12,15]*[9], Chih-Hung Lee[13][9], Tomomitsu Hirota[1]*, Li-Fang Wang[14], Satoru Doi[2], Akihiko Miyatake[3], Tadao Enomoto[4], Kaori Tomita[5], Masafumi Sakashita[5], Takechiyo Yamada[5], Shigeharu Fujieda[5], Koji Ebe[6], Hidehisa Saeki[7], Satoshi Takeuchi[8], Masutaka Furue[8], Wei-Chiao Chen[10], Yi-Ching Chiu[10], Wei Pin Chang[11], Chien-Hui Hong[13], Edward Hsi[16], Suh-Hang Hank Juo[10,16], Hsin-Su Yu[13], Yusuke Nakamura[9], Mayumi Tamari[1]

1 Laboratory for Respiratory Diseases, Center for Genomic Medicine, The Institute of Physical and Chemical Research (RIKEN), Kanagawa, Japan, 2 Department of Pediatric Allergy, Osaka Prefectural Medical Center for Respiratory and Allergic Diseases, Osaka, Japan, 3 Miyatake Asthma Clinic, Osaka, Japan, 4 NPO Japan Health Promotion Supporting Network, Wakayama, Japan, 5 Division of Otorhinolaryngology Head and Neck Surgery, University of Fukui, Fukui, Japan, 6 Takao Hospital, Kyoto, Japan, 7 Department of Dermatology, The Jikei University School of Medicine, Tokyo, Japan, 8 Department of Dermatology, Graduate School of Medical Sciences, Kyushu University, Fukuoka, Japan, 9 Laboratory of Molecular Medicine, The Institute of Medical Science, The University of Tokyo, Tokyo, Japan, 10 Department of Medical Genetics, College of Medicine, Kaohsiung Medical University, Kaohsiung, Taiwan, 11 Department of Healthcare Management, Yuanpei University, HsinChu, Taiwan, 12 Cancer Center, Kaohsiung Medical University Hospital, Kaohsiung, Taiwan, 13 Department of Dermatology, Graduate Institute of Medicine, Kaohsiung Medical University, Kaohsiung, Taiwan, 14 Department of Dermatology, National Taiwan University College of Medicine, Taipei, Taiwan, 15 Center for Resources, Research, and Development, Kaohsiung Medical University, Kaohsiung, Taiwan, 16 Department of Medical Research, Kaohsiung Medical University Hospital, Kaohsiung, Taiwan

Abstract

Atopic dermatitis is a chronic inflammatory skin disease. Multiple genetic and environmental factors are thought to be responsible for susceptibility to AD. In this study, we collected 2,478 DNA samples including 209 AD patients and 729 control subjects from Taiwanese population and 513 AD patients and 1027 control subject from Japanese population for sequencing and genotyping ORAI1. A total of 14 genetic variants including 3 novel single-nucleotide polymorphisms (SNPs) in the ORAI1 gene were identified. Our results indicated that a non-synonymous SNP (rs3741596, Ser218Gly) associated with the susceptibility of AD in the Japanese population but not in the Taiwanese population. However, there is another SNP of ORAI1 (rs3741595) associated with the risk of AD in the Taiwanese population but not in the Japanese population. Taken together, our results indicated that genetic polymorphisms of ORAI1 are very likely to be involved in the susceptibility of AD.

Editor: Amanda Ewart Toland, Ohio State University Medical Center, United States of America

Funding: The authors are grateful to the members of The Rotary Club of Osaka-Midosuji District 2660 Rotary International in Japan for supporting our study. This work was supported in part by grants from the Ministry of Education, Culture, Sports, Science, and Technology, Japan, and from the Ministry of Health, Labor, and Welfare, Japan. This study was also partly supported by funding from NHRI-100A1-PDCO-03000001, Excellence for Cancer Research Center grant, Department of Health, Executive Yuan, Taiwan, ROC (NO. DOH100-TD-C-111-002) and from the National Science Council, Taiwan, ROC (NSC 98-2320-B-037-028-MY2; 100-2320-B-037-002). The funders had no role in study design, data collection and analysis, decision to publish, or preparation of the manuscript.

Competing Interests: The authors have declared that no competing interests exist.

* E-mail: wcc@kmu.edu.tw (W-C. Chang); thirota@src.riken.jp (TH)

[9] These authors contributed equally to this work.

Introduction

Atopic dermatitis (AD) or childhood eczema is a chronic relapsing inflammatory skin disease [1] that usually associated with a family history of atopic disorders such as allergic rhinitis and bronchial asthma [2,3,4]. There has been a dramatic increase in the prevalence of AD in the last decade. Although the pathogenesis of AD remains elusive, multiple genetic and environmental factors are thought to contribute to the disease onset [2,3,4]. Genes associated with skin-barrier formation and adaptive immunity have been implicated in the development of AD. For example, filaggrin (FLG) is essential for the maintenance of the skin-barrier function. Genetic mutations in FLG are significantly associated with the risk of AD and elevated

immunoglobulin E (IgE) levels [5]. In addition, single nucleotide polymorphisms (SNPs) in Toll-like receptors (TLRs), ST2, IL-3, IL-4, IL-5, IL12RB1, and IL-13 have been shown to be associated with the pathogenesis of AD [6,7,8,9,10,11,12]. The results from a genome-wide association study (GWAS) have indicated the complex involvement of multiple loci in the susceptibility of human AD [13].

Despite all the knowledge, the treatment of severe AD remains a challenge. Clinical trials have indicated that cyclosporine is an effective treatment option in children with AD. Short-term treatment with cyclosporine has shown to alleviate disease activity [14]. Cyclosporine, an immunosuppressant, functions as a phosphatase inhibitor that prevents the translocation of calcium-dependent transcription factor—nuclear factor of activated T cells

(NFAT). The influx of calcium through store-operated calcium (SOC) channels is one of the major pathways to increase the intracellular calcium concentration in non-excitable cells such as the mast cells and T lymphocytes [15]. In mast cells, short-term SOC influx has been shown to result in the secretion of inflammatory molecules such as arachidonic acids and leukotriene C_4 [16,17]. In T lymphocytes, the nuclear translocation of NFAT could be driven by the SOC-mediated calcineurin signaling pathway in order to control immune responses [18]. The molecular components of the SOC channels were first identified in patients with severe combined immune deficiency (SCID) syndrome [19]. *ORAI1* gen encoding Orai1 protein is one of the major proteins of SOC channels. A point mutation created in the *ORAI1* gene resulted in the reduction of calcium influx through the SOC channels and dysfunction of the immune system. *ORAI1*-knockout mice exhibited defective mast cells and attenuated cytokine release [20].

In our study, we first conducted LD (linkage disequilibrium) mapping of the *ORAI1* gene, performed a case-control association study and showed a haplotype analysis. We then tested the correlation between the *ORAI1* genetic polymorphisms and the expression level of the *ORAI1* transcript. Our results support a functional role of *ORAI1* polymorphisms in the susceptibility of human AD in both Japanese and Taiwanese population.

Materials and Methods

Subjects

A total of 513 atopic dermatitis patients were recruited in Takao Hospital and the University of Tokyo. All subjects with atopic dermatitis were diagnosed according to the criteria of Hannifin and Rajka [21]. There are four major criteria, including pruritus, chronic or relapsing dermatitis, dermatitis affecting flexural surfaces in adults, and a personal or family history of cutaneous or respiratory atopy. There are 23 minor criteria, such as hypopigmented patch, infraorbital darkening,

cheilitis, hyperlinerized palm, and elevated IgE, etc. To be included, the patients had to meet three major criteria plus at least one minor criterion or two major criteria plus at least three minor criteria. Japanese subjects with AD were recruited from several hospitals and diagnosed according to the criteria of Hanifin and Rajka by dermatologists. A total of 839 adult control individuals who had no history of bronchial asthma, allergic rhinitis and atopic dermatitis were recruited by detailed doctors' interviews. A total of 188 healthy individuals who had no history of atopic dermatitis based on a questionnaire were recruited in Fukui University (3).

Information of these participants is provided in Table S1. All individuals were unrelated Japanese and gave written informed consent to participate in the study according to the rules of the process committee at the Center for Genomic Medicine, The Institute of Physical and Chemical Research (RIKEN).

A total of 209 AD patients were recruited from a dermatological clinic at Kaohsiung Medical University hospital and National Taiwan University hospital in Taiwan from January 1st to December 15th in 2008. A diagnosis of AD patients was also based on criteria proposed by Hanifin and Rajka [21]. Information of these participants is provided in Table S2. We took a medical history and performed physical examinations and blood biochemistry exams to exclude other diseases causing pruritus, such as contact dermatitis, asteatotic dermatitis, and metabolic diseases. Suspected cases were biopsied to exclude other mimicking cutaneous diseases, including cutaneous T cell lymphoma. Patients were excluded if they had received any topical treatments for at least 2 weeks or systemic treatment for 2 months prior to the study. Patients were excluded if they had active skin diseases other than AD, including HIV infection and cancers of any origin. Patients visiting the same hospital in the Department of Preventive Medicine for medical diseases other than atopic diseases were referred to the Department of Dermatology were hospital-based controls. They were excluded if they had active skin diseases, past history of AD, allergic asthma, allergic rhinitis, allergic

Table 1. Locations and allele frequencies of polymorphisms in *ORAI1*.

	SNP[a]	Location	Amino acid	Allele frequency(%)	NCBI[b]
Marker 1	−979G/A	5′ flanking region		2	
Marker 2	−410G/A	5′ flanking region		2	rs116376569
Marker 3	−244GTCCAGGCCCCGGGG×1/×2	5′ flanking region		4	
Marker 4[c]	14542C/T	exon2	I182I	33	rs3741595
Marker 5[c]	14648A/G	exon2	S218G	17	rs3741596
Marker 6	14701T/C	exon2	A235A	17	rs3741597
Marker 7	14782T/C	exon2	V262V	17	rs3825174
Marker 8[c]	14794C/T	exon2	T266T	33	rs3825175
Marker 9	14952T/A	3′ UTR		17	rs11548651
Marker 10	14988C/T	3′ UTR		17	rs76753792
Marker 11[c]	1502A/G	3′ UTR		33	rs712853
Marker 12	15036insT	3′ UTR		33	rs35558190
Marker 13	15123T/C	3′ UTR		2	
Marker 14	15375A/G	3′ flanking region		17	rs74808898

[a]Numbering according to the genomic sequence of *ORAI1* (AC140062.11).
Position 1 is the A of the initiation codon.
[b]NCBI, Number from the dbSNP of NCBI (http://www.ncbi.nlm.nih.gov/SNP/).
[c]SNPs were genotyped in both Taiwanese and Japanese population.

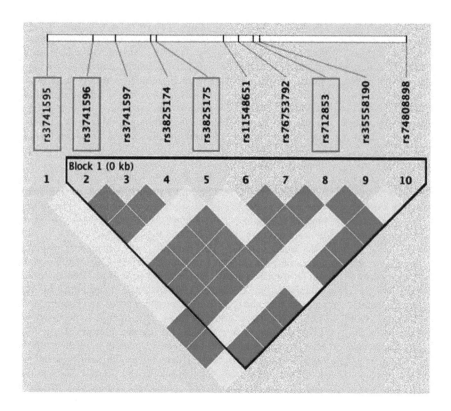

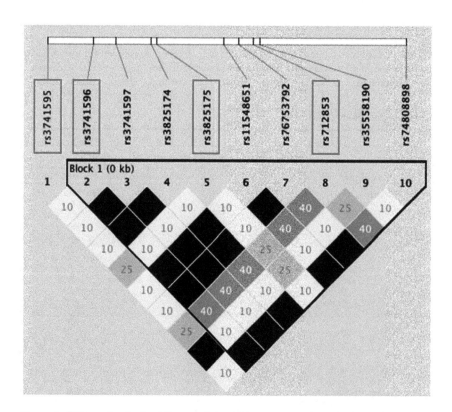

Figure 1. SNPs and pairwise LD map of the *ORAI1* gene. Four boxed polymorphisms were genotyped in the Japanese population. Pairwise D′/ LOD (upper) and r² (lower) for all combinations of SNP pairs are shown.

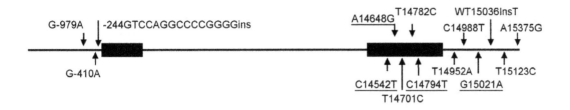

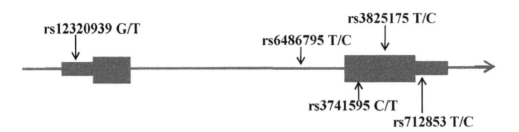

Figure 2. A graphical overview of *ORAI1* gene polymorphisms identified in in the Japanese population (upper). A graphical overview of tSNPs of *ORAI1* gene selected for genotyping in the Taiwanese population.

conjuntivitis, cancers of any origin, or HIV infection or were taking oral corticosteroids. A board-certified dermatologist took a medical history, examined the whole surface the body, and assigned a SCORAD severity index score for each subject. Venous peripheral blood was drawn and the serum was stored at −70°C until assayed. IgE levels from AD patients were measured in a College of American Pathologists (CAP) accredited laboratory in the same hospital. The study was approved by the Institutional Review Board of the Hospital. All clinical assessments and specimen collections were conducted according to Declaration of Helsinki principles. Each participant signed an informed written consent form before entering the study. Patients or controls who did not sign the inform consent were excluded.

Selection of human *ORAI1* polymorphisms for genotyping

Genomic DNA was prepared from peripheral blood samples using standard protocols. To identify SNPs in the human *ORAI1* gene, we sequenced all exons, including a minimum of 200 bases of the flanking intronic sequence, 2 kb of the 5′ flanking region, and a 2 kb continuous 3′ flanking region of the last exon except for regions with interspersed repeats from 24 subjects as described in Japanese population. Pairwise LD was calculated as D′/LOD and r^2 and the Tag SNPs were selected among 10 SNPs with a frequency of greater than 10% by using the Haploview 4.2 program (http://www.broad.mit.edu/mpg/haploview/). Genotyping of SNPs was performed by the TaqMan allele-specific amplification (TaqMan-ASA) method (Applied Biosystems, Foster City, CA).

Table 2. Genotype counts for *ORAI1* and atopic dermatitis susceptibility in Japanese and Taiwanese population.

| db SNP ID | Allele 1/2 | Subjects | Japanese (case-control association analysis) | | | | | Taiwanese (case-control association analysis) | | | | | |
| | | | Genotype[a] | | | Allele*2 | | Genogype | | | Allele*2 | | |
			1/1	1/2	2/2	Frequency of allele 2	P^a	OR (95% c.i.)	1/1	1/2	2/2	Frequency of allele 2	P	OR (95% c.i.)
rs12320939	G/T	AD							50	90	67	0.54	0.050	1.25 (1.00–1.55)
		Control							184	341	165	0.49		
rs6486795	T/C	AD							59	93	47	0.47	0.0004	1.50 (1.20–1.88)
		Control							277	320	98	0.37		
rs3741595	C/T	AD	323	160	25	0.21	0.275	0.90 (0.75–1.08)	83	93	31	0.37	0.0001	1.59 (1.27–2.01)
		Control	622	343	58	0.22			370	275	53	0.27		
rs3741596	A/G	AD	315	177	19	0.21	0.002	1.36 (1.12–1.64)						
		Control	717	283	27	0.16								
rs3825175	C/T	AD	197	243	71	0.38	0.245	0.91 (0.78–1.06)	89	81	37	0.37	0.187	0.86 (0.69–1.08)
		Control	379	476	171	0.40			239	346	114	0.41		
rs712853	G/A	AD	165	266	80	0.42	0.027	1.19 (1.02–1.38)	26	71	109	0.70	0.035	1.29 (1.02–1.64)
		Control	397	479	144	0.38			97	303	301	0.65		

[a]*P* values represent the Cochran-Armitage trend *P* for case-control comparisons.

Table 3. Haplotype frequency of four SNPs in *ORAI1* in Japanese population.

	rs3741595	rs3741596	rs3825175	rs712853	n AD	Control	Frequency AD	Control	*P* value	Odds ratio (95% c.i.)
Haplotype 1	C	A	T	G	386	819	0.38	0.40		
Haplotype 2	T	A	C	G	212	459	0.21	0.22		
Haplotype 3	C	A	C	A	211	435	0.20	0.21		
Haplotype 4	C	G	C	A	216	337	0.21	0.16	0.0017	1.36 (1.12–1.64)
					1026	2050	1.00	1.00		

In Taiwanese population, we sequenced all exons of *ORAI1* gene in 10 subjects, however, none of SNP was found. We further choose five *ORAI1* tagging SNPs (rs12320939, rs6486795, rs3741595, rs3825175 and rs712853) with a minor allele frequency >10% in the Han Chinese population were selected from the HapMap database (http://www.hapmap.org). Genotyping was performed using the TaqMan Allelic Discrimination Assay (Applied Biosystems, Foster city, CA, USA). The polymerase chain reaction (PCR) was carried out using the ABI7900 Thermal Cycler. After PCR, fluorescence from reaction products was measured and analyzed using the System SDS software version 1.2.3.

Real-time quantitative RT-PCR

Total RNA from normal human tissues was purchased from Clontech (Mountain View, CA). Each RNA was reverse transcribed with Superscript III reverse transcriptase and oligo dT primers (Invitrogen, Carlsbad, CA). The expression of *ORAI1* transcripts was determined by real-time quantitative reverse transcription polymerase chain reaction (RT-PCR) using SYBR Premix Ex Taq (Takara, Shiga, Japan) with specific primers (5'-ACCTCGGCTCTGCTCTCC -3' and 5'- GATCATGAGCGCAAACAGG -3'). In all experiments, the amounts of cDNA were standardized by quantification of the housekeeping gene glyceraldehyde-3-phosphate dehydrogenase (*GAPDH*).

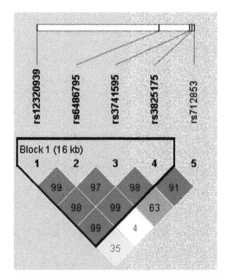

Figure 3. *ORAI1* gene LD and haplotype block structure in AD. The number on the cell is the LOD score of D'.

Statistical analysis

We tested agreement with Hardy-Weinberg Equilibrium using a χ^2 goodness-of-fit test at each locus in both populations. In Japanese population, we then compared differences in genotype frequencies of the polymorphisms between case and control subjects by the Cochran-Armitage trend test, and calculated odds ratios (ORs) with 95 percent confidence intervals (95% CI). We applied Bonferroni correction; the multiplication of the *P* values by four, the number of tag SNPs. In the association study, *P* values of less than 0.05 were considered to be statistically significant. Haplotype frequencies for three loci were estimated, and haplotype association tests were performed using Haploview 4.2. Total IgE levels and expression levels of *ORAI1* transcripts between genotypic groups were tested with the Jonckheere-Terpstra test. Chi-square test was then used to compare differences in allele frequencies and genotype distribution of the polymorphisms between AD and controls.

Results

Association of *ORAI1* SNPs with susceptibility to atopic dermatitis

After extensive examination of *ORAI1* by direct sequencing, we identified 14 polymorphisms (three SNPs in promoter region and five SNPs within the transcript) (Table 1). Eight polymorphisms were contained in the available public databases, NCBI dbSNP (http://www.ncbi.nlm.nih.gov/SNP/). We calculated pairwise linkage disequilibrium (LD) as r^2 and selected four tag SNPs with a minor allele frequency (MAF) of >10% using the Haploview 4.2 program (http://www.broad.mit.edu/mpg/haploview/). The four tag SNPs captured 10 of the 10 alleles with a mean r^2 of 0.98 (r^2>0.76) (Figure 1 and Table S3). The locations of these four SNPs are shown in Figure 2 (upper). In Taiwanese population, five *ORAI1* tagging SNPs with a minor allele frequency >10% in the Han Chinese population were selected from the HapMap database (http://www.hapmap.org). A graphical overview of the genotyped polymorphism is shown in Figure 2 (Lower).

We next carried out case-control association studies of the four and five SNPs in the 1540 Japanese subjects and 938 Taiwanese subjects. The control genotypes did not deviate from Hardy-Weinberg equilibrium. As shown in Table 2, a nonsynonymous *ORAI1* SNP (rs3741596, Ser218Gly) showed significant associations with susceptibility to atopic dermatitis (*P*= 0.002, OR = 1.36, 95% CI 1.12–1.64) by the Cochran-Armitage trend test in Japanese population. Other variants did not show a significant association after Bonferroni correction. In Taiwanese population, rs6486795 and rs3741595 were significantly associated with susceptibility to atopic dermatitis under the dominant and allelic models.

Table 4. Haplotype frequency of four SNPs in *ORAI1* in Taiwanese population.

	rs12320939	rs6486795	rs3741595	rs3825175	n AD	Control	Frequency AD	Control	P value	Odds ratio (95% c.i.)
Haplotype 1	T	C	T	C	148	370	0.38	0.27	0.0014	1.54 (1.18–2.01)
Haplotype 2	T	C	C	C	36	130	0.09	0.10		
Haplotype 3	T	T	C	C	33	154	0.08	0.11		
Haplotype 4	G	T	C	C	30	142	0.08	0.10		
Haplotype 5	G	T	C	T	143	550	0.36	0.41		
					390	1346	0.99	0.99		

If the frequencies less than 1% were excluded.

Haplotypes of *ORAI1* and their association with the disease occurrence of atopic dermatitis

To further identify the effects of Haplotypes of *ORAI1* to atopic dermatitis, we constructed the haplotypes of the three SNPs to estimate the frequency of each haplotype in controls in the Japanese population (Table 3). Three common haplotypes were identified in the Japanese population. Haplotype C-G-C-A (rs3741595, rs3741596, rs3825175, and rs712853) of *ORAI1* was significantly associated with atopic dermatitis. A *P* value of 0.0017 was obtained by using the Haploview 4.2 program. In the Taiwanese population, the haplotype block structure of *ORAI1* was shown in Figure 3. Among five haplotypes, subjects with T-C-T-C haplotype (rs12320939, rs6486795, rs3741595 and rs3825175) have a significant risk to AD (OR = 1.54, 95% CI = 1.18–2.01, P = 0.0014) (Table 4).

Expression of *ORAI1* mRNA in skin, immune tissues

To investigate the *ORAI1* mRNA expression in various human tissues, we conducted real-time quantitative RT-PCR. As shown in Figure 4, *ORAI1* mRNA was expressed abundantly in all tissues examined, especially in the tissues of lung, spleen, and skin.

rs3741597 is associated with the expression level of the *ORAI1* transcript

We next assessed whether the rs3741597 genotype correlated with the mRNA levels of *ORAI1* transcript (NM_032790). The *ORAI1* mRNA expression data for the EBV-transformed lymphoblastoid cell lines from 42 JPT HapMap subjects were analyzed by the Jonckheere-Terpstra trend test. As shown in Figure 5, the expression level of transcripts of NM_032790 was positively correlated with the rs3741597 genotype (*P* = 0.040). These results suggested that rs3741597 or other SNPs, 14648A/G (rs3741596), 14782T/C (rs3825174), 14952T/A (rs11548651), 14988C/T (rs76753792), and 15375A/G (rs74808898), in strong linkage disequilibrium with rs3741597 might influence susceptibility to atopic dermatitis through higher expression of an *ORAI1* transcript.

Discussion

We screened the polymorphisms of *ORAI1* and performed a case-control association study and a haplotype analysis. A total of 14 genetic variants was identified from Japanese population, 3 SNPs are novel. Our results showed a significant association between AD and a non-synonymous SNP (rs3741596, Ser218Gly)

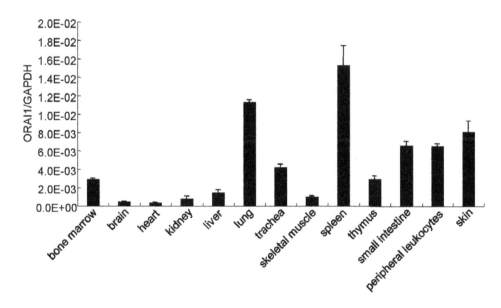

Figure 4. Expression of *ORAI1* mRNA in different tissues. Quantities of total RNA extracted from normal human tissues were determined by real-time quantitative reverse transcription polymerase chain reaction (RT-PCR). The results were normalized to GAPDH transcripts.

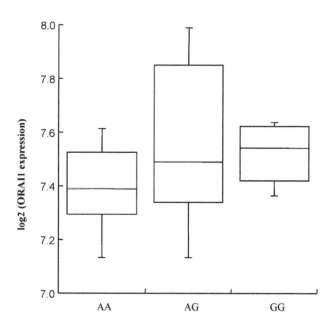

Figure 5. Differential expression of an *ORAI1* transcript (NM_032790) of EBV-transformed lymphoblastoid cell lines from HapMap-JPT (Japanese in Tokyo) subjects for each rs3741597 genotype. *P* value was calculated by the Jonckheere-Terpstra test.

in the human *ORAI1* gene in the Japanese population. rs3741596 was genotyped in the Taiwanese population, however, the MAFs of this SNP is less than 1% which is different from the allele frequency of Japanese population (data not shown). In addition, rs3741595 of *ORAI1* is associated with the risk of AD in the Taiwanese population but not in the Japanese population. We also performed I^2 index to assess heterogeneity on three SNPs which were genotyped in both Taiwan and Japan. The I^2 indexes of rs3825175 and rs712853 showed no heterogeneity on these locus. The heterogeneity only occurred on rs3741595 (I^2 Index = 93%) We attribute this to the different genetic backgrounds in the populations, due to variation in allele frequencies, population admixture, heterogeneity of the phenotype between populations.

The rs3741597 genotype correlated with the mRNA levels of the *ORAI1* transcript. Another three SNPs (14952T/A, 14988C/T, and 15375A/G) located in the 3′ flanking region, which are in strong LD with rs3741597, may influence higher expression of an *ORAI1* transcript. MicroRNAs (miRNA) are small non-coding RNAs that control gene expression by preferentially binding to the 3′-untranslated regions (3′-UTR) of the target genes [22]. Therefore, further functional analysis of the 3′-UTR of the *ORAI1* gene should be conducted in order to clarify the mechanism underlying this susceptibility.

Several diseases have been linked to the *ORAI1*-mediated calcium influx. Feske et al. identified a mutation in the Orai1 from SCID patients. This missense mutation caused a reduction in the SOC influx and a decrease in immune response [19]. Studies from the Orai1-knockout mice have shown an important role of this gene in the activation of inflammatory reactions in mast cells [20,23]. To study the role of *ORAI1*, we analyzed the tissue distribution of ORAI1. The highest expression of ORAI1 was found in the spleen, an organ involved in immune function. The tissue distribution of ORAI1 in our study revealed the potential importance of ORAI1 in the regulation of immune system—a finding consistent with that reported previously. In addition, the

expression of ORAI1 was found to be higher in the proliferative vascular smooth muscle cells [24]. Furthermore, results obtained from ORAI1 knockdown cells indicated a reduction of cell proliferation in both endothelial and breast cancer cells [25,26]. Studies using keratinocytes have shown that calcium is an important regulator of cell proliferation and differentiation [27]. Dysregulated apoptosis in keratinocytes contributes to the progress of AD [28]. Hence, genetic polymorphisms may result in the changes of gene expression level of *ORAI1* that further contribute to the dysregulated growth in keratinocytes, leading to a defective skin-barrier formation. Cell-based physiological studies in the keratinocytes are required to identify the role of *ORAI1* in AD.

STIM1 and ORAI1 are the two major components in the regulation of calcium entry through store-operated calcium channels. Co-expression of STIM1 and Orai1/CRACM1 results in the amplification of store-operated Ca^{2+} influx signals [1,29,30]. The SOC entry pathway is influenced by ORAI1 or STIM1 knockdown [31,32]. Importantly, the overexpression of orai1 also causes the attenuation of store-operated Ca^{2+} influx [33]. Two possible mechanisms were proposed. The oligomers formed by the overexpressed ORAI1 may lose sensitivity to the signals released from calcium store [34]. Soboloff et al. suggested that the coupling stoichiometry between Orai1 and STIM1 is not unity, therefore, overexpression of Orai1 may influence the functional compositions of SOC [30]. Combined the findings from other groups [34], our results propose that the genetic polymorphisms in the 3′-UTR of the *ORAI1* gene may change the expression level of Orai1, which, in turn, may cause dysfunction of calcium channels and immune responses. However, the coupling stoichiometry between the different expression levels of ORAI1 should also be further considered.

Previous studies have revealed the significant association between genetic polymorphisms of *ORAI1* and inflammatory diseases such as ankylosing spondylitis and calcium nephrolithiasis [35,36]. In this study, we identified 14 genetic variants including 3 novel SNPs in the *ORAI1* gene. In a total of 2,478 subjects (938 Taiwanese and 1540 Japanese), our results indicated that different genetic polymorphisms of *ORAI1* are associated with AD susceptibility in the Japanese, and Taiwanese populations. This is the first report to state the relationship between the genetic polymorphisms of *ORAI1* and allergic diseases. Given the polygenic nature of allergic diseases such as AD, the susceptibility gene *ORAI1* could provide a new clue in the pathogenesis of AD. The prevalence of atopic dermatitis in Taiwan is around 6.7%, therefore, this study should reach a power level of 0.97 (case 209; control 729). Although further replication studies in larger Taiwanese population is needed, it is likely to variants in the ORAI1 gene play a role in susceptibility to AD in both Japanese and Taiwanese populations. Further study on the relationship between the genotype of *ORAI1* and the downstream functional relevance during dermal inflammation should be conducted in order to understand the etiology of AD.

Supporting Information

Table S1 Basal characteristics of patients with Atopic Dermatitis (AD) and of normal controls in Japanese population.

Table S2 Basal characteristics of patients with Atopic Dermatitis (AD) and of normal controls in Taiwanese population.

Table S3   Pairwise linkage disequilibrium for all possible two-way comparisons among 10 polymorphisms in *ORAI1* with 24 Japanese volunteers.

Acknowledgments

We thank Makiko T. Shimizu, Hiroshi Sekiguchi, Aya I. Jodo and Nami Kawaraichi for technical assistance. We are grateful to Prof. Anant Parekh (University of Oxford) for the functional study.

Author Contributions

Conceived and designed the experiments: W-C. Chang CHL TH LFW SD AM TE KT MS TY SF KE HS ST MF W-C. Chen SHHJ CHH HSY WPC YN MT. Performed the experiments: W-C. Chang TH W-C. Chen. Analyzed the data: W-C. Chang CHL TH YCC W-C. Chen EH WPC MT. Contributed reagents/materials/analysis tools: W-C. Chang MT CHL TH SD AM TE KT MS TY SF KE HS ST MF SHHJ CHH HSY YN. Wrote the paper: W-C. Chang CHL TH YCC W-C. Chen MT.

References

1. Peinelt C, Vig M, Koomoa DL, Beck A, Nadler MJ, et al. (2006) Amplification of CRAC current by STIM1 and CRACM1 (Orai1). Nat Cell Biol 8: 771–773.
2. Hill PB, Hillier A, Olivry T (2001) The ACVD task force on canine atopic dermatitis (VI): IgE-induced immediate and late-phase reactions, two inflammatory sequences at sites of intradermal allergen injections. Vet Immunol Immunopathol 81: 199–204.
3. Olivry T, Hill PB (2001) The ACVD task force on canine atopic dermatitis (XVIII): histopathology of skin lesions. Vet Immunol Immunopathol 81: 305–309.
4. Vickery BP (2007) Skin barrier function in atopic dermatitis. Curr Opin Pediatr 19: 89–93.
5. Enomoto H, Hirata K, Otsuka K, Kawai T, Takahashi T, et al. (2008) Filaggrin null mutations are associated with atopic dermatitis and elevated levels of IgE in the Japanese population: a family and case-control study. J Hum Genet 53: 615–621.
6. Akdis M (2006) Healthy immune response to allergens: T regulatory cells and more. Curr Opin Immunol 18: 738–744.
7. Oh DY, Schumann RR, Hamann L, Neumann K, Worm M, et al. (2009) Association of the toll-like receptor 2 A-16934T promoter polymorphism with severe atopic dermatitis. Allergy 64: 1608–1615.
8. Oiso N, Fukai K, Ishii M (2000) Interleukin 4 receptor alpha chain polymorphism Gln551Arg is associated with adult atopic dermatitis in Japan. Br J Dermatol 142: 1003–1006.
9. Rafatpanah H, Bennett E, Pravica V, McCoy MJ, David TJ, et al. (2003) Association between novel GM-CSF gene polymorphisms and the frequency and severity of atopic dermatitis. J Allergy Clin Immunol 112: 593–598.
10. Shimizu M, Matsuda A, Yanagisawa K, Hirota T, Akahoshi M, et al. (2005) Functional SNPs in the distal promoter of the ST2 gene are associated with atopic dermatitis. Hum Mol Genet 14: 2919–2927.
11. Takahashi N, Akahoshi M, Matsuda A, Ebe K, Inomata N, et al. (2005) Association of the IL12RB1 promoter polymorphisms with increased risk of atopic dermatitis and other allergic phenotypes. Hum Mol Genet 14: 3149–3159.
12. Tsunemi Y, Saeki H, Nakamura K, Sekiya T, Hirai K, et al. (2002) Interleukin-13 gene polymorphism G4257A is associated with atopic dermatitis in Japanese patients. J Dermatol Sci 30: 100–107.
13. Wood SH, Ke X, Nuttall T, McEwan N, Ollier WE, et al. (2009) Genome-wide association analysis of canine atopic dermatitis and identification of disease related SNPs. Immunogenetics 61: 765–772.
14. Berth-Jones J, Finlay AY, Zaki I, Tan B, Goodyear H, et al. (1996) Cyclosporine in severe childhood atopic dermatitis: a multicenter study. J Am Acad Dermatol 34: 1016–1021.
15. Parekh AB, Putney JW, Jr. (2005) Store-operated calcium channels. Physiol Rev 85: 757–810.
16. Chang WC, Nelson C, Parekh AB (2006) Ca2+ influx through CRAC channels activates cytosolic phospholipase A2, leukotriene C4 secretion, and expression of c-fos through ERK-dependent and -independent pathways in mast cells. FASEB J 20: 2381–2383.
17. Chang WC, Parekh AB (2004) Close functional coupling between Ca2+ release-activated Ca2+ channels, arachidonic acid release, and leukotriene C4 secretion. J Biol Chem 279: 29994–29999.
18. Gwack Y, Feske S, Srikanth S, Hogan PG, Rao A (2007) Signalling to transcription: store-operated Ca2+ entry and NFAT activation in lymphocytes. Cell Calcium 42: 145–156.
19. Feske S, Gwack Y, Prakriya M, Srikanth S, Puppel SH, et al. (2006) A mutation in Orai1 causes immune deficiency by abrogating CRAC channel function. Nature 441: 179–185.
20. Vig M, DeHaven WI, Bird GS, Billingsley JM, Wang H, et al. (2008) Defective mast cell effector functions in mice lacking the CRACM1 pore subunit of store-operated calcium release-activated calcium channels. Nat Immunol 9: 89–96.
21. Hanifin J, Rajka G (1980) Diagnostic features of atopic dermatitis. Acta Dermatol Venereol (Stockh) 92: 44–47.
22. Fabian MR, Sonenberg N, Filipowicz W (2010) Regulation of mRNA translation and stability by microRNAs. Annu Rev Biochem 79: 351–379.
23. Gwack Y, Srikanth S, Oh-Hora M, Hogan PG, Lamperti ED, et al. (2008) Hair loss and defective T- and B-cell function in mice lacking ORAI1. Mol Cell Biol 28: 5209–5222.
24. Potier M, Gonzalez JC, Motiani RK, Abdullaev IF, Bisaillon JM, et al. (2009) Evidence for STIM1- and Orai1-dependent store-operated calcium influx through ICRAC in vascular smooth muscle cells: role in proliferation and migration. FASEB J 23: 2425–2437.
25. Abdullaev IF, Bisaillon JM, Potier M, Gonzalez JC, Motiani RK, et al. (2008) Stim1 and Orai1 mediate CRAC currents and store-operated calcium entry important for endothelial cell proliferation. Circ Res 103: 1289–1299.
26. Yang S, Zhang JJ, Huang XY (2009) Orai1 and STIM1 are critical for breast tumor cell migration and metastasis. Cancer Cell 15: 124–134.
27. Korkiamaki T, Yla-Outinen H, Koivunen J, Karvonen SL, Peltonen J (2002) Altered calcium-mediated cell signaling in keratinocytes cultured from patients with neurofibromatosis type 1. Am J Pathol 160: 1981–1990.
28. Trautmann A, Akdis M, Blaser K, Akdis CA (2000) Role of dysregulated apoptosis in atopic dermatitis. Apoptosis 5: 425–429.
29. Mercer JC, Dehaven WI, Smyth JT, Wedel B, Boyles RR, et al. (2006) Large store-operated calcium selective currents due to co-expression of Orai1 or Orai2 with the intracellular calcium sensor, Stim1. J Biol Chem 281: 24979–24990.
30. Soboloff J, Spassova MA, Tang XD, Hewavitharana T, Xu W, et al. (2006) Orai1 and STIM reconstitute store-operated calcium channel function. J Biol Chem 281: 20661–20665.
31. Liou J, Kim ML, Heo WD, Jones JT, Myers JW, et al. (2005) STIM is a Ca2+ sensor essential for Ca2+-store-depletion-triggered Ca2+ influx. Curr Biol 15: 1235–1241.
32. Roos J, DiGregorio PJ, Yeromin AV, Ohlsen K, Lioudyno M, et al. (2005) STIM1, an essential and conserved component of store-operated Ca2+ channel function. J Cell Biol 169: 435–445.
33. DeHaven WI, Smyth JT, Boyles RR, Putney JW, Jr. (2007) Calcium inhibition and calcium potentiation of Orai1, Orai2, and Orai3 calcium release-activated calcium channels. J Biol Chem 282: 17548–17556.
34. Li Z, Lu J, Xu P, Xie X, Chen L, et al. (2007) Mapping the interacting domains of STIM1 and Orai1 in Ca2+ release-activated Ca2+ channel activation. J Biol Chem 282: 29448–29456.
35. Chou YH, Juo SH, Chiu YC, Liu ME, Chen WC, et al. (2011) A Polymorphism of ORAI1 Gene is Associated with the Risk and Recurrence of Calcium Nephrolithiasis. Journal of Urology 185(5): 1742–6.
36. Wei CC, Yen JH, Juo SH, Chen WC, Wang YS, et al. (2011) Association of ORAI1 haplotypes with the Risk of HLA-B27 positive Ankylosing Spondylitis. PLos ONE 6(6): e20426.

11

Health Outcome Measures in Atopic Dermatitis: A Systematic Review of Trends in Disease Severity and Quality-of-Life Instruments 1985–2010

Balvinder Rehal, April Armstrong*

Department of Dermatology, University of California Davis, Davis, California, United States of America

Abstract

Background: A number of disease-severity and quality-of-life (QoL) instruments have emerged in atopic dermatitis (AD) in the last decade.

Objectives: To identify trends in outcomes instruments used in AD clinical trials and to provide a useful summary of the dimensions and validation studies for the most commonly used measures.

Method: All randomized control trials (RCTs) from 1985 to 2010 in the treatment of AD were examined.

Results: Among the 791 RCTs reviewed, we identified 20 disease-severity and 14 QoL instruments. Of these outcomes instruments, few have been validated. SCORAD, EASI, IGA and SASSAD were the most commonly used disease-severity instruments and CDLQI, DFI, DLQI and IDQOL were the most frequently used QoL measures.

Limitations: The small number of RCTs using QoL scales makes identifying trends for QoL instruments difficult.

Conclusion: Overall, there is an increase in the use of disease-severity and QoL instruments in AD clinical trials.

Editor: Lise Lotte Gluud, Copenhagen University Hospital Gentofte, Denmark

Funding: These authors have no support or funding to report.

Competing Interests: The authors have declared that no competing interests exist.

* E-mail: aprilarmstrong@post.harvard.edu

Introduction

Atopic dermatitis is a chronic, inflammatory skin disease that affects patients' physical and psychosocial wellbeing. The burden of atopic dermatitis has been documented in the medical literature [1,2]. Patients suffering from atopic dermatitis often experience embarrassment from the skin lesions, and severe disease can adversely affect social interactions and personal relationships. The symptoms of atopic dermatitis, notably pruritus, can be intractable and lead to significant emotional distress and sleep loss [3].

Despite continuing efforts in developing new treatments for atopic dermatitis, scarce literature exists that evaluates disease-severity and quality-of-life (QoL) outcome measures in AD [4,5,6,7]. This systematic review examines the trends in outcomes instruments, specifically disease-severity and QoL instruments, in randomized controlled trials (RCT) in the treatment of AD published between 1985 to 2010. We discuss the most frequently used disease-severity and QoL measures in terms of their dimensions (aspects of AD that the instrument measures) and validation studies that have supported their increased use in clinical trials.

Methods

To examine the disease and QoL outcome measures used in atopic dermatitis trials, we conducted a systematic review of RCTs for AD from 1985 to 2010 in the U.S. National Library of Medicine using the Medline search engine and in the electronic database, Scopus, which includes the EMBASE database. In Medline we applied the Medical Subject Headings search terms "atopic dermatitis" and "treatment" and limited the search to human RCTs published in the English language from January 1, 1985 to July 14, 2010. In Scopus, we searched for RCTs in atopic dermatitis using the search "TITLE-ABS-KEY(atopic dermatitis) AND (TITLE-ABS-KEY(randomized control trial*) OR TITLE-ABS-KEY(RCT))."

Results

In Medline, our search identified an initial group of 552 studies published between 1985 and 20010 in AD. Of these 552 studies, 195 were excluded either because they were not RCTs, not pertaining to atopic dermatitis studies, not in English, or no outcome measures were used (Figure 1). In Scopus our search generated 239 studies from 1985–2010. After cross-referencing the list of studies with our Medline search, we were left with 141 articles. Of these, 116 were excluded for the reasons listed above. After exclusion, 382 studies were reviewed from both Medline and Scopus.

A total of 20 disease-severity scales and 14 QoL scales were used in the RCTs for the treatment of atopic dermatitis. We list the

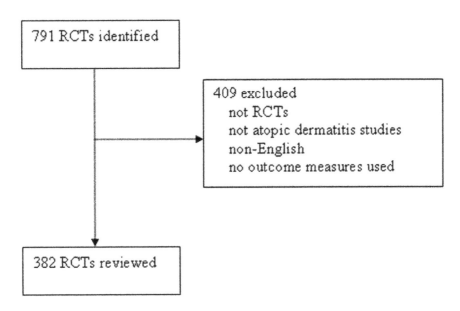

Figure 1. Excluded studies.

disease-severity instruments and QoL measures in Tables 1 and 2, respectively.

The most frequently used disease-severity instruments from 1985 to 2010 were the Severity scoring of atopic dermatitis (SCORAD), Eczema Area and Severity Index (EASI), Investiga- tors' Global Assessment (IGA) and Six Area, Six Sign Atopic Dermatitis (SASSAD) (Table 1). SCORAD was the most frequently used scale; it was used in 113 out of 382 RCTs (30%). The next most frequently used scale was the EASI, which was used in 63 out of 382 RCTs (16%), followed by the IGA that

Table 1. Severity of disease scales.

Scale	Clinical signs						Disease extent	Subjective Sx	# of studies used in
	Erythema	Edema/ papulation	oozing/ crusts	excoriation	lichenification	dryness/ scaling			
Severity scoring of atopic dermatitis (SCORAD)	*	*	*	*	*		*	*	76
Eczema Area and Severity Index (EASI)	*	*		*	*		*		51
Investigators' Global Assessment (IGA)	*	*	*						41
Six Area, Six Sign Atopic Dermatitis (SASSAD)	*		*	*	*	*	*	*	14
Investigators' Global Atopic Dermatitis Assessment (IGADA)	*	*	*	*	*	*	*		4
Costa et al	*	*	*	*	*	*	*	*	3
Leiciester Sign Score (LSS)	*		*	*	*	*	*		2
Visual Analogue Scale (VAS) pruritus								*	2
Total Severity Score (TSS)	*	*	*	*	*		*		2
Physicians Global Assessment (PGA)	*					*	*		2
Intensity Item Score Aggregate (IISA)	*	*	*	*	*	*	*	*	1
Atopic Dermatitis Severity Index (ADSI)	*		*	*	*		*	*	1
Investigators' Static Global Assessment (ISGA)	*	*	*		*	*		*	1
Nottingham Eczema Severity Score (NESS)							*	*	1
Investigators' Global Assessment Score (IGAS)	*	*						*	1
Dry skin are and severity index (DASI)	*					*	*	*	1
Atopic Dermatitis Area and Severity Index (ADASI)	*	*	*	*	*	*	*		1
Total body severity assessment (TBSA)	*	*	*	*			*	*	1

Table 2. Quality of life scales.

Scale	Questions										# Studies used in
	Severity	itching	mood	sleep	dressing/ clothes	leisure activities	treatment	Parent mood	Parent sleep	family disruption/ tension	
Children's Dermatology Life Quality Index (CDLQI)		*	*	*	*	*	*				13
Dermatology Life Quality Index (DLQI)		*	*		*	*	*				8
Infant's Dermatology Quality of Life (IDQOL)	*	*	*	*	*	*	*				7
Dermatitis Family Impact (DFI)				*		*		*	*	*	6
Parent's Index of Quality of Life in Atopic Dermatitis (PIQoL-AD)				*		*	*	*	*	*	2
Quality of Life Index for Atopic Dermatitis (QoLIAD)		*			*	*					2
Short Form Health Survey (SF-36)		*			*	*					2
Parents of Children with Atopic Dermatitis (PQoL–AD)								*	*		1
German Instrument for the assessment of Quality of Life in Skin Diseases (DIELH)		*	*			*	*				1
Eczema Disability Index (EDI)						*	*				1
Skindex-29		*	*	*		*					1

was used in 48 out of 382 RCTs (13%). SASSAD was used in 18 out of 382 RCTs (5%). The four most commonly used scales, SCORAD, EASI, IGA and SASSAD, were used in the majority of RCTs: 242 out of 382 (63%). The remaining 14 scales were used in 57 out of 382 RCTs (15%).

The trend for disease-severity scales showed that the number of disease-severity instruments used in clinical trials increased dramatically from 1985 to 2010 (Figure 2). Specifically, SCORAD was used in 4% of RCTs from 1985–1997 and 40% RCTs from 1998–2010. SCORAD had its peak usage from 2005 to 2010.

EASI, IGA and SASSAD were also used more commonly from 1985–2010 (Figure 2). From 1985–1997, no RCTs used EASI, IGA or SASSAD. EASI also had its peak usage from 2005 to 2010. To our knowledge, IGA has not been validated to date, but its usage has been nearly identical to that of EASI (Figure 2). Out of the 48 RCTs that used IGA, 32 trials used IGA in conjunction with EASI (67%).

Among the 382 RCTs, 67 studies employed QoL instruments. Of the studies that used QoL outcomes measures, the Children's Dermatology Life Quality Index (CDLQI) was the most frequently used (33%), followed by the Dermatitis Family Impact (DFI) (15%), the Dermatology Life Quality Index (DLQI) (13%) and the Infant's Dermatology Life Quality Index.

(IDQOL) (12%) (Table 2). Overall, the use of QoL scales in RCTs has increased from 1985 to 2010 (Figure 3). None of the four most commonly used QoL instruments, CDLQI, DFI, DLQI or IDQOL were used between 1985–1997.

Common Disease-Severity Scales in Atopic Dermatitis: Dimensions and Evidence for Validation

Severity Scoring of Atopic Dermatitis (SCORAD). From 1985 to 2010, SCORAD was the most widely used disease-severity scale in atopic dermatitis. SCORAD was used in 113 out of the 382 studies that met our search criteria (30%). It was developed in

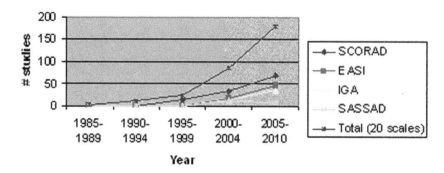

Figure 2. Trends in Disease Severity Instruments 1985–2010.

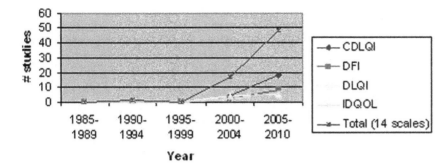

Figure 3. Trends in Quality of Life Instruments 1985–2010.

1993 by the European Task Force on Atopic Dermatitis [8]. The SCORAD index uses the rule of nines to assess disease extent and evaluates five clinical characteristics to determine disease severity: (1) erythema, (2) edema/papulation, (3) oozing/crusts, (4) excoriation and (5) lichenification. SCORAD also assesses subjective symptoms of pruritus and sleep loss with Visual Analogue Scales (VAS) [8]. These three aspects: extent of disease, disease severity and subjective symptoms combine to give a maximum possible score of 103. Although it is a combined score, the three aspects can be separated and used individually if necessary. Of all the severity scales used in atopic dermatitis, it is the most widely validated disease-severity instrument [9]. SCORAD has been found to be valid and reliable, and it has shown excellent agreement with global assessments of disease severity [8,9,10,11,12,13,14,15,16,17,18,19,20,21,22]. However, some studies have shown interobserver variation in scoring lichenification and extent of disease [8,9,10,18,20,23].

Eczema Area and Severity Index (EASI). EASI was the second most commonly used scale in our review of the literature. It was used in 63 out of 382 RCTs (16%). EASI was developed by modifying the PASI (Psoriasis Area and Severity Index), a widely accepted and standardized scoring system for psoriasis [24]. EASI assesses extent of disease at four body sites and measures four clinical signs: (1) erythema, (2) induration/papulation, (3) excoriation, and (4) lichenification each on a scale of 0 to 3. EASI confers a max score of 72 [25]. EASI evaluates two dimensions of atopic dermatitis: disease extent and clinical signs. Unlike the SCORAD, it does not assess symptoms like pruritus and sleep loss. Some investigators express that subjective symptoms may be the most important marker for assessing patient morbidity and they may also be a good indicator for disease severity. In a large validation study with a cohort of 1550 pediatric patients, EASI was found to have excellent validity, internal consistency and sensitivity to change [26]. While EASI is a valid and reliable instrument, most interobserver variability lies in the dimension of induration/papulation [13,21,25,26,27].

Investigators' Global Assessment (IGA). IGA was the third most common scale, used in 48 out of 382 RCTs (13%). IGA allows investigators to assess overall disease severity at one given time point, and it consists of a 6-point severity scale from clear to very severe disease (0 = clear, 1 = almost clear, 2 = mild disease, 3 = moderate disease, 4 = severe disease and 5 = very severe disease) [28]. IGA uses clinical characteristics of erythema, infiltration, papulation, oozing and crusting as guidelines for the overall severity assessment [28]. To our knowledge, IGA has not been validated as an outcome measure [7]. However, IGA has been used to validate other outcome scales as one "gold standard." [9,26] While the combined use of IGA with another validated

scale does not make IGA itself a stand-alone, validated instrument, IGA appears to correlate well with the EASI and is considered an instrument with reasonable face validity. Potential weaknesses of IGA include lack of responsiveness and discrimination for disease severity and lack of subjective symptoms.

Six-Area, Six-Sign Atopic Dermatitis (SASSAD). SASSAD was used in 18 out of 382 RCTs (5%), which ranks SASSAD as the fourth most commonly used scale. SASSAD assesses six clinical signs of disease severity (erythema, exudation, dryness, cracking, excoriation, and lichenification) at six body sites (head/neck, trunk, arms, hands, legs and feet). Each clinical sign on a given body site is graded on a scale of 0–3, and the scale confers a maximum score of 108 [29]. SASSAD does not assess subjective symptoms. The SASSAD is sensitive to changes in topical steroid requirements, pruritus, and sleep loss [30,31,32,33,34]. In a small reliability study involving 6 patients, there was interobserver variation for dryness and lichenification [35].

Quality-of-Life Instruments in Atopic Dermatitis: Dimensions and Evidence for Validation

Children's Dermatology Life Quality Index (CDLQI). CDLQI was the most common QoL instrument from our search, used in 22 out of 382 RCTs (6%). Drs. Lewis-Jones and Finlay developed and validated CDLQI in 1995, with the purpose of measuring the QoL in children with skin disease [36]. The questionnaire was designed for children ages 4 through 16. CDLQI is completed by the child with the help of an adult if necessary, preferably a parent. The questionnaire consists of 10 questions that encompass different aspects of a child's life that could be affected by their skin disease. The instrument includes physical symptoms, such as itching and sleep loss, as well as psychosocial questions regarding friendships, bullying, school performance, sports participation, and enjoyment of vacation. The questions are graded from 0–3, with a possible maximum score of 30 with higher scores representing worse QoL. [36]. In the initial validation study, children with atopic eczema accounted for 20% of all patients [36]. To determine test-retest repeatability, CDLQI was used in a population of children without skin disease [36].

Since its validation, CDLQI has been used in numerous studies to determine the effectiveness of interventions in children with AD [37,38]. CDLQI has been translated and validated in Cantonese [39,40,41]. A cartoon version of CDLQI was validated in 2003, which appears to be quicker and preferred by children [42].

Dermatitis Family Impact (DFI). The DFI questionnaire was used in 10 out of 382 RCTs (2.6%), making it the second most common quality of life scale used in our review. It was developed in 1998 by Drs. Lawson, Lewis-Jones, Finlay, Reid and Owens to help measure how family life is affected by a child suffering from atopic dermatitis [43]. It is designed to be completed by a caretaker of the child, usually a parent, and consists of 10 questions related to housework, food preparation and feeding, sleep, family leisure activity, shopping, expenditure, fatigue, emotional distress and relationships [43]. Each question is graded from 0–3 with a maximum possible score of 30. DFI has been found to be valid, reliable, and sensitive to change in multiple studies [6,39,43,44,45,46,47,48]. Two studies that assessed validity of the instrument were based on using separate components of the DFI, as opposed to using the total score as was originally intended by creators of the scale [43,46]. DFI has also been validated in Malay and Portuguese [39,44,45,48].

Dermatology Life Quality Index (DLQI). DLQI was the third most common QoL scale that was used in 9 out of 382 RCTs (2.4%) in our review. DLQI was developed in 1994 by Drs. Finlay and Khan to measure quality of life in routine clinical practice in adults over age of 18 [49]. DLQI is a 10-item questionnaire that inquires about skin symptoms, feelings of embarrassment, and how skin disease has affected day-to-day activities, working and social life. Similar to CDLQI, each question on DLQI is scored from 0 to 3 with a maximum score of 30 and high scores representing worse QoL.

Both DLQI and CDLQI are specialty-specific but not disease-specific QoL instruments. In the original article by Finlay and Khan, patients with atopic dermatitis had the worst QoL as measured by DLQI compared to the other skin diseases assessed in the study [49]. DLQI has been extensively validated in multiple studies [49,50,51]. A 10-year review of the literature found that DLQI is highly specific for assessing decrements in QoL in patients with atopic dermatitis compared with the general population [51]. Specifically, patients with atopic eczema had a mean score of 4.2 compared to 0.3 in a normal population [50,51]. DLQI has high repeatability, internal consistency, and sensitivity to change [51].

Infants' Dermatitis Quality of Life Index (IDQOL). IDQOL was the fourth most common scale found in our review, used in 8 out of 382 RCTs (2.1%) examined. It was developed in 2001 by Drs. Lewis-Jones, Finlay, and Dykes to assess QoL in infants with AD [52]. IDQOL is completed by the parents of infants from birth to 4 years. The instrument consists of 10 questions regarding an infant or young child's difficulties with mood, sleep, bathing, dressing, play, mealtimes, other family activities, and treatment [52]. Each question is graded from 0–3 with a maximum total score of 30. A higher number correlates with a greater impairment of quality of life. An additional question exists that is scored separately on a scale of 0–4 that asks for the parents' overall assessment of eczema severity. In the original article the scale was validated with repeatability and sensitivity to change confirmed [52]. The scale was further validated with sensitivity to change confirmed and has been used in over 15 studies [43,53].

Discussion

Effective management of skin diseases begins with evaluation of both clinical disease severity and health-related QoL. In dermatology, the assessment of disease severity is frequently condition-specific and uses defined, observable parameters [54,55,56,57]. QoL refers to the impact of a disease on a patient's overall function and wellbeing [58]. While disease severity is central for clinical evaluation and monitoring treatment response, QoL measures are as important for determining the effect of a disease or intervention on a patient's general welfare.

In the last 25 years, 20 disease-severity scales and 14 QoL instruments have been used in clinical trials involving patients with atopic dermatitis. Despite the emergence of multiple disease-severity and QoL instruments, few instruments have been validated. The four most commonly used disease-severity scales SCORAD, EASI, IGA, and SASSAD were used in 242 out of the 382 RCTs reviewed (63%). SCORAD, EASI, and SASSAD have been extensively validated [7]. The four most commonly used QoL instruments were DLQI, CDLQI, IDQOL, and DFI. All four scales have demonstrated validity, reliability, and sensitivity to change [36,47,51,52].

The use of four top disease-severity instruments in AD has increased from 1985 to 2010 (Figure 2). For example, when we compared instrument usage patterns between the period from 2000–2004 with that from 2005–2010, we found that SCORAD usage increased by 106%; EASI usage increased by 165%; IGA usage increased by 169%, and SASSAD usage decreased by 20%. Over this ten-year period, IGA had the greatest rate of increase. The greater increased rate of IGA usage may be attributed to its ease of administration. Compared to IGA, EASI also experienced a higher rate of adoption in clinical trials since 1985. The usage patterns of EASI and IGA appear to parallel with each other, which suggests researchers' preference for both scales as objective measures of AD.

The increased usage of disease severity scales appeared to coincide with the publication of validation studies. SCORAD had its peak usage from 2005 to 2010, which corresponded closely to the publication of its validation studies from 2004 to 2006. EASI also had its peak usage from 2005 to 2010, which coincided with the publication of its validation studies in 2004 and 2005.

Among the four most commonly used QoL instruments, all were used more commonly as the years progressed. One possible explanation for this trend is that QoL measures have become as important as disease-severity instruments for patient evaluation and management. Of note, the four most common quality of life scales were developed by the same group of physicians and are similar in format and design. This may limit the diversity of the scale and the variety of characteristics that are used when assessing QoL in patients with atopic dermatitis. Additionally, our search of the literature was limited to randomized controlled trials. Other disease-specific quality of life instruments may exist that have not been used in randomized control trials.

Another limitation of our review is that, out of 382 RCTs examined, we identified 67 RCTs that used QoL measurements (18%), which makes identifying trends for individual QoL instruments difficult.

In this review, we identified trends for disease-severity and QoL outcomes measurements in atopic dermatitis from 1985–2010. We also summarized dimensions of the most commonly used scales and cited evidence for their validation. Although the consistent use of validated measures assessing disease severity and QoL in AD was not observed 20 years ago, this study found a promising trend of increased usage of validated instruments in clinical trials that measure AD disease severity and QoL in the past decade. Outcomes researchers in dermatology are encouraged to select validated outcomes measures that provide accurate measurement of disease dimensions and allow for comparison among studies.

This is the first systematic analysis of trends in the usage of outcomes measures in dermatological research. We anticipate that similar studies will be forthcoming in other disease areas within dermatology that assess the use of outcomes instruments. This type of study depicts the progression of a field's research quality and validity, and it encourages future outcomes researchers to devise instruments that will be streamlined, valid, and reliable.

Author Contributions

Conceived and designed the experiments: AA BR. Analyzed the data: AA BR. Contributed reagents/materials/analysis tools: AA BR. Wrote the paper: AA BR.

References

1. Holm EA, Wulf HC, Stegmann H, Jemec GB (2006) Life quality assessment among patients with atopic eczema. Br J Dermatol 154: 719–725.
2. Chamlin SL, Frieden IJ, Williams ML, Chren MM (2004) Effects of atopic dermatitis on young American children and their families. Pediatrics 114: 607–611.
3. Hanifin JM, Rajka G (1980) Diagnostic features of atopic dermatitis. Acta derm venereol (Stockh). pp 44–47.
4. Dohil MA, Eichenfield LF (2005) A treatment approach for atopic dermatitis. Pediatr Ann 34: 201–210.
5. Finlay AY (1998) Quality of life assessments in dermatology. Semin Cutan Med Surg 17: 291–296.
6. McKenna SP, Doward LC (2008) Quality of life of children with atopic dermatitis and their families. Curr Opin Allergy Clin Immunol 8: 228–231.
7. Schmitt J, Langan S, Williams HC (2007) What are the best outcome measurements for atopic eczema? A systematic review. J Allergy Clin Immunol 120: 1389–1398.
8. Kunz B, Oranje AP, Labreze L, Stalder JF, Ring J, et al. (1997) Clinical validation and guidelines for the SCORAD index: consensus report of the European Task Force on Atopic Dermatitis. Dermatology 195: 10–19.
9. Charman C, Williams H (2000) Outcome measures of disease severity in atopic eczema. Arch Dermatol 136: 763–769.
10. (1993) Severity scoring of atopic dermatitis: the SCORAD index. Consensus Report of the European Task Force on Atopic Dermatitis. Dermatology 186: 23–31.
11. Angelova-Fischer I, Bauer A, Hipler UC, Petrov I, Kazandjieva J, et al. (2005) The objective severity assessment of atopic dermatitis (OSAAD) score: validity, reliability and sensitivity in adult patients with atopic dermatitis. Br J Dermatol 153: 767–773.
12. Ben-Gashir MA, Seed PT, Hay RJ (2004) Quality of life and disease severity are correlated in children with atopic dermatitis. Br J Dermatol 150: 284–290.
13. Breuer K, Braeutigam M, Kapp A, Werfel T (2004) Influence of pimecrolimus cream 1% on different morphological signs of eczema in infants with atopic dermatitis. Dermatology 209: 314–320.
14. Charman CR, Venn AJ, Williams H (2005) Measuring atopic eczema severity visually: which variables are most important to patients? Arch Dermatol 141: 1146–1151; discussion 1151.
15. Hon KL, Kam WY, Lam MC, Leung TF, Ng PC (2006) CDLQI, SCORAD and NESS: are they correlated? Qual Life Res 15: 1551–1558.
16. Hon KL, Leung TF, Wong Y, Fok TF (2006) Lesson from performing SCORADs in children with atopic dermatitis: subjective symptoms do not correlate well with disease extent or intensity. Int J Dermatol 45: 728–730.
17. Hon KL, Ma KC, Wong E, Leung TF, Wong Y, et al. (2003) Validation of a self-administered questionnaire in Chinese in the assessment of eczema severity. Pediatr Dermatol 20: 465–469.
18. Oranje AP, Stalder JF, Taieb A, Tasset C, de Longueville M (1997) Scoring of atopic dermatitis by SCORAD using a training atlas by investigators from different disciplines. ETAC Study Group. Early Treatment of the Atopic Child. Pediatr Allergy Immunol 8: 28–34.
19. Pucci N, Novembre E, Cammarata MG, Bernardini R, Monaco MG, et al. (2005) Scoring atopic dermatitis in infants and young children: distinctive features of the SCORAD index. Allergy 60: 113–116.
20. Schafer T, Dockery D, Kramer U, Behrendt H, Ring J (1997) Experiences with the severity scoring of atopic dermatitis in a population of German pre-school children. Br J Dermatol 137: 558–562.
21. Staab D, Kaufmann R, Brautigam M, Wahn U (2005) Treatment of infants with atopic eczema with pimecrolimus cream 1% improves parents' quality of life: a multicenter, randomized trial. Pediatr Allergy Immunol 16: 527–533.
22. Wolkerstorfer A, de Waard van der Spek FB, Glazenburg EJ, Mulder PG, Oranje AP (1999) Scoring the severity of atopic dermatitis: three item severity score as a rough system for daily practice and as a pre-screening tool for studies. Acta Derm Venereol 79: 356–359.
23. Sprikkelman AB, Tupker RA, Burgerhof H, Schouten JP, Brand PL, et al. (1997) Severity scoring of atopic dermatitis: a comparison of three scoring systems. Allergy 52: 944–949.
24. Fredriksson T, Pettersson U (1978) Severe psoriasis–oral therapy with a new retinoid. Dermatologica 157: 238–244.
25. Hanifin JM, Thurston M, Omoto M, Cherill R, Tofte SJ, et al. (2001) The eczema area and severity index (EASI): assessment of reliability in atopic dermatitis. EASI Evaluator Group. Exp Dermatol 10: 11–18.
26. Barbier N, Paul C, Luger T, Allen R, De Prost Y, et al. (2004) Validation of the Eczema Area and Severity Index for atopic dermatitis in a cohort of 1550 patients from the pimecrolimus cream 1% randomized controlled clinical trials programme. Br J Dermatol 150: 96–102.
27. Belloni G, Pinelli S, Veraldi S (2005) A randomised, double-blind, vehicle-controlled study to evaluate the efficacy and safety of MAS063D (Atopiclair) in the treatment of mild to moderate atopic dermatitis. Eur J Dermatol 15: 31–36.
28. Siegfried E, Korman N, Molina C, Kianifard F, Abrams K (2006) Safety and efficacy of early intervention with pimecrolimus cream 1% combined with corticosteroids for major flares in infants and children with atopic dermatitis. J Dermatolog Treat 17: 143–150.
29. Berth-Jones J (1996) Six area, six sign atopic dermatitis (SASSAD) severity score: a simple system for monitoring disease activity in atopic dermatitis. Br J Dermatol 135 Suppl 48: 25–30.
30. Berth-Jones J, Finlay A, Zaki I, Tan B, Goodyear H, et al. (1996) Cyclosporine in severe childhood atopic dermatitis: A multicenter study* 1. Journal of the American Academy of Dermatology 34: 1016–1021.
31. Granlund H, Erkko P, Sinisalo M, Reitamo S (1995) Cyclosporin in atopic dermatitis: time to relapse and effect of intermittent therapy. Br J Dermatol 132: 106–112.
32. Berth-Jones J, Graham-Brown RA, Marks R, Camp RD, English JS, et al. (1997) Long-term efficacy and safety of cyclosporin in severe adult atopic dermatitis. Br J Dermatol 136: 76–81.
33. Jenner N, Campbell J, Marks R (2004) Morbidity and cost of atopic eczema in Australia. Australas J Dermatol 45: 16–22.
34. Sowden JM, Berth-Jones J, Ross JS, Motley RJ, Marks R, et al. (1991) Double-blind, controlled, crossover study of cyclosporin in adults with severe refractory atopic dermatitis. Lancet 338: 137–140.
35. Charman CR, Venn AJ, Williams HC (2002) Reliability testing of the Six Area, Six Sign Atopic Dermatitis severity score. Br J Dermatol 146: 1057–1060.
36. Lewis-Jones MS, Finlay AY (1995) The Children's Dermatology Life Quality Index (CDLQI): initial validation and practical use. Br J Dermatol 132: 942–949.
37. Emerson RM, Lawson S, Williams HC (1998) Do specialist eczema clinics benefit children with atopic dermatitis? British Journal of Dermatology 139: 46.
38. Harper JI, Ahmed I, Barclay G, Lacour M, Hoeger P, et al. (2000) Cyclosporin for severe childhood atopic dermatitis: short course versus continuous therapy. Br J Dermatol 142: 52–58.
39. Aziah MS, Rosnah T, Mardziah A, Norzila MZ (2002) Childhood atopic dermatitis: a measurement of quality of life and family impact. Med J Malaysia 57: 329–339.
40. Chuh AA (2003) Validation of a Cantonese version of the Children's Dermatology Life Quality Index. Pediatr Dermatol 20: 479–481.
41. Clayton TH, Clark SM, Britton J, Pavlov S, Radev S (2007) A comparative study of the Children's Dermatology Life Quality Index (CDLQI) in paediatric dermatology clinics in the UK and Bulgaria. J Eur Acad Dermatol Venereol 21: 1436–1437.
42. Holme SA, Man I, Sharpe JL, Dykes PJ, Lewis-Jones MS, et al. (2003) The Children's Dermatology Life Quality Index: validation of the cartoon version. Br J Dermatol 148: 285–290.
43. Beattie PE, Lewis-Jones MS (2006) An audit of the impact of a consultation with a paediatric dermatology team on quality of life in infants with atopic eczema and their families: further validation of the Infants' Dermatitis Quality of Life Index and Dermatitis Family Impact score. Br J Dermatol 155: 1249–1255.
44. Lewis-Jones M, Finlay A (2006) Quality of life research. In: Medicine WCo, ed.
45. Alvarenga TM, Caldeira AP (2009) Quality of life in pediatric patients with atopic dermatitis. J Pediatr (Rio J) 85: 415–420.
46. Grimalt R, Mengeaud V, Cambazard F (2007) The steroid-sparing effect of an emollient therapy in infants with atopic dermatitis: a randomized controlled study. Dermatology 214: 61–67.
47. Lewis-Jones MS, Finlay AY, Dykes PJ (2001) The Infants' Dermatitis Quality of Life Index. Br J Dermatol 144: 104–110.
48. Weber MB, Fontes Neto Pde T, Prati C, Soirefman M, Mazzotti NG, et al. (2008) Improvement of pruritus and quality of life of children with atopic dermatitis and their families after joining support groups. J Eur Acad Dermatol Venereol 22: 992–997.
49. Finlay AY, Khan GK (1994) Dermatology Life Quality Index (DLQI)–a simple practical measure for routine clinical use. Clin Exp Dermatol 19: 210–216.
50. Badia X, Mascaro JM, Lozano R (1999) Measuring health-related quality of life in patients with mild to moderate eczema and psoriasis: clinical validity, reliability and sensitivity to change of the DLQI. The Cavide Research Group. Br J Dermatol 141: 698–702.
51. Lewis V, Finlay AY (2004) 10 years experience of the Dermatology Life Quality Index (DLQI). J Investig Dermatol Symp Proc 9: 169–180.
52. Lewis-Jones MS, Finlay AY, Dykes PJ (1999) Measurement of the impact of atopic dermatitis on infant's and their families lives. British Journal of Dermatology 141: 105–106.
53. Department of Dermatology WCoM, Cardiff University The Infant's Dermatitis Quality of Life Index (IDQOL).

54. Chren MM (2000) Giving "scale" new meaning in dermatology: measurement matters. Arch Dermatol 136: 788–790.
55. Williams H (1997) Is a simple generic index of dermatologic disease severity an attainable goal? Archives of Dermatology 133: 1451.
56. Chen SC (2007) Dermatology quality of life instruments: sorting out the quagmire. J Invest Dermatol 127: 2695–2696.

57. Barzilai DA, Weinstock MA, Mostow EN (2007) Practicing evidence-based dermatology: a short guide. Skinmed 6: 122–127.
58. Finlay AY (1997) Quality of life measurement in dermatology: a practical guide. Br J Dermatol 136: 305–314.

12

Alcohol Intake in Pregnancy Increases the Child's Risk of Atopic Dermatitis. The COPSAC Prospective Birth Cohort Study of a High Risk Population

Charlotte Giwercman Carson, Liselotte Brydensholt Halkjaer, Signe Marie Jensen, Hans Bisgaard*

Copenhagen Prospective Studies on Asthma in Childhood, Health Sciences, University of Copenhagen, Copenhagen University Hospital, Gentofte, Copenhagen, Denmark

Abstract

Background: Atopic dermatitis has increased four-fold over the recent decades in developed countries, indicating that changes in environmental factors associated with lifestyle may play an important role in this epidemic. It has been proposed that alcohol consumption may be one contributing risk factor in this development.

Objective: To analyze the impact of alcohol intake during pregnancy on the development of atopic dermatitis during the first 7 years of life.

Method: The COPSAC cohort is a prospective, longitudinal, birth cohort study of 411 children born to mothers with a history of asthma, followed up for 7 years with scheduled visits every 6 months as well as visits for acute exacerbations of atopic dermatitis. Risk of atopic dermatitis from any alcohol consumption during pregnancy was analyzed as time-to-diagnosis and adjusted for known risk factors.

Results: 177 of 411 children developed atopic dermatitis before age 7 years. We found a significant effect of alcohol intake during pregnancy on atopic dermatitis development (HR 1.44, 95% CI 1.05–1.99 p = 0.024). This conclusion was unaffected after adjustment for smoking, mother's education and mother's atopic dermatitis.

Limitations: The selection of a high-risk cohort, with all mothers suffering from asthma, and all children having a gestational age above 35 weeks with no congenital abnormality, systemic illness, or history of mechanical ventilation or lower airway infection.

Conclusion: Alcohol intake by pregnant women with a history of asthma, is significantly associated with an increased risk for the child for developing atopic dermatitis during the first 7 years of life.

Editor: Claire Thorne, UCL Institute of Child Health, University College London, United Kingdom

Funding: Copenhagen Prospective Studies on Asthma in Childhood is funded by private and public research funds. The Lundbeck Foundation; the Pharmacy Foundation of 1991; Augustinus Foundation; the Danish Medical Research Council and The Danish Pediatric Asthma Centre provided the core funding. The funders had no role in study design, data collection and analysis, decision to publish, or preparation of the manuscript.

Competing Interests: The authors have declared that no competing interests exist.

* E-mail: bisgaard@copsac.com

Introduction

Atopic dermatitis (AD) has increased fourfold over the last five decades in western countries[1–4], indicating that changes in environmental factors associated with western lifestyle may play an important role[4–6]. It has been proposed that alcohol consumption may be one contributing factor to the rise in atopic diseases[7,8] as alcohol consumption is part of the western lifestyle and has increased in the same period with an annual consumption nearly tripling in Denmark since 1955[9,10]. Also, alcohol consumption during pregnancy is frequent in westernized countries[11–14].

We previously reported a cross-sectional analysis of a comprehensive range of potential risk factors for the development of AD by age 3 suggesting mother's AD, father's allergic rhinitis, child's FLG status, dog exposure at birth and baby's birth length as significant risk factors. Furthermore, breast feeding and mother's intake of alcohol during pregnancy was found to be marginally significant risk factors for AD in the child[15]. Recently, we reported a longitudinal analysis of age-at-onset showing that breast feeding increased the risk of AD[16].

In this 7-year follow-up study we have used close longitudinal observations to re-test our initial observation of a borderline significant risk from alcohol intake by the pregnant mother on the development of AD in the child.

Methods

Ethics Statement

The Copenhagen Study on Asthma in Childhood (COPSAC) was conducted in accordance with the guiding principles of the Declaration of Helsinki, approved by the Ethics Committee for

Copenhagen (KF 01–289/96) and The Danish Data Protection Agency (2002–41–2434), and in compliance with "Good Clinical Practice" (GCP) guidelines. Informed, written consent was obtained from all parents.

Participants

The COPSAC cohort is a prospective longitudinal birth cohort, including 411 children born to mothers with asthma. Mother's asthma was defined as doctor diagnosed asthma with a history of medication during two seasons[17]. The main recruiting area of the cohort was greater Copenhagen, Denmark and all children were born between August 1998 and December 2001. The children were enrolled at one month of age and visited the COPSAC clinic at scheduled visits every six months thereafter, as well as for any acute complaints from skin or airways. Skin examinations, diagnoses and treatment of AD were handled in accordance with predefined standard operating procedures by trained medical doctors employed for this purpose in the COPSAC clinic. The enrolled children were primarily cared for at the COPSAC clinic. Data validity was assured by quality control procedures. Data were collected on-line and locked after external monitoring and with an automated audit trail showing operations on the database after locking. The study was previously described in details elsewhere[17,18]. See Table S1 for baseline characteristics.

Risk assessments

COPSAC provides comprehensive assessments of the prenatal, perinatal and postnatal milieu, aiming to elucidate critical factors driving atopic disease expression. In this study we analyzed alcohol intake during pregnancy for development of AD during the first 7 years of life.

AD was defined based on the criteria of Hanifin and Rajka[19] as previously detailed[20], with age at first AD diagnosis used as outcome.

Childhood asthma was diagnosed based on preasthma (recurrent episodes of troublesome wheezing, breathlessness and/or cough) and the response and subsequent relapse to a 3-month trial of inhaled corticosteroids[17].

Rhinitis was defined as troublesome sneezing, blocked or runny nose in the past 12 months in periods without accompanying cold or flu[21]. All diagnoses were performed by the doctors in the COPSAC clinic.

Alcohol intake during pregnancy was determined at the interview at the 1-month visit. The mothers were interviewed about their drinking habits, and the average alcohol intake pr. week pr. trimester was entered online. Mothers drinking minimum one unit of alcohol pr. week in minimum one of the 3 trimesters were defined as having an intake of alcohol during pregnancy. One unit of alcohol was defined as 15 ml or 12 g of alcohol, explained to the mothers as e.g. one beer or one glass of wine. Information about mother's education (high school/medium-long education/university), smoking habits in the 3rd trimester (smoking yes/no) and AD (doctor diagnosed) was also recorded at the 1-month scheduled visits in the COPSAC clinic.

Statistical analysis

The association between alcohol intake during pregnancy and development of AD during the first 7 years of life was examined by survival analysis. The children were retained in the analysis from birth, until age at first diagnosis of AD, drop-out, or 7 years of age whichever came first.

Kaplan-Meier curves were estimated for alcohol drinking during pregnancy. The plots were used as a descriptive presentation of the results, illustrating the cumulative risk of developing AD with respect to mother's alcohol intake during pregnancy. Survival analyses were performed by use of Cox proportional-hazards regression, supporting the Kaplan-Meier curves with information about hazard ratios (HR), 95% confidence intervals (CI) and p-values. The dependent variable was the time to first event (AD diagnosis, dropout or 7 years). The confounders, mother's education, smoking habits in 3rd trimester and AD, were placed in the regression models simultaneously. Tests for functional form and proportional hazards were based on martingales.

The overall significance level used was 0.05. The analyses were done using PROC TPHREG in SAS version 9.1 as well as R version 2.6.1.

Results

COPSAC enrolled 411 infants out of which 77 were lost to follow-up before debut of AD symptoms and/or before the age of 7 years. There was no difference in alcohol consumption between the group lost to follow-up and the remaining families (Table S1). Forty eight percent of the mothers had a history of AD, 16% and 13% of the fathers had a history of asthma and AD, respectively. There were 16 siblings and 18 twins in the cohort, thus totaling 8.3% of the participants. All 411 children were included in the univariate analysis. Data for mother's education were missing for 34 children, leaving 377 children for the confounder adjusted analysis (92% of the enrolled cohort).

108 mothers in the cohort (26%) had an intake of one or more units of alcohol pr. week in minimum one of the 3 trimesters, respectively 88, 73 and 73 women in the 1st, 2nd and 3rd trimester. The quantity of alcohol intake was distributed as follows (in units of alcohol pr. trimester):

1st trimester: range 1–7, median: 1, mean: 1.55, interquartile range: 1–2

2nd trimester: range 1–7, median: 1, mean: 1.44, interquartile range: 1–2

3rd trimester: range 1–7, median: 1, mean: 1.51, interquartile range: 1–2

One hundred seventy-seven children of the 411 participating infants (43%) had an AD diagnosis before age 7 years. In the group of children developing AD 31% (55) of the mothers had been drinking alcohol at some point during pregnancy, i.e. more than an average of one unit of alcohol pr. week in minimum one of the three trimesters. Of the 234 children who did not develop AD, 23% (53) of the mothers had been drinking alcohol at some point during pregnancy. This difference in prevalence of mother's alcohol drinking in the two groups of children (31% vs. 23%) was marginally statistically significant (p = 0.055)

The age-at-onset analysis confirmed an increased risk of AD associated with alcohol intake during pregnancy, with the effect persisting throughout the whole 7 years follow-up period (Figure 1) (HR 1.44, 95% CI 1.05–1.99, p = 0.024).

The hazard ratio from the univariate analysis was largely unchanged after confounder adjusted analysis adjusting for mother's education, smoking habits 3rd trimester and AD (HR 1.45, 95% CI 1.04–2.02, p = 0.029).

There was no association between alcohol intake during pregnancy and other atopic endpoints (wheeze episodes, asthma, allergic rhinitis, blood eosinophil count, total IgE, sensitization (specific IgE≥0.35 kU/L), nasal eosinophilia and cord blood IgE (IgE≥0.5 kU/L)). Results are not shown.

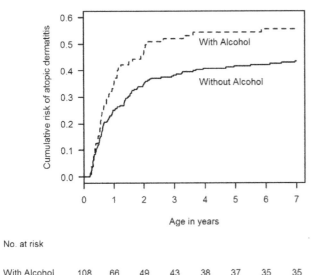

No. at risk

With Alcohol	108	66	49	43	38	37	35	35
Without Alcohol	303	215	173	153	136	128	125	122

Figure 1. Kaplan-Meier plots for the effect of alcohol intake during pregnancy on subsequent atopic dermatitis development in the offspring during the first 7 years of life.

Discussion

Main finding

In this prospective, longitudinal, birth cohort study we find alcohol intake during pregnancy to be associated with an increased risk of developing AD in the first 7 years of life, adjusted for possible confounders. The increased risk was persistent throughout the whole 7 years follow-up period.

Strengths and limitations

Recall bias is reduced from the prospective data collection, with half-yearly clinic visits and visits at any acute symptoms from the skin. The alcohol related questions were recorded before any onset of atopic diseases including AD.

Misclassification of AD is reduced by the participants being diagnosed and treated at the COPSAC clinic and not by their general practitioner. Furthermore, all mothers in the cohort have personal experience with atopic diseases, and should therefore be expected to be better at reporting symptoms. Ambiguities over the definition of AD, especially during infancy and early childhood, make the estimates of prevalence unreliable and render comparisons between studies difficult. In this cohort study the specificity of the AD diagnosis is high, since the diagnosis, detailed phenotype and management of skin lesions were controlled solely by the COPSAC clinic physicians from predefined standard operating procedures and included assessment of localization and severity at each visit. This reduces the risk of misclassification and is of particular importance in the clinical evaluation of AD where inter-observer variation is a problem[22]. The specificity of the diagnosis in this study is illustrated by the observation that the cumulative incidence of seborrheic dermatitis capitis was not significantly different in children with AD and in children with skin lesions not fulfilling AD diagnosis, suggesting that there was no misclassification between AD and seborrheic dermatitis capitis.

We have used predefined questions concerning alcohol consumption, recording average alcohol intake per week per trimester. We are aware that alcohol histories are notoriously

unreliable. However, this unreliability is not biased as it must be expected to be equal among mothers to children later developing AD and not. Therefore, it can only result in a type 2 and not a type 1 error, i.e. it could have obscured an effect but it could not cause a false effect to be seen.

We have chosen to present data as a binary variable just to determine whether alcohol intake during pregnancy correlates to AD at all. We found similar estimates in sub-analyses stratifying for alcohol amount or onset/duration of alcohol intake, but the number of individuals in each group was very small. Therefore, these results are not included in the article. This narrow definition of alcohol intake limits our results and future studies designed to determine quantity of alcohol ingested should be sought. The external validity of our study is limited from the selection of a high-risk cohort, with all mothers suffering from asthma, and all children having a gestational age above 35 weeks with no congenital abnormality, systemic illness, or history of mechanical ventilation or lower airway infection. Therefore, our results need replication in an unselected population.

Interpretation

We have previously demonstrated risk factors in the development of AD in a cross-sectional analysis by age 3 in this birth cohort[15]. We found that mother's AD, father's allergic rhinitis, child's FLG status, dog exposure at birth and higher birth length were significant factors predicting AD by 3 years of age. Duration of breastfeeding and mother's alcohol consumption during pregnancy also increased the risk of AD but were not statistical significant in this cross-sectional analysis. However, age-of-onset survival statistics was used in subsequent analyses to show, that both breast feeding[16] and now also mother's alcohol intake in pregnancy were significant risk factors for AD in the off-spring.

AD has increased dramatically since the 1960's in Western countries[1–3,23] and genetic factors only cannot explain the recent rapid increase in the incidence. The exposure to early life style factors is thought to be crucial for the later development of AD, and suggestions about factors influencing the intra uterine milieu have been made[24–30]. A questionnaire based cohort study, reported a significant and dose-dependent effect from the mother's intake of alcohol during pregnancy in the risk of developing AD during the first 2 months of child life, but not beyond this period. This effect was mainly seen in high-risk infants (two parents with allergic disease)[31].The authors interpreted their observations to be indirectly supported by a study investigating the influence of environmental factors on levels of total IgE in cord blood of 2631 newborn infants[32]. They found an independent positive dose–response relationship between maternal alcohol consumption during pregnancy and the levels of cord blood IgE, and hypothized that the increased IgE synthesis may contribute to the immunologic sensitization. However, increased IgE is generally not believed to be directly associated to AD, but rather to illustrate a common mechanism for the atopic diseases. This is also supported by the paradox, that alcohol consumption is found associated with an increased risk of developing perennial allergic rhinitis, but not seasonal allergic rhinitis[33]. In our study we do not find any association to other atopic diseases, including cord blood IgE, allergic rhinitis, total IgE and sensitization, and can therefore not support the hypothesis that the association between alcohol and AD are caused by a higher level of IgE.

In this study we adjusted for reasonable confounders including mother's education, smoking habits in 3rd trimester and AD. These confounders were chosen, because we believe them to be the only factors both affecting the child's risk of developing AD and the mother's alcohol intake. Other factors, such as prenatal behavior, pets in home at birth and breastfeeding were not included in the analysis as confounders, because we do not believe them to affect both the exposure (mother's alcohol intake during pregnancy) and the outcome (AD). We detect an association between alcohol intake during pregnancy and the child's risk of developing AD, but the underlying causal relationship is not clear and further studies are needed to confirm our findings and explore the reasons for our observed associations.

It has been suggested that factors, which influence cytokine production by the feto-placental unit, may be important determinants of atopic disease[34]. This is further supported by findings that the effect of the maternal line on childhood AD is greater than that of the paternal line[35–38], which are, however, not confirmed in all studies[39,40]. Alcohol may trigger hypersensitivity reactions, i.e. allergic, asthmatic or eczematous symptoms. The mechanisms underlying these reactions are unknown, but are hypothesized to be due to a histamine-releasing effect of acetaldehyde[41–46]. Gonzalez-Quintela et al[47] have reported that alcohol intake may induce changes in the cytokine profile, including increasing level of some Th2-associated cytokines, and impairment of the Th1 lymphocyte response. This is supported by other studies[45,46]. However, such differences in cytokine profiles are most often found in alcohol abusers, and one should therefore be cautious in transferring these findings to our cohort's pregnant women. Still, it could be worth considering as a possible explanation for our observed association between mother's alcohol intake and the offspring's risk of developing AD, although further studies are needed to clarify this.

Conclusion

We found that alcohol intake during pregnancy in asthmatic women is associated with a statistically significantly higher risk of developing AD in the offspring. The increased risk is still significant after confounder adjustment for other known risk factors. However, the underlying mechanism is not clear.

Acknowledgments

The authors wish to thank the children and parent participating in the COPSAC cohorts as well as the COPSAC study teams.

The abstract from this manuscript has been presented as a poster at the European Respiratory Society's annual congress in Barcelona, September 2010. Data will not be presented in any other official form.

Author Contributions

Conceived and designed the experiments: HB LBH CGC. Performed the experiments: HB LBH CGC. Analyzed the data: SMJ CGC HB. Contributed reagents/materials/analysis tools: SMJ CGC HB. Wrote the paper: SMJ CGC HB LBH.

References

1. Schultz LF, Hanifin JM (1992) Secular change in the occurrence of atopic dermatitis. Acta Derm Venereol Suppl (Stockh) 176: 7–12.
2. Schultz LF, Diepgen T, Svensson A (1996) The occurrence of atopic dermatitis in north Europe: an international questionnaire study. J Am Acad Dermatol 34: 760–764.
3. Olesen AB, Ellingsen AR, Olesen H, Juul S, Thestrup-Pedersen K (1997) Atopic dermatitis and birth factors: historical follow up by record linkage. BMJ 314: 1003–1008.
4. Law M, Morris JK, Wald N, Luczynska C, Burney P (2005) Changes in atopy over a quarter of a century, based on cross sectional data at three time periods. BMJ 330: 1187–1188.
5. Krause T, Koch A, Friborg J, Poulsen LK, Kristensen B, et al. (2002) Frequency of atopy in the Arctic in 1987 and 1998. Lancet 360: 691–692.
6. Von Hertzen LC, Haahtela T (2004) Asthma and atopy - the price of affluence? Allergy 59: 124–137.
7. Vally H, Thompson PJ (2003) Alcoholic drink consumption: a role in the development of allergic disease? Clin Exp Allergy 33: 156–158.
8. Linneberg A, Petersen J, Nielsen NH, Madsen F, Frolund L, et al. (2003) The relationship of alcohol consumption to total immunoglobulin E and the development of immunoglobulin E sensitization: the Copenhagen Allergy Study. Clin Exp Allergy 33: 192–198.
9. Fagt S, Trolle E (2001) [The supply of food in 1955–1999. Development in Danish Diet - consumption, food, purchases and eating habits] (danish). 38–40.
10. Academy of Medical Sciences (2004) Calling Time - The Nation's drinking as a major health issue.
11. Olsen J, Frische G, Poulsen AO, Kirchheiner H (1989) Changing smoking, drinking, and eating behaviour among pregnant women in Denmark. Evaluation of a health campaign in a local region. Scand J Soc Med 17: 277–280.
12. Ogston SA, Parry GJ (1992) EUROMAC. A European concerted action: maternal alcohol consumption and its relation to the outcome of pregnancy and child development at 18 months. Results–strategy of analysis and analysis of pregnancy outcome. Int J Epidemiol 21 Suppl 1: S45–S71.
13. Kesmodel U, Wisborg K, Olsen SF, Henriksen TB, Secher NJ (2002) Moderate alcohol intake during pregnancy and the risk of stillbirth and death in the first year of life. Am J Epidemiol 155: 305–312.
14. Ebrahim SH, Luman ET, Floyd RL, Murphy CC, Bennett EM, et al. (1998) Alcohol consumption by pregnant women in the United States during 1988–1995. Obstet Gynecol 92: 187–192.
15. Bisgaard H, Halkjaer LB, Hinge R, Giwercman C, Palmer C, et al. (2009) Risk analysis of early childhood eczema. J Allergy Clin Immunol 123: 1355–1360.

16. Giwercman C, Halkjaer LB, Jensen SM, Bonnelykke K, Lauritzen L, et al. (2010) Increased risk of eczema but reduced risk of early wheezy disorder from exclusive breast-feeding in high-risk infants. J Allergy Clin Immunol 125: 866–871.
17. Bisgaard H (2004) The Copenhagen Prospective Study on Asthma in Childhood (COPSAC): design, rationale, and baseline data from a longitudinal birth cohort study. Ann Allergy Asthma Immunol 93: 381–389.
18. Bisgaard H, Hermansen MN, Loland L, Halkjaer LB, Buchvald F (2006) Intermittent inhaled corticosteroids in infants with episodic wheezing. N Engl J Med 354: 1998–2005.
19. Hanifin JM, Rajka G (1980) Diagnostic features of atopic dermatitis. Acta Derm Venereol 92: 44–47.
20. Halkjaer LB, Loland L, Buchvald FF, Agner T, Skov L, et al. (2006) Development of atopic dermatitis during the first 3 years of life: the Copenhagen prospective study on asthma in childhood cohort study in high-risk children. Arch Dermatol 142: 561–566.
21. Chawes BL, Kreiner-Moller E, Bisgaard H (2009) Objective assessments of allergic and nonallergic rhinitis in young children. Allergy 64: 1547–1553.
22. Williams HC, Burney PG, Strachan D, Hay RJ (1994) The U.K. Working Party's Diagnostic Criteria for Atopic Dermatitis. II. Observer variation of clinical diagnosis and signs of atopic dermatitis. Br J Dermatol 131: 397–405.
23. Law M, Morris JK, Wald N, Luczynska C, Burney P (2005) Changes in atopy over a quarter of a century, based on cross sectional data at three time periods. BMJ 330: 1187–1188.
24. Jones CA, Holloway JA, Warner JO (2000) Does atopic disease start in foetal life? Allergy 55: 2–10.
25. Bjorksten B (1999) The intrauterine and postnatal environments. J Allergy Clin Immunol 104: 1119–1127.
26. Bjorksten B (1999) Environment and infant immunity. Proc Nutr Soc 58: 729–732.
27. Xu B, Jarvelin MR, Pekkanen J (1999) Prenatal factors and occurrence of rhinitis and eczema among offspring. Allergy 54: 829–836.
28. Kurzius-Spencer M, Halonen M, Carla L, I, Martinez FD, Wright AL (2005) Prenatal factors associated with the development of eczema in the first year of life. Pediatr Allergy Immunol 16: 19–26.
29. Prescott SL (2003) Early origins of allergic disease: a review of processes and influences during early immune development. Curr Opin Allergy Clin Immunol 3: 125–132.
30. Bjorksten B (1999) Allergy priming early in life. Lancet 353: 167–168.
31. Linneberg A, Petersen J, Gronbaek M, Benn CS (2004) Alcohol during pregnancy and atopic dermatitis in the offspring. Clin Exp Allergy 34: 1678–1683.

32. Bjerke T, Hedegaard M, Henriksen TB, Nielsen BW, Schiotz PO (1994) Several genetic and environmental factors influence cord blood IgE concentration. Pediatr Allergy Immunol 5: 88–94.

33. Bendtsen P, Gronbaek M, Kjaer SK, Munk C, Linneberg A, et al. (2008) Alcohol consumption and the risk of self-reported perennial and seasonal allergic rhinitis in young adult women in a population-based cohort study. Clin Exp Allergy 38: 1179–1185.

34. Macaubas C, de Klerk NH, Holt BJ, Wee C, Kendall G, et al. (2003) Association between antenatal cytokine production and the development of atopy and asthma at age 6 years. Lancet 362: 1192–1197.

35. Bradley M, Kockum I, Soderhall C, Van Hage-Hamsten M, Luthman H, et al. (2000) Characterization by phenotype of families with atopic dermatitis. Acta Derm Venereol 80: 106–110.

36. Ruiz RG, Kemeny DM, Price JF (1992) Higher risk of infantile atopic dermatitis from maternal atopy than from paternal atopy. Clin Exp Allergy 22: 762–766.

37. Moore MM, Rifas-Shiman SL, Rich-Edwards JW, Kleinman KP, Camargo CA, Jr., et al. (2004) Perinatal predictors of atopic dermatitis occurring in the first six months of life. Pediatrics 113: 468–474.

38. Harris JM, Cullinan P, Williams HC, Mills P, Moffat S, et al. (2001) Environmental associations with eczema in early life. Br J Dermatol 144: 795–802.

39. Bohme M, Wickman M, Lennart NS, Svartengren M, Wahlgren CF (2003) Family history and risk of atopic dermatitis in children up to 4 years. Clin Exp Allergy 33: 1226–1231.

40. Wadonda-Kabondo N, Sterne JA, Golding J, Kennedy CT, Archer CB, et al. (2004) Association of parental eczema, hayfever, and asthma with atopic dermatitis in infancy: birth cohort study. Arch Dis Child 89: 917–921.

41. Vally H, Thompson PJ (2003) Allergic and asthmatic reactions to alcoholic drinks. Addict Biol 8: 3–11.

42. Linneberg A, Berg ND, Gonzalez-Quintela A, Vidal C, Elberling J (2008) Prevalence of self-reported hypersensitivity symptoms following intake of alcoholic drinks. Clin Exp Allergy 38: 145–151.

43. Vally H, de KN, Thompson PJ (2000) Alcoholic drinks: important triggers for asthma. J Allergy Clin Immunol 105: 462–467.

44. Nihlen U, Greiff LJ, Nyberg P, Persson CG, Andersson M (2005) Alcohol-induced upper airway symptoms: prevalence and co-morbidity. Respir Med 99: 762–769.

45. Cook RT (1998) Alcohol abuse, alcoholism, and damage to the immune system–a review. Alcohol Clin Exp Res 22: 1927–1942.

46. Kazbariene B, Kalibatas J, Krikstaponiene A, Zabulyte D, Monceviciute-Eringiene E (2007) Alterations of human immune system functions in relation to environmental contamination, gender and alcohol consumption intensity. Cent Eur J Public Health 15: 13–17.

47. Gonzalez-Quintela A, Vidal C, Lojo S, Perez LF, Otero-Anton E, et al. (1999) Serum cytokines and increased total serum IgE in alcoholics. Ann Allergy Asthma Immunol 83: 61–67.

13

Investigating International Time Trends in the Incidence and Prevalence of Atopic Eczema 1990–2010: A Systematic Review of Epidemiological Studies

Ivette A. G. Deckers[1,2]*, Susannah McLean[1], Sanne Linssen[2], Monique Mommers[2], C. P. van Schayck[3], Aziz Sheikh[1,2]

1 Allergy and Respiratory Research Group, Centre for Population Health Sciences, The University of Edinburgh, Edinburgh, United Kingdom, 2 CAPHRI, Department of Epidemiology, Maastricht University Medical Centre+, Maastricht, The Netherlands, 3 CAPHRI, Department of General Practice, Maastricht University Medical Centre+, Maastricht, The Netherlands

Abstract

The prevalence of atopic eczema has been found to have increased greatly in some parts of the world. Building on a systematic review of global disease trends in asthma, our objective was to study trends in incidence and prevalence of atopic eczema. Disease trends are important for health service planning and for generating hypotheses regarding the aetiology of chronic disorders. We conducted a systematic search for high quality reports of cohort, repeated cross-sectional and routine healthcare database-based studies in seven electronic databases. Studies were required to report on at least two measures of the incidence and/or prevalence of atopic eczema between 1990 and 2010 and needed to use comparable methods at all assessment points. We retrieved 2,464 citations, from which we included 69 reports. Assessing global trends was complicated by the use of a range of outcome measures across studies and possible changes in diagnostic criteria over time. Notwithstanding these difficulties, there was evidence suggesting that the prevalence of atopic eczema was increasing in Africa, eastern Asia, western Europe and parts of northern Europe (i.e. the UK). No clear trends were identified in other regions. There was inadequate study coverage worldwide, particularly for repeated measures of atopic eczema incidence. Further epidemiological work is needed to investigate trends in what is now one of the most common long-term disorders globally. A range of relevant measures of incidence and prevalence, careful use of definitions and description of diagnostic criteria, improved study design, more comprehensive reporting and appropriate interpretation of these data are all essential to ensure that this important field of epidemiological enquiry progresses in a scientifically robust manner.

Editor: Martyn Kirk, The Australian National University, Australia

Funding: The authors have no support or funding to report.

Competing Interests: The authors have declared that no competing interests exist.

* E-mail: Ivette.deckers@maastrichtuniversity.nl

Introduction

Atopic eczema is a very common inflammatory skin disorder [1]. Its prevalence appears to vary across the world as noted in key international epidemiological studies [2–5]. Such variation has been found in both children and adults and points to the likely importance of environmental risk factors. In addition, atopic eczema has been shown to cluster in families and there is growing evidence that it is an herald condition in many people who go on to develop allergic problems affecting other organ systems (e.g. food allergy) [6,7]. Genetics are important in the aetiology of atopic eczema: in particular, recent genetic epidemiological studies found a strong association between filaggrin gene defects (present in 1 in 10 Europeans and North Americans), and atopic eczema [7]. Filaggrin plays a role in maintaining the epidermal skin barrier function, whereby it helps to retain moisture in the skin and limits penetration by allergens. These functions can be impaired in filaggrin loss-of-function mutations, this resulting in dry, scaly skin, which increases the risk of allergic sensitisation and disease [7–9].

Monitoring disease trends over time aids aetiological understanding and helps with the planning of health services nationally and internationally. Building on our previous work on asthma, we sought to describe international trends in the incidence and prevalence of atopic eczema [10]. We aimed to draw preferentially on high quality studies using appropriate study designs and, in particular, studies using validated instruments [such as the International Study of Asthma and Allergies in Childhood (ISAAC) or the European Community Respiratory Health Survey (ECRHS)] [11,12].

Methods

This review is reported using the Preferred Reporting Items for Systematic Reviews and Meta-Analyses (PRISMA) statement as a guide (see Appendix S1) [13]. The methods for this review were specified in advance and documented in a study protocol.

Our full search strategy is given in Appendix S2. In short, we searched seven electronic databases, namely Medline, CINAHL, Embase, Global Health, Global Health Library, Google Scholar and Web of Knowledge, from 1 January 1990 to 19 May 2010 (date of last search). We used both Medical Subject Headings (MeSH) and free text terms of the following concepts: (atopic

Table 1. Inclusion criteria.

1. Epidemiological design (e.g. cohort, repeated cross-sectional or routine health care)
2. Estimates of eczema incidence and or prevalence at least twice within the period 1990–2010
3. Use of a comparable approach and instrument to measure eczema at each time point.

eczema OR atopic dermatitis) AND (cohort studies OR cross-sectional studies OR ISAAC OR ECRHS) AND (incidence OR prevalence OR trend). The searches were not limited by age, sex, ethnicity or language. Furthermore, bibliographies of key reports were scanned and a citation search was conducted for any additional papers of interest. We only included full-text reports of cohort studies, repeated cross-sectional surveys or analyses of routine healthcare datasets, as we considered these appropriate designs for the assessment of disease trends. Studies were required to present at least two estimates of atopic eczema incidence and/or prevalence within the period 1990 to 2010 and, at each assessment time point, they needed to use a similar approach and instrument (see Table 1). The screening of titles and abstracts and the eligibility assessment of full-text reports was independently performed by two reviewers. Disagreements were resolved by discussion or by a third reviewer if agreement could not be reached. Similarly, to establish the methodological quality of each study, the internal and external validity was examined using the Critical Appraisal Skills Programme (CASP) tool [14] and scored as 'good', 'moderate' or 'poor'. This methodological assessment included for example an appraisal of whether validated instruments were used [i.e. at least one of the ISAAC key questions (see Table 2)]. Reviewers were not masked when assessing study quality. Incidence and/or prevalence data as well as study and participant characteristics were extracted onto a customised data extraction sheet by one reviewer and thoroughly checked by the second reviewer.

To compare disease trends, our primary outcome measure was the lifetime prevalence of symptoms suggestive of atopic eczema or the incidence of atopic eczema (see Table 3). We also collected data on the secondary outcomes, such as the lifetime prevalence of physician-diagnosed eczema or 12-month prevalence measures. There was too much heterogeneity of populations studied and methods employed to undertake meta-analysis.

Results

Our searches retrieved 2,464 titles from which we identified 70 papers that satisfied our inclusion criteria (see Figure 1). We excluded one of these studies because the full-text paper was only available in Korean [15] and we were unable to procure a translation; there were therefore 69 papers in our final dataset. Data from included studies judged to be of moderate or good quality are summarised in Table 4 and explored descriptively by region (see Tables 5, 6, 7, 8 and 9) [16]. Data from the primary outcomes are additionally represented on a map (see Figure 2). Data from studies judged to be at greater risk of bias are available from the corresponding author [17–22]. Nearly all studies had prevalence data, while incidence data were only reported in three European studies [23–25]. Prevalence data are described using lifetime prevalence of atopic eczema symptoms.

Africa

As presented in Table 4, we found four studies on atopic eczema trends for Africa [26–29]. Incidence was not measured in any of these studies. Prevalence was measured based on parental- or self-report as assessed by ISAAC-based questions (see Table 5). Data were mainly from 13–14 year old children and in these children the general trend in Africa (Kenya, Morocco and South Africa) for the prevalence of atopic eczema was increasing [25,27,28] [26,27,29]. In these children, an approximate doubling of the lifetime prevalence of atopic eczema symptoms was found for Morocco [e.g. flexural rash in Marrakech, Morocco – from 9.9% (1995) to 20.9% (2001–02) [26], for South Africa [e.g. flexural rash – from 10.2% (1995) to 16.5% (2002)] [29] and for Kenya [e.g. itchy recurrent rash in flexural areas – from 11.4% (1995) to 19.8% (2001)] [27]. In Nigeria in children of this age group, the lifetime prevalence of itchy rash decreased from a high baseline prevalence [from 26.1% (1995) to 18.0% (2001–02)] [28]. Prevalence estimates in 2001–02 were, however, comparable for all countries. An approximate doubling was also seen in the lifetime prevalence of physician-diagnosed atopic eczema in 13–14 year olds in South Africa and Kenya [27,29]. In contrast, the prevalence of physician-diagnosed atopic eczema in Nigeria considerably decreased over a 5-year period from 1995 to 2001 in 6–7 year olds [from 9.4% to 6.8%] and in 13–14 year olds [from 38.4% to 19.4%] [28]. The baseline estimate for 13–14 year

Table 2. Key question for atopic eczema from the ISAAC questionnaire.

Have you *ever* had an itchy rash which was coming and going for at least six months?
Have you had this itchy rash at any time *in the last 12 months?*
Has this itchy rash *at any time* affected any of the following places: the folds of the elbows, behind the knees, in front of the ankles, under the buttocks, or around the neck, ears or eyes?
At what age did this itchy rash first occur; under 2 years, age 2-4 years or age 5 or more?
Has this rash cleared completely at any time *during the last 12 months?*
In the last 12 months, how often, on average, have you been kept awake at night by this itchy rash; never in the last 12 months, less than one night per week or one or more nights per week?
Have you *ever* had eczema?

Table 3. Primary and secondary outcomes measures.

Primary outcomes	Lifetime prevalence of atopic eczema symptoms
	Incidence of atopic eczema
Secondary outcomes	Lifetime prevalence of physician diagnosis of atopic eczema
	12-month prevalence of atopic eczema symptoms
	12-month prevalence of physician diagnosis of atopic eczema

olds was again extremely high. In other African countries, single estimates of atopic eczema prevalence may have been reported, but we were unable to locate any serial data on trends.

Asia

For Asia, we summarised 20 papers representing 61 measures of trends in Table 4. The majority of data came from eastern Asia [30–39], whereas south-eastern Asia [40–43] and western Asia [44–49] were represented to a lesser extent. For other regions in Asia, we found no relevant data. Here too no study assessed trends in incidence; rather, each study measured prevalence as based on parental- or self-report by questionnaires (see Tables 6). Trends were found for different age groups in 12 different countries and showed no overall pattern.

In eastern Asia, the general trend for atopic eczema prevalence was mainly increasing across different age groups. Lee et al. (2007) reported an increase in the sex- and age-standardised lifetime prevalence of ISAAC-based parental-report of atopic eczema symptoms in Taiwan among 12–15 year olds [from 2.4% (1995–96) to 4.0% (2001)] [32]. The lifetime prevalence of atopic eczema symptoms also increased in Korea in the same age group [from

7.2% (1995) to 9.3% (2000)] [36], in China (Guangzhou city) in a similar age group 13–14 [from 1.7% (1994–95) to 3.0% (2001)] [37] and in Japan in a wider-ranged age group 7–15 [from 10.1% (1996) to 13.6% (2006)] [39]. Moreover, baseline prevalences were low, but considerably higher in Korea and Japan, compared to Taiwan and China. In a slightly younger age group 6–12 in Korea, atopic eczema symptoms showed a modest increase from a substantially higher baseline prevalence [from 15.3% (1995) to 17.0% (2000)] [36]. In the youngest children aged 6–7, the prevalence of atopic eczema symptoms was stable in Hong Kong [e.g. chronic rash – from 5.7% (1995) to 5.4% (2001)] [31], whilst a modest increase was seen in a later study in Taiwan in a similar age group 6–8 [e.g. chronic rash - from 5.8% (2002) to 7.7% (2007)] [34]. Trends in the lifetime prevalence of physician-diagnosed atopic eczema followed nearly the same pattern as the lifetime prevalence of atopic eczema symptoms; trends were increasing in most countries among different age groups with only few exceptions.

In south-eastern Asia, the prevalence of different atopic eczema symptoms showed mixed trends. For chronic rash, the lifetime prevalence was stable in 6–7 year olds in Singapore [10.5% (1994) and 12.5% (2001)] [42] and in north-eastern Thailand [18.0%

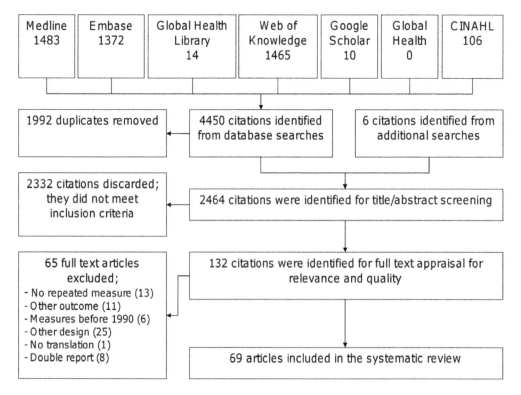

Figure 1. PRISMA flow diagram.

Table 4. Summary of trends in different atopic eczema outcomes between 1990 and 2010 by region*.

Region	Papers (n)	Trends (n)	Incidence			Lifetime prevalence						12-month prevalence					
						symptoms			diagnosis			symptoms			diagnosis		
			↑	↔	↓	↑	↔	↓	↑	↔	↓	↑	↔	↓	↑	↔	↓
Africa	4	20	0	0	0	9	0	1	2	0	2	4	1	1	0	0	0
Asia	20	61															
eastern	10	27	0	0	0	7	2	0	7	1	1	7	1	0	0	0	1
south-eastern	4	20	0	0	0	2	4	0	1	3	0	4	6	0	0	0	0
western	6	14	0	0	0	1	0	3	0	3	2	0	2	2	0	0	1
Americas	5	21															
North	0	0	0	0	0	0	0	0	0	0	0	0	0	0	0	0	0
Central	1	6	0	0	0	0	0	2	2	0	0	0	0	2	0	0	0
South	4	15	0	0	0	0	5	0	0	1	3	0	5	1	0	0	0
Europe	31	101															
western	10	42	1	1	0	4	2	0	12	5	0	4	9	0	0	0	4
southern	4	15	0	0	0	1	1	0	4	1	0	5	1	0	2	0	0
northern	15	41	1	1	0	9	1	1	15	1	0	8	2	1	0	1	0
eastern	2	3	0	0	0	0	0	0	1	2	0	0	0	0	0	0	0
Oceania	3	4	0	0	0	1	0	0	1	1	0	1	0	0	0	0	0

*Based on UN classification [16].

(1998–99) and 17.2% (2003)] [41]. Moreover, this prevalence also remained stable in older children (aged 12–15) in Singapore and, even though the baseline prevalence was appreciably lower, in 13–14 year olds in north-eastern Thailand. For chronic rash with a typical distribution, however, the lifetime prevalence was increasing in Singapore in children of both age groups [e.g. in 6–7 year olds – from 6.1% (1994) to 9.8% (2001)] [43]. In Malaysia and two specific geographical areas in Thailand (Chiang Mai and Bangkok) only data regarding the 12-month prevalence of atopic eczema symptoms were available [40,41]. In Malaysia and Chiang Mai, the 12-month prevalence of atopic eczema symptoms increased in 6–7 year olds, but was stable in 13–14 year olds, whereas the opposite was seen in Bangkok.

In western Asia, data were found for Georgia, Kuwait, Turkey and Israel [44–49]. In Georgia, the lifetime prevalence of atopic eczema symptoms was found to be decreasing in two different geographical areas among 6–7 year olds: in Tbilisi [from 4.5% (1996) to 3.4% (2003)] and in Kutaisi [from 5.2% (1996) to 2.4% (2003)] [44]. This trend was additionally apparent in the lifetime prevalence of physician-diagnosed atopic eczema in these children. There was also a decrease in the prevalence of atopic eczema symptoms in 13–14 year old children from Kuwait [from 17.5% (1995–96) to 10.6% (2001–02)], but the baseline prevalence was much higher [48]. In Israel, the lifetime prevalence of itchy rash in a distribution suggestive of atopic eczema was found to be increasing [from 5.9% (1997) to 8.7% (2003)] [49]. In Turkey, two measures of the prevalence of physician-diagnosed atopic eczema were reported. The lifetime prevalence was stable in 6–13 year old children [6.1% (1992) and 6.5% (2007)] [47], whilst the 12-month prevalence was reported to have decreased over a 15-year period in 7–12 year old children [from 4.0% (1992) to 1.2% (2007)] [46].

The Americas
We found no studies on atopic eczema trends for North America, one study for Central America [50] and four studies for South America [51–54] (see Table 4). No studies reported an incidence trend. The study from Central America, which was conducted in Mexico in 6–8 and 11–14 year old children (see Table 7) [50]. This study showed a sharply decreasing lifetime (and 12-month) prevalence of itchy rash in both age groups [e.g. in 6–8 year olds – from 15.0% (1995) to 7.3% (2002)] and, conversely, a from low baseline increasing lifetime prevalence of physician-diagnosed atopic eczema in both age groups [e.g. in 6–8 year olds – from 3.9% (1995) to 6.1% (2002)].

All four studies from South America were from Brazil and each study included only trends in prevalence as based on parental- or self-report by questionnaires (see Table 7) [51–54]. Two studies measured the lifetime prevalence of atopic eczema symptoms and showed a stable trend among 6–7 and 13–14 year olds [e.g. itchy rash in São Paulo in 6–7 year olds - 13.6% (1996) and 15.0% (1999)] [51,52]. In another study, the 12-month prevalence of itchy rash remained stable in children aged 13–14 years old [6.3% (1995) and 6.0% (2001)] [53], whereas in the last study both the lifetime prevalence of physician-diagnosed atopic eczema and the 12-month prevalence of atopic eczema symptoms were decreasing in 13–14 year olds across five centres [e.g. physician-diagnosed atopic eczema - from 5.3% (1994–95) to 4.5% (2001–03)] [54].

Europe
The largest set of reports (n = 31) on atopic eczema trends is for Europe. The majority of all trends were increasing, although decreasing and stable trends were found in some areas (see Table 4).

Incidence. Three studies reported on incidence trends in atopic eczema in Europe [23–25]. In Denmark, the adjusted cumulative incidence of the UK Working Party-based parental-report of physician-diagnosed atopic eczema in 7 year olds was 18.9% in 1993 and 19.6% in 1998 (see Table 8). Compared to the survey of 1993 the sample size was over nine times larger in the survey of 1998 [23]. Further, the cumulative incidence of parental-

Table 5. Good and moderate quality studies reporting the prevalence of parental- or self-report of atopic eczema between 1990 and 2010 in Africa.

Study	Geographic area	Age range (y)	Outcome	Time period	Baseline estimate N	Baseline estimate % (95%CI)/(SE)**	Final estimate N	Final estimate % (95%CI)/(SE)**	Summary measures	Conclusion	Quality
Measures of symptoms of atopic eczema											
Falade et al. (2009) [28]	Nigeria (Ibadan)	6–7	ISAAC-based parental-report of:	1995/2001–02	1,696		2,396		% change (S.E.)		Moderate
			lifetime prevalence of itchy rash			7.7 (0.7)		10.2 (0.6)	2.5 (0.9), P = 0.007	Increase	
			12-month prevalence of itchy rash			4.5 (0.5)		5.0 (0.5)	0.5 (0.7), P = 0.437	Stable	
Falade et al. (2009) [28]	Nigeria (Ibadan)	13–14	ISAAC-based parental-report of:	1995/2001–02	3,057		3,142		% change (S.E.)		Moderate
			lifetime prevalence of itchy rash			26.1 (0.8)		18.0 (0.7)	−8.1 (1.0), P<0.001	Decrease	
			12-month prevalence of itchy rash			17.7 (0.7)		7.7 (0.5)	−10.0 (0.8), P<0.001	Decrease	
Bouayad et al. (2006) [26]	Morocco (Casablanca)	13–14	ISAAC-based self-report of:	1995/2001–02	3,178		1,744		% change per year		Moderate
			lifetime prevalence of rash			20.5		34.2 (33.4–35.0)	2.28, P<0.001	Increase	
			lifetime prevalence of flexural rash			12.6		23.9 (23.2–24.6)	1.88, P<0.001	Increase	
			12-month prevalence of rash			14.2		26.1 (25.3–26.8)	1.98, P<0.001	Increase	
Bouayad et al. (2006) [26]	Morocco (Marrakech)	13–14	ISAAC-based self-report of:	1995/2001–02	2,896		1,677		% change per year		Moderate
			lifetime prevalence of rash			20.4		33.9 (33.1–34.7)	2.20, P<0.001	Increase	
			lifetime prevalence of flexural rash			9.9		20.9 (20.2–21.7)	1.79, P<0.001	Increase	
			12-month prevalence of rash			13.1		23.1 (22.3–23.8)	1.63, P<0.001	Increase	
Esamai et al. (2002) [27]	Kenya (Uasin Gishu)	13–14	ISAAC-based self-report of:	1995/2001	3,018		3,258				Moderate
			lifetime prevalence of itchy recurrent rash			23.8		28.5	P = 0.001	Increase	
			lifetime prevalence of itchy recurrent rash in flexural areas			11.4		19.8	P = 0.001	Increase	
			12-month prevalence itchy recurrent rash			14.4		21.3	P = 0.001	Increase	
Zar et al. (2007) [29]	South Africa (Cape Town)	13–14	ISAAC-based self-report of:	1995/2002	5,161		5,019		OR (95%CI)		Moderate
			lifetime prevalence of itchy rash			15.5		26.2	1.93 (1.75–2.14), P<0.001	Increase	
			lifetime prevalence of flexural rash			10.2		16.5	1.75 (1.56–1.97), P<0.001	Increase	
			12-month prevalence itchy rash			11.8		19.4	1.77 (1.56–1.97), P<0.001	Increase	
Measures of physician-diagnosed atopic eczema											
Falade et al. (2009) [28]	Nigeria (Ibadan)	6–7	ISAAC-based parental-report of:	1995/2001–02	1,696		2,396		% change (S.E.)		Moderate
			lifetime prevalence of physician-diagnosed atopic eczema			9.4 (0.7)		6.8 (0.5)	−2.6 (0.9), P = 0.003	Decrease	
Falade et al. (2009) [28]	Nigeria (Ibadan)	13–14	ISAAC-based self-report of:	1995/2001–02	3,057		3,142		% change (S.E.)		Moderate

Table 5. Cont.

Study	Geographic area	Age range (y)	Outcome	Time period	Baseline estimate N	Baseline estimate % (95%CI)/(SE)**	Final estimate N	Final estimate % (95%CI)/(SE)**	Summary measures	Conclusion	Quality
			lifetime prevalence of physician-diagnosed atopic eczema			38.4 (0.9)		19.4 (0.7)	−19.0 (1.1), P<0.001	Decrease	Moderate
Esamai et al. (2002) [27]	Kenya (Uasin Gishu)	13–14	ISAAC-based self-report of: lifetime prevalence of atopic eczema	1995/2001	3,018	13.9	3,258	28.5	P=0.001	Increase	
Zar et al. (2007) [29]	South Africa (Cape Town)	13–14	ISAAC-based self-report of: lifetime prevalence of physician-diagnosed atopic eczema	1995/2002	5,161	9.6	5,019	16.7	OR (95% CI) 1.88 (1.67–2.12), P<0.001	Increase	Moderate

Abbreviations – CI: confidence intervals; SE: standard error; OR: odds ratio.
*Based on UN classification [16].
**95% CI and SE are only reported if included in original report.

report of history of physician-diagnosed atopic eczema in 5–6 year olds was stable in West Germany [12.5% (1991) and 12.8% (1997)], whilst it increased sharply in East Germany [from 9.6% (1991) to 23.4% (1997)] [24]. Finally, the age- and sex-standardised incidence of physicians' recorded atopic eczema diagnosis as based on secondary analysis of QRESEARCH, a large primary care dataset (n = 333,294) in England, increased from 9.6% (2001) to 13.6% (2005) per 1000 patient-years [25].

Prevalence. Prevalence data on trends in atopic eczema for western Europe are shown in Table 9 [24,55–63]. Parental- and self-report of atopic eczema symptoms were reported in five countries [55,56,59,60,62,63]. The lifetime prevalence of atopic eczema symptoms increased in 5–7 year old children in Switzerland [from 11.7% (1992) to 17.4% (2001)] [56] and in slightly older children (aged 6–9) in Austria, but from a lower baseline [from 9.2% (1995–97) to 11.0% (2001–03)] [63]. This lifetime prevalence of atopic eczema symptoms also increased in Belgium, both in boys and girls aged 6–7 [e.g. in boys - from 12.9% (1995–96) to 18.4% (2002)], whilst in 13–14 year old boys and girls it remained stable [e.g. in boys −15.7% (1995–96) and 13.3% (2002)] [62]. We found no data on the lifetime prevalence of atopic eczema symptoms for Germany and France. In France, the lifetime prevalence of physician-diagnosed atopic eczema increased in 13–14 year olds [from 25.8% (1995) to 30.4% (2002)] [55]. In Germany (Münster), this prevalence also increased in 13–14 year olds [e.g. in boys - from 8.2% (1994–95) to 10.9% (1999–2000)], whilst it showed a stable trend in 6–7 year olds [e.g. in boys −14.3% (1994–95) and 13.6% (1999–2000)] [60].

In southern Europe, the lifetime prevalence of atopic eczema symptoms remained stable in the Maltese Islands in 5–8 year olds [7.0% (1994–95) and 6.7% (2001–02)] [64] and increased in Greece in older children (aged 8–10) [from 4.5% (1991) to 9.5% (2003)] [65]. Here, the trend was measured over a longer time period and started at a lower baseline level. In Italy and Portugal, no lifetime prevalence trends for atopic eczema symptoms were reported. The lifetime prevalence of physician-diagnosed atopic eczema showed an increasing trend in 6–7 year olds in Italy [from 14.3% (1994–95) to 17.0% (2002)] [66] and in the same age group in Portugal [from 18.6% (1993–94) to 21.0% (2002)] [67]. Compared to Italy and Portugal, the increase of physician-diagnosed atopic eczema in the Maltese Islands in a similar age group of 5–8 year olds was considerably larger and more than doubled over a 7-year period, as it originated from a low baseline [from 4.4% (1994–95) to 11.2% (2001–02)] [64].

For northern Europe, 15 papers reported on trends in atopic eczema [23,25,68–80]. The prevalence of rash and rash with a typical distribution was overall increasing in boys and girls and in 6–7 and 13–14 year olds in the UK [e.g. in 6–7 year old boys – from 17.8% (1995–96) to 21.0% (2001–02)], although not all trends reached significance [80]. Several other studies, which measured the lifetime prevalence of physician-diagnosed atopic eczema [68,71,75–77] or the lifetime prevalence of physicians' recorded atopic eczema diagnosis [25,73] in the UK, also showed increasing trends confirming patterns of atopic eczema prevalence in the UK in children and across all age-groups over time. An increasing trend for atopic eczema symptoms was also found in Estonia in 6–7 year olds [from 16.9% (1993–94) to 22.0% (2001–02)] [69]. However, in Sweden in slightly older children (aged 7–8), the lifetime prevalence of atopic eczema symptoms was decreasing [from 29.3% (1996) to 26.5% (2006)] [78]. Despite this decrease, prevalence estimates remained higher as compared to Estonia. There was no data on the lifetime prevalence of atopic eczema symptoms available in Lithuania and Norway. In Lithuania in 6–7 year olds, the prevalence of physician-diagnosed

Table 6. Good and moderate quality studies reporting the prevalence of parental- or self-report of atopic eczema between 1990 and 2010 in Asia.

Study	Geographic area	Age range (y)	Outcome	Time period	Baseline estimate N	Baseline estimate % (95%CI)/(SE)**	Final estimate N	Final estimate % (95%CI)/(SE)**	Summary measures	Conclusion	Quality
Eastern Asia*											
Measures of symptoms of atopic eczema											
Liao MF et al. (2009) [34]	Central Taiwan (Changhwa County)	6-8	ISAAC-based parental-report of:	2002/2007	7,040		4,622		POR (95% CI)		Good
			lifetime prevalence of chronic rash			5.8		7.7	1.39 (1.20-1.61), P<0.001	Increase	
			lifetime prevalence of chronic rash with typical distribution			5.9		8.9	1.56 (1.34-1.83), P<0.001	Increase	
			12-month prevalence of chronic rash			7.0		9.7	1.45 (1.25-1.67), P<0.001	Increase	
Liao PF et al. (2009) [35]	Taiwan	6-15	ISAAC-based parental-report of:	1994/2002	75,960		11,580		No formal test		Moderate
			12-month prevalence of current atopic eczema symptoms			1.5		2.8	—	Increase	
Lee et al. (2007) [32]	Taiwan	12-15	ISAAC-based parental-report of:	1995-96/2001	42,919		10,215		Adjusted PR (95% CI)		Good
			Sex- and age-standardised lifetime prevalence of atopic eczema symptoms			2.4		4.0	1.61 (1.42-1.81), P<0.001	Increase	
Yan et al. (2005) [38]	Taiwan (Taipei)	13-14	ISAAC-based self-report of:	1994-95/2001-02	11,400		6,303				Moderate
			12-month prevalence of recurrent itchy rash in a typical distribution			1.4 (1.1-1.6)		4.1 (3.6-4.6)	P<0.001	Increase	
Lee et al. (2004) [31]	China (Hong Kong)	6-7	ISAAC-based parental-report of:	1995/2001	3,618		4,448		OR (95% CI)		Moderate
			lifetime prevalence of chronic rash			5.7		5.4	0.95 (0.79-1.15), P=0.56	Stable	
			lifetime prevalence of chronic rash at typical areas			4.2		3.6	0.85 (0.68-1.07), P=0.18	Stable	
			12-month prevalence of chronic rash			4.2		4.2	1.00 (0.80-1.25), P=1.00	Stable	
Wang et al. (2006) [37]	China (Guangzhou city)	13-14	ISAAC-based self-report of:	1994-95/2001	3,855		3,516				Moderate
			lifetime prevalence of flexural atopic eczema symptoms			1.7 (1.3-2.1)		3.0 (2.4-3.6)	P<0.05	Increase	
			12-month prevalence of flexural atopic eczema symptoms			1.3 (0.9-1.7)		2.2 (1.7-2.7)	P=0.002	Increase	
Oh et al. (2004) [36]	Korea	6-12	ISAAC-based parental-report of:	1995/2000	25,361		27,425		No formal test		Moderate
			lifetime prevalence of itchy atopic eczema symptoms			15.3 (14.9-15.8)		17.0 (16.5-17.4)		Increase	
			12-month prevalence of itchy flexural atopic eczema symptoms			7.3 (7.0-7.6)		10.7 (10.4-11.1)		Increase	

Table 6. Cont.

Study	Geographic area	Age range (y)	Outcome	Time period	Baseline estimate N	Baseline estimate % (95%CI)/(SE)**	Final estimate N	Final estimate % (95%CI)/(SE)**	Summary measures	Conclusion	Quality
Oh et al. (2004) [36]	Korea	12–15	ISAAC-based parental-report of:	1995/2000	15,068		14,777		No formal test		Moderate
			lifetime prevalence of itchy atopic eczema symptoms			7.2 (6.8–7.7)		9.3 (8.8–9.8)		Increase	
			12-month prevalence of itchy flexural atopic eczema symptoms			3.9 (3.6–4.3)		6.1 (5.7–6.5)		Increase	
Kusunoki et al. (2009) [30]	Japan (Kyoto)	7–15	Parental-report of:	1996/2006	16,176		13,215				Moderate
			lifetime prevalence of symptoms of atopic dermatitis			10.1		13.6	P<0.0001	Increase	
			12-month prevalence of symptoms of atopic dermatitis			4.2		5.6	P<0.0001	Increase	
Measures of physician-diagnosed atopic eczema											
Liao MF et al. (2009) [34]	Taiwan (Changhwa County)	6–8	ISAAC-based parental-report of:	2002/2007	7,040		4,622		POR (95% CI)		Good
			lifetime prevalence of physician-diagnosed atopic eczema			18.0		23.9	1.44 (1.31–1.57), P<0.001	Increase	
Liao PF et al. (2009) [35]	Taiwan	6–15	ISAAC-based parental-report of:	1994/2002	75,960		11,580		No formal test		Moderate
			lifetime prevalence of atopic eczema			1.9		3.4		Increase	
Lee et al. (2005) [33]	Taiwan	12–15	ISAAC-based parental-report of:	1995–96/2001	44,104		11,048		No formal test		Moderate
			lifetime prevalence of physician-diagnosed atopic eczema			1.6		2.8		Increase	
Yan et al. (2005) [38]	Taiwan (Taipei)	13–14	ISAAC-based self-report of:	1994–95/2001–02	11,400		6,303				Moderate
			lifetime prevalence of atopic eczema			11.8 (11.2–12.4)		17.4 (16.4–18.3)	P<0.001	Increase	
Lee et al. (2004) [31]	China (Hong Kong)	6–7	ISAAC-based parental-report of:	1995/2001	3,618		4,448		OR (95% CI)		Moderate
			lifetime prevalence of atopic eczema			28.1		30.7	1.13 (1.03–1.25), P=0.01	Increase	
Wang et al. (2006) [37]	China (Guangzhou city)	13–14	ISAAC-based self-report of:	1994–95/2001	3,855		3,516				Moderate
			lifetime prevalence of physician-diagnosed atopic eczema			18.3 (17.1–19.5)		17.6 (16.3–18.9)	P=0.462	Stable	
Oh et al. (2004) [36]	Korea	6–12	ISAAC-based parental-report of:	1995/2000	25,361		27,425		No formal test		Moderate
			lifetime prevalence of physician-diagnosed atopic eczema			16.6 (16.2–17.1)		24.9 (24.4–25.4)		Increase	

Table 6. Cont.

Study	Geographic area	Age range (y)	Outcome	Time period	Baseline estimate N	% (95%CI)/(SE)**	Final estimate N	% (95%CI)/(SE)**	Summary measures	Conclusion	Quality
Oh et al. (2004) [36]	Korea	12–15	ISAAC-based parental-report of:	1995/2000	15,068		14,777		No formal test		Moderate
			lifetime prevalence of physician-diagnosed atopic eczema			7.3 (6.9–7.7)		12.8 (12.3–13.3)		Increase	
Yura et al. (2001) [39]	Japan (Osake Prefecture)	7–12	Parental-report of:	1993/1997	514,656		458,284		No formal test		Moderate
			lifetime prevalence of physician-diagnosed atopic dermatitis			24.1		22.9		Decrease	
			12-month prevalence of physician-diagnosed atopic dermatitis			6.8		5.7		Decrease	
South-eastern Asia*											
Measures of symptoms of atopic eczema											
Wang et al. (2004) [43]	Singapore	6–7	ISAAC-based parental-report of:	1994/2001	2,030		5,305		% Change (S.E.)		Good
			lifetime prevalence of chronic rash			10.5 (1.2)		12.5 (0.5)	2.0 (1.3), P=0.194	Stable	
			lifetime prevalence of chronic rash with typical distribution			6.1 (0.9)		9.8 (0.4)	3.7 (1.0), P=0.028	Increase	
			12-month prevalence of chronic rash			8.9 (1.1)		11.0 (0.4)	2.1 (1.2), P=0.155	Stable	
Wang et al. (2004) [43]	Singapore	12–15	ISAAC-based parental-report of:	1994/2001	4,208		4,058		% Change (S.E.)		Good
			lifetime prevalence of chronic rash			12.3 (0.5)		14.9 (0.6)	2.6 (0.8), P=0.056	Stable	
			lifetime prevalence of chronic rash with typical distribution			7.0 (0.4)		10.2 (0.5)	3.2 (0.6), P<0.001	Increase	
			12-month prevalence of chronic rash			9.5 (0.5)		11.6 (0.5)	2.1 (0.7), P=0.034	Increase	
Quah et al. (2005) [40]	Malaysia (Kota Bharu)	6–7	ISAAC-based parental-report of:	1995/2001	3,939		3,157		% Change (95% CI)		Good
			12-month prevalence of flexural itchy rash			14.0		17.6	3.6 (1.3–5.9), P=0.004	Increase	
Quah et al. (2005) [40]	Malaysia (Kota Bharu)	13–14	ISAAC-based parental-report of:	1995/2001	3,116		3,004		% Change (95% CI)		Good
			12-month prevalence of flexural itchy rash			12.1		13.4	1.3 (-4.6–7.1), P=0.11	Stable	
Trakultivakorn et al. (2007) [42]	Thailand (Chiang Mai)	6–7	ISAAC-based parental-report of:	1995/2001	3,828		3,106				Moderate
			12-month prevalence of atopic eczema symptoms			11.4		16.3	P<0.01	Increase	
Trakultivakorn et al. (2007) [42]	Thailand (Bangkok)	6–7	ISAAC-based parental-report of:	1995/2001	3,628		3,430				Moderate
			12-month prevalence of atopic eczema symptoms			12.5		13.3	P=0.33	Stable	

Table 6. Cont.

Study	Geographic area	Age range (y)	Outcome	Time period	Baseline estimate N	Baseline estimate % (95%CI)/(SE)**	Final estimate N	Final estimate % (95%CI)/(SE)**	Summary measures	Conclusion	Quality
Teeratakulpisarn et al. (2004) [41]	Thailand (Northeast)	6–7	parental-report of:	1998-99/2003	2,658		2,119		No formal test		Moderate
			lifetime prevalence of rash			18.0		17.2		Stable	
			12-month prevalence of rash			15.2		14.7		Stable	
Trakultivakorn et al. (2007) [41]	Thailand (Chiang Mai)	13–14	ISAAC-based parental-report of:	1995/2001	3,927		3,538				Moderate
			12-month prevalence of atopic eczema symptoms			9.6		8.6	P = 0.63	Stable	
Trakultivakorn et al. (2007) [41]	Thailand (Bangkok)	13–14	ISAAC-based parental-report of:	1995/2001	3,713		4,669				Moderate
			12-month prevalence of atopic eczema symptoms			6.8		10.4	P<0.01	Increase	
Teeratakulpisarn et al. (2004) [41]	Thailand (Northeast)	13–14	parental-report of:	1998-99/2003	3,410		2,956		No formal test		Moderate
			lifetime prevalence of rash			9.9		10.9		Stable	
			12-month prevalence of rash			7.4		8.7		Stable	
Measures of physician-diagnosed atopic eczema											
Wang et al. (2004) [43]	Singapore	6–7	ISAAC-based parental-report of:	1994/2001	2,030		5,305		% Change (S.E.)		Good
			lifetime prevalence of physician-diagnosed atopic eczema			3.0 (0.7)		8.8 (0.4)	5.8 (0.8), P<0.001	Increase	
Wang et al. (2004) [43]	Singapore	12–15	ISAAC-based parental-report of:	1994/2001	4,208		4,058		% Change (S.E.)		Good
			lifetime prevalence of physician-diagnosed atopic eczema			4.1 (0.3)		5.8 (0.4)	1.7 (0.5), P = 0.810	Stable	
Teeratakulpisarn et al. (2004) [41]	Thailand (Northeast)	6–7	Parental-report of:	1998-99/2003	2,658		2,119		No formal test		Moderate
			lifetime prevalence of atopic eczema			30.5		29.2		Stable	
Teeratakulpisarn et al. (2004) [41]	Thailand (Northeast)	13–14	Self-report of:	1998-99/2003	3,410		2,956		No formal test		Moderate
			lifetime prevalence of atopic eczema			24.4		26.8		Stable	
Western Asia*											
Measures of symptoms of atopic eczema											
Abramidze et al. (2006) [44]	Georgia (Tbilisi)	6–7	ISAAC-based parental-report of:	1996/2003	6,770		6,002		% Change		Moderate
			lifetime prevalence of symptoms of flexural dermatitis			4.5		3.4	−1.1, P<0.05	Decrease	
			current prevalence of itchy rash			5.3		5.8	0.5, P = not significant	Stable	

Table 6. Cont.

Study	Geographic area	Age range (y)	Outcome	Time period	Baseline estimate N	Baseline estimate % (95%CI)/(SE)**	Final estimate N	Final estimate % (95%CI)/(SE)**	Summary measures	Conclusion	Quality
Abramidze et al. (2006) [44]	Georgia (Kutaisi)	6–7	ISAAC-based parental-report of:	1996/2003					% Change		Moderate
			lifetime prevalence of symptoms of flexural dermatitis			5.2		2.4	−2.8, P<0.05	Decrease	
			current prevalence of itchy rash			6.1		3.4	−2.7, P<0.05	Decrease	
Abramidze et al. (2007) [45]	Georgia (Tbilisi and Kutaisi)	13–14	ISAAC-based self-report of:	1996/2003	6,746		5,653		% Change		Moderate
			current prevalence of itchy rash			4.1		4.3	0.2, P=not significant	Stable	
Owayed et al. (2008) [48]	Kuwait	13–14	ISAAC-based self-report of:	1995–96/2001–02	3,110		2,822		% Change		Moderate
			lifetime prevalence itchy rash			17.5 (16.2–18.8)		10.6 (9.5–11.7)	P<0.001	Decrease	
			12-month prevalence of itchy rash			12.6 (11.4–13.8)		8.3 (7.3–9.3)	P<0.001	Decrease	
Romano-Zelekha et al. (2007) [49]	Israel	13–14	ISAAC-based self-report of:	1997/2003	10,057		8,978				Moderate
			lifetime prevalence of itchy rash in a typical distribution			5.9		8.7	P<0.05	Increase	

Measures of physician-diagnosed atopic eczema

Study	Geographic area	Age range (y)	Outcome	Time period	Baseline estimate N	Baseline estimate % (95%CI)/(SE)**	Final estimate N	Final estimate % (95%CI)/(SE)**	Summary measures	Conclusion	Quality
Abramidze et al. (2006) [44]	Georgia (Tbilisi)	6–7	ISAAC-based parental-report of:	1996/2003	6,770		6,002		% Change		Moderate
			lifetime prevalence of physician-diagnosed atopic eczema			11.6		3.6	−8, P<0.05	Decrease	
Abramidze et al. (2006) [44]	Georgia (Kutaisi)	6–7	ISAAC-based parental-report of:	1996/2003					% Change		Moderate
			lifetime prevalence of physician-diagnosed atopic eczema			4.7		1.8	−2.9, P<0.05	Decrease	
Abramidze et al. (2007) [45]	Georgia (Tbilisi and Kutaisi)	13–14	ISAAC-based self-report of:	1996/2003	6,746		5,653		% Change		Moderate
			lifetime prevalence of physician-diagnosed atopic eczema			3.0		2.6	−0.4, P=not significant	Stable	
Owayed et al. (2008) [48]	Kuwait	13–14	ISAAC-based self-report of:	1995–96/2001–02	3,110		2,822		P=0.101		Moderate
			lifetime prevalence of physician-diagnosed atopic eczema			11.3 (10.2–12.4)		12.8 (11.6–14)		Stable	
Kalyoncu et al. (1999) [47]	Turkey (Ankara)	6–13	ISAAC-based self-report of:	1992/1997	1,036		738		P=not significant		Moderate
			lifetime prevalence of physician-diagnosed atopic dermatitis			6.1 (4.7–7.7)		6.5 (4.8–8.5)		Stable	
Demir et al. (2010) Turkey (Ankara) [46]		7–12	Parental-report of:	1992/2007	1,036		442		Adjusted POR		Moderate

Table 6. Cont.

Study	Geographic area	Age range (y)	Time period	Baseline estimate N	Baseline estimate % (95%CI)/(SE)**	Final estimate N	Final estimate % (95%CI)/(SE)**	Summary measures % (95%CI)/(SE)**	Conclusion	Quality
			current prevalence of atopic eczema		4.0 (2.8–5.2)		1.2 (0.2–2.2)	0.4 (0.2–1.0), P trend = 0.004	Decrease	

Abbreviations – CI: confidence intervals, SE: standard error, OR: odds ratio, POR: prevalence odds ratio, PR: prevalence ratio.
*Based on UN classification [16].
**95% CI or SE are only reported if included in original report.
#Point estimate extracted from graph or chart.

atopic eczema was increasing from an extremely low baseline [from 1.4% (1994–95) to 3.5% (2002–03)] [72]. In Norway, this prevalence was stable in 9–11 year olds [21.1% (1995) and 20.8% (2000)] [79].

Two studies yielded relevant data in relation to eastern Europe. In Poland, the lifetime prevalence of parental-reported physician-diagnosed atopic eczema increase over a decade in children aged 7–10 [from 2.3% (1993) to 8.1% (2002)] [81]. Later, this same prevalence, measured with a different questionnaire in both 7–9 and 7–14 year olds, remained stable in Hungary over a relatively short time period [e.g. for 7–9 year olds –15.1% (2002) and 17.1% (2005)] [82]. In Europe, there were many other countries with single measurements of any atopic eczema outcome, but serial data were not yet available.

Oceania

For Oceania, we found three papers from Australia with prevalence data on atopic eczema trends (see Table 4) [83–85]. As shown in Table 10, the lifetime prevalence of atopic eczema symptoms was measured in Melbourne in 6–7 year olds, where it markedly increased from 22.6% in 1993 to 32.3% in 2002 [84]. Two other studies measured trends in lifetime prevalence of atopic eczema diagnosis. In one study this was increasing in 4–6 year olds, even though the baseline prevalence was high [from 31.0% (2000) to 37.0% (2005)] [83] and in another study, using a non-validated questionnaire, it was stable in 8–11 year olds [85].

Discussion

The considerable body of international literature identified by this systematic review was heterogeneous in many respects rendering it difficult to directly compare different regions. That said, there was no obvious consistent overall global trend in the incidence or prevalence of atopic eczema symptoms and diagnosis. Nevertheless, in Africa and eastern Asia there was an increasing trend for both the lifetime prevalence of parental- and self-reported atopic eczema symptoms and physician-diagnosed atopic eczema. In western Europe and parts of northern Europe (i.e. the UK), these trends were also mainly increasing. There were extremely diverse trends among different age groups and countries in south-eastern Asia, western Asia and southern Europe. In addition, data for the Americas, eastern Europe and Oceania were limited. The heterogeneous findings in some regions and the limited data available for other regions have precluded conclusions regarding a global atopic eczema trend and atopic eczema trends in major parts of the world.

We found that many outcome measures are used across studies to determine changes in atopic eczema prevalence. Although we found that trends of all outcomes generally pointed in the same direction, we considered the lifetime prevalence of parental- or self-report of atopic eczema symptoms the optimal outcome for the purpose of comparing disease trends between regions within our highly heterogeneous dataset. As atopic eczema occurs in episodes and may be season-related it is particularly difficult to compare studies measuring current or 12-month symptomatology or if patient- and/or study- characteristics, such as age group, do not match. Furthermore, there are marked differences per region in current medical practice, including prevention strategies, national guidelines and physician's awareness of the problem, that make prevalence estimates and trends of physician-diagnosed atopic eczema difficult to compare across the globe. Even though the diagnostic process of a physician is overall likely to be standardised, there is no objective gold standard. This is highlighted in the ENRIECO project which shows that different countries use

Table 7. Good and moderate quality studies reporting the prevalence of parental- or self-report of atopic eczema between 1990 and 2010 in the Americas.

Study	Geographic area	Age range (y)	Outcome	Time period	Baseline estimate N	Baseline estimate % (95%CI)/ (SE)**	Final estimate N	Final estimate % (95%CI)/(SE)**	Summary measures	Conclusion	Quality
Central America *											
Measures of symptoms of atopic eczema											
Barraza-villareal et al. (2007) [50]	Mexico (Cuernavaca)	6–8	ISAAC-based parental-report of:	1995/2002	2,770		2,633				Good
			lifetime prevalence of dry itchy skin spots			15.0 (13.8–16.4)		7.3 (6.3–8.4)	P = 0.000	Decrease	
			12-month prevalence of dry itchy skin spots			10.1 (9.1–11.3)		5.8 (4.9–6.8)	P = 0.000	Decrease	
Barraza-villareal et al. (2007) [50]	Mexico (Cuernavaca)	11–14	ISAAC-based parental-report of:	1995/2002	2,795		2,605				Good
			lifetime prevalence of dry itchy skin spots			17.0 (15.6–18.4)		7.0 (6.0–8.1)	P = 0.000	Decrease	
			12-month prevalence of dry itchy skin spots			10.5 (9.5–11.7)		5.4 (4.5–6.3)	P = 0.000	Decrease	
Measures of physician-diagnosed atopic eczema											
Barraza-villareal et al. (2007) [50]	Mexico (Cuernavaca)	6–8	ISAAC-based parental-report of:	1995/2002	2,770		2,633				Good
			lifetime prevalence of physician-diagnosed atopic eczema			3.9 (3.2–4.7)		6.1 (5.2–7.2)	P = 0.000	Increase	
Barraza-villareal et al. (2007) [50]	Mexico (Cuernavaca)	11–14	ISAAC-based parental-report of:	1995/2002	2,795		2,605				Good
			lifetime prevalence of physician-diagnosed atopic eczema			4.2 (3.5–5.0)		6.9 (6.0–8.0)	P = 0.000	Increase	
South America *											
Measures of symptoms of atopic eczema											
Camelo-Nunes et al. (2004) [52]	Brazil (São Paulo)	6–7	ISAAC-based parental-report of:	1996/1999	3,005		3,033				Moderate
			lifetime prevalence of itchy rash			13.6		15.0	P = not significant	Stable	
			lifetime prevalence of lesions in skin-folds			7.5		6.6	P = not significant	Stable	
			12-month prevalence of itchy rash			10.6		9.9	P = not significant	Stable	
Camelo-Nunes et al. (2004) [52]	Brazil (São Paulo)	13–14	ISAAC-based self-report of:	1996/1999	3,008		3,487				Moderate
			lifetime prevalence of itchy rash			12.6		14.0	P = not significant	Stable	
			lifetime prevalence of lesions in skin-folds			4.8		4.6	P = not significant	Stable	
			12-month prevalence of itchy rash			8.1		8.8	P = not significant	Stable	
Borges et al. (2008) [51]	Brazil (Federal district of Brasilia)	13–14	ISAAC-based self-report of:	1996/2002	3,254		3,009				Moderate
			lifetime prevalence of itchy rash			15.5		16.8	P = 0.185	Stable	

Table 7. Cont.

Study	Geographic area	Age range (y)	Outcome	Time period	Baseline estimate N	Baseline estimate % (95%CI)/(SE)**	Final estimate N	Final estimate % (95%CI)/(SE)**	Summary measures	Conclusion	Quality
			12-month prevalence of itchy rash			9.2		10.2	P=0.202	Stable	
Solé et al (2007) [54]	Brazil (5 centres)	13-14	ISAAC-based self-report of:	1994-95/2001-03	15,419		15,684		OR (95% CI)		Moderate
			12-month prevalence of itchy rash			10.3		8.4	0.80 (0.74–0.86), P<0.05	Decrease, not uniform among centres	
Riedi et al. (2005) [53]	Brazil (Curitiba)	13-14	ISAAC-based self-report of:	1995/2001	3,008		3,628				Moderate
			12-month prevalence of Itchy rash			6.3		6.0	P=not significant	Stable	
			12-month prevalence of Intermittent itchy rash in skin creases			3.7		3.7	P=not significant	Stable	

Measures of physician-diagnosed atopic eczema

Study	Geographic area	Age range (y)	Outcome	Time period	Baseline estimate N	Baseline estimate % (95%CI)/(SE)**	Final estimate N	Final estimate % (95%CI)/(SE)**	Summary measures	Conclusion	Quality
Camelo-Nunes et al. (2004) [52]	Brazil (São Paulo)	6-7	ISAAC-based parental-report of:	1996/1999	3,005		3,033				Moderate
			lifetime prevalence of physician-diagnosed atopic eczema			13.2		11.4	P<0.05	Decrease	
Camelo-Nunes et al (2004) [52]	Brazil (São Paulo)	13-14	ISAAC-based parental-report of:	1996/1999	3,008		3,487				Moderate
			lifetime prevalence of physician-diagnosed atopic eczema			14.0		15.0	P=not significant	Stable	
Borges et al. (2008) [51]	Brazil (Federal district of Brasilia)	13-14	ISAAC-based self-report of:	1996/2002	3,254		3,009				Moderate
			lifetime prevalence of physician-diagnosed atopic eczema			9.8		13.6	P=0.0002	Decrease	
Solé et al (2007) [54]	Brazil (5 centres)	13-14	ISAAC-based self-report of:	1994-95/2001-03	15,419		15,684		OR (95% CI)		Moderate
			lifetime prevalence of physician-diagnosed atopic eczema			5.3		4.5	0.84 (0.76–0.93), P<0.05	Decrease, not uniform among centres	

Abbreviations – CI: confidence intervals, SE: standard error, OR: odds ratio.

*Based on UN classification [16].

**95% CI and SE are only reported if included in original report.

Table 8. Good and moderate quality studies reporting the incidence of parental- or self-report of atopic eczema between 1990 and 2010 in Europe.

Study	Geographic area	Age range (y)	Outcome	Time period	Baseline estimate N	Baseline estimate % (95%CI)/(SE)**	Final estimate N	Final estimate % (95%CI)/(SE)**	Summary measures	Conclusion	Quality
Schäfer et al. (2000) [24]	Germany (west)	5–6	Parental-report of:	1991/1997	4,001		4,001		No formal test		Moderate
			cumulative incidence of history of physician-diagnosed atopic eczema			12.5		12.8		Stable	
Schäfer et al. (2000) [24]	Germany (east)	5–6	Parental-report of:	1991/1997					No formal test		Moderate
			cumulative incidence of history of physician-diagnosed atopic eczema			16.0		23.4		Increase	
Olesen et al. (2005) [23]	Denmark	7	UK working party-based parental-report of:	1993/1998	1,060		9,744		No formal test		Moderate
			adjusted cumulative incidence of physician-diagnosed atopic dermatitis			18.9		19.6		Stable	
Simpson et al. (2009) [25]	UK	all	QRESEARCH-based physicians' recorded:	2001–05	>30 million py		>30 million py		Relative % Change		Moderate
			age- and sex-standardised incidence of atopic eczema diagnosis (per 1000 patient years (py))			9.6 (9.5–9.7)		13.6 (13.5–13.7)	41.8, P<0.001	Increase	

Abbreviations – CI: confidence intervals, SE: standard error.
*Based on UN classification [16].
**95% CI and SE are only reported if included in original report.

Table 9. Good and moderate quality studies reporting the incidence and prevalence of parental- or self-report of atopic eczema between 1990 and 2010 in Europe.

Study	Geographic area	Age range (y)	Outcome	Time period	Baseline estimate N	% (95%CI)/(SE)**	Final estimate N	% (95%CI)/(SE)**	Summary measures	Conclusion	Quality
Western Europe*											
Measures of symptoms of atopic eczema											
Grize et al. (2006) [56]	Switzerland	5–7	ISAAC-based parental-report of:	1992/2001	988		1,274				Good
			adjusted lifetime prevalence of skin rash			11.7 (9.7–14.0)		17.4 (15.3–19.7)	P=0.0014	Increase	
			adjusted 12-month prevalence of atopic eczema specific skin rash			4.6 (3.4–6.2)		7.6 (6.2–9.2)	P=0.0090	Increase	
Vellinga et al. (2005) [62]	Belgium (Antwerp)	6–7	ISAAC-based parental-report of:	1995–96/2002					POR (95% CI)		Good
			lifetime prevalence of rash in boys		2,313	12.9	2,225	18.4	1.5 (1.3–1.8), P=0.00	Increase	
			lifetime prevalence of rash in girls		2,359	15.7	2,196	19.8	1.3 (1.1–1.5), P=0.00	Increase	
			12-month prevalence of rash in boys		2,313	8.5	2,225	11.4	1.4 (1.1–1.7), P=0.00	Increase	
			12-month prevalence of rash in girls		2,359	11.9	2,196	14.7	1.3 (1.1–1.5), P=0.01	Increase	
Vellinga et al. (2005) [62]	Belgium (Antwerp)	13–14	ISAAC-based parental-report of:	1995–96/2002					POR (95% CI)		Good
			lifetime prevalence of rash in boys		1,240	15.7	1,215	13.3	0.9 (0.7–1.1), P=0.17	Stable	
			lifetime prevalence of rash in girls		1,150	19.0	1,318	20.3	1.1 (0.9–1.3), P=0.30	Stable	
			12-month prevalence of rash in boys		1,240	9.7	1,215	8.5	0.9 (0.7–1.1), P=0.30	Stable	
			12-month prevalence of rash in girls		1,150	13.3	1,318	13.6	1.0 (0.8–1.3), P=0.84	Stable	
Krämer et al. (2009) [59]	Germany (west)	6	ISAAC-based parental-report of:	1994–95/1996–2000	4,761		3,654		Area-adjusted trend	Stable	Good
			12-month prevalence of itchy skin rash			4.6		4.5	0.89 (0.41–1.92)		
Krämer et al. (2009) [59]	Germany (east)	6	ISAAC-based parental-report of:	1994–95/1996–2000	114,457		9,031		Area-adjusted trend	Stable	Good
			12-month prevalence of itchy skin rash			6.3		6.2	0.96 (0.66–1.39)		
Maziak et al. (2003) [60]	Germany (Münster)	6–7	ISAAC-based parental-report of:	1994–95/1999–2000					POR (95% CI)		Good
			12-month prevalence of atopic eczema symptoms in boys		1,754	7.3	1,863	6.6	0.9 (0.69–1.17)	Stable	
			12-month prevalence of atopic eczema symptoms in girls		1,713	6.7	1,666	9.8	1.5 (1.18–1.97)	Increase	
Maziak et al. (2003) [60]	Germany (Münster)	13–14	ISAAC-based self-report of:	1994–95/1999–2000					POR (95% CI)		Good
			12-month prevalence of atopic eczema symptoms in boys		1,865	5.0	1,894	4.5	0.9 (0.66–1.22)	Stable	
			12-month prevalence of atopic eczema symptoms in girls		1,892	9.4	1,922	11.1	1.2 (0.98–1.50)	Stable	

Table 9. Cont.

Study	Geographic area	Age range (y)	Outcome	Time period	Baseline estimate N	Baseline estimate % (95%CI)/(SE)**	Final estimate N	Final estimate % (95%CI)/(SE)**	Summary measures	Conclusion	Quality
Weber et al. (2010) [63]	Austria (Upper)	6–9	ISAAC-based parental-report of:	1995–97/ 2001–03	12,115		11,468		No formal test		Moderate
			lifetime prevalence of rash			9.2		11.0		Increase	
			12-month prevalence of rash			6.0		6.7		Stable	
Annesi-Maesano et al. (2009) [55]	France (Languedoc Roussillon)	13–14	ISAAC-based self-report of:	1995/2002	3,383		1,642		Absolute/relative % Change		Moderate
			12-month prevalence of atopic eczema symptoms			12.5		14.3	1.78/0.14, P = not significant	Stable	
Measures of physician-diagnosed atopic eczema											
Grize et al. (2006) [56]	Switzerland	5–7	ISAAC-based parental-report of:	1992/2001	988		1,274				Good
			adjusted lifetime prevalence of physician-diagnosed atopic eczema			18.4 (15.8–21.2)		15.2 (13.2–17.4)	P trend = 0.1065	Stable	
Vellinga et al. (2005) [62]	Belgium (Antwerp)	6–7	ISAAC-based parental-report of:	1995–96/ 2002					POR (95% CI)		Good
			lifetime prevalence atopic eczema in boys		2,313	18.5	2,225	20.8	1.2(1.0–1.3), P = 0.06	Increase	
			lifetime prevalence atopic eczema in girls		2,359	19.1	2,196	22.4	1.2(1.1–1.4), P = 0.01	Increase	
Vellinga et al. (2005) [62]	Belgium (Antwerp)	13–14	ISAAC-based parental-report of:	1995–96/ 2002					POR (95% CI)		Good
			lifetime prevalence atopic eczema in boys		1,240	23.4	1,215	21.1	0.9(0.7–1.1), P = 0.17	Stable	
			lifetime prevalence atopic eczema in girls		1,150	27.8	1,318	29.7	1.1(0.9–1.3), P = 0.30	Stable	
Schäfer et al. (2000) [24]	Germany (west)	5–6	Report of:	1991/1997	801		771		No formal test		Moderate
			current prevalence of physician-diagnosed atopic eczema			11.2		4.5		Decrease	
Schäfer et al. (2000) [24]	Germany (east)	5–6	Report of:	1991/1997	285		633		No formal test		Moderate
			current prevalence of physician-diagnosed atopic eczema			17.5		11.2		Decrease	
Krämer et al. (2009) [59]	Germany (west)	6	Report of:	1991–95/ 1996–2000	4,761		3,654		Area-adjusted trend (10 y)		Good
			current prevalence of physician-diagnosed atopic eczema			10.5		5.2	0.30 (0.17–0.53)	Decrease	
Krämer et al. (2009) [59]	Germany (east)	6	Report of:	1991–1995/ 1996–2000	114,457		9,031		Area-adjusted trend (10 y)		Good
			current prevalence of physician-diagnosed atopic eczema			14.3		10.5	0.36 (0.17–0.61)	Decrease	

Table 9. Cont.

Study	Geographic area	Age range (y)	Outcome	Time period	Baseline estimate N	% (95%CI)/(SE)**	Final estimate N	% (95%CI)/(SE)**	Summary measures % (95%CI)/(SE)**	Conclusion	Quality
Maziak et al. (2003) [60]	Germany (Münster)	6–7	ISAAC-based parental-report of:	1994–95/ 1999–2000					POR (95% CI)		Good
			lifetime prevalence of physician-diagnosed atopic eczema in boys		1,754	14.3	1,863	13.6	0.9 (0.77–1.13)	Stable	
			lifetime prevalence of physician-diagnosed atopic eczema in girls		1,713	14.6	1,666	16.9	1.2 (0.99–1.44)	Stable	
Maziak et al. (2003) [60]	Germany (Münster)	13–14	ISAAC-based parental-report of:	1994–95/ 1999–2000					POR (95%CI)		Good
			lifetime prevalence of physician-diagnosed atopic eczema in boys		1,865	8.2	1,894	10.9	1.4 (1.09–1.71)	Increase	
			lifetime prevalence of physician-diagnosed atopic eczema in girls		1,892	12.3	1,922	17.4	1.5 (1.22–1.77)	Increase	
Heinrich et al. (2002) [58]	Germany (east)		Parental-report of:	1992–1993/ 1998–1999	2,773		3,092		No formal test		Moderate
		6	adjusted lifetime prevalence of physician-diagnosed atopic eczema			8.6		13.0		Increase	
		9	adjusted lifetime prevalence of physician-diagnosed atopic eczema			8.6		11.8		Increase	
		12	adjusted lifetime prevalence of physician-diagnosed atopic eczema			9.6		10.2		Increase	
Schernhammer et al. (2008) [61]	Austria (Upper)	6–7	ISAAC-based parental-report of:	1995–97/ 2001–03	13,399		12,784		P<0.001		Moderate
			lifetime prevalence of physician-diagnosed atopic eczema			10.1		13.8		Increase	
Haidinger et al. (2008) [57]	Austria (Upper)	6–7	ISAAC-based parental-report of:	1995–97/ 2001–03	35,238		12,541		% Change		Moderate
			lifetime prevalence of physician-diagnosed atopic eczema			9.9		13.6	3.7	Increase	
Weber et al. (2010) [63]	Austria (Upper)	6–9	ISAAC-based parental-report of:	1995–97/ 2001–03	12,115		11,468		No formal test		Moderate
			lifetime prevalence of physician-diagnosed atopic dermatitis			9.6		13.4		Increase	
Schernhammer et al. (2008) [61]	Austria (Upper)	12–14	ISAAC-based self-report of:	1995–97/ 2001–03	1,516		1,443		P<0.001		Moderate
			lifetime prevalence of physician-diagnosed atopic eczema			6.3		12.1		Increase	
Annesi-Maesano et al. (2009) [55]	France (Languedoc Roussillon)	13–14	ISAAC-based self-report of:	1995/2002	3,383		1,642		Absolute/relative % Change		Moderate
			lifetime prevalence of physician-diagnosed atopic dermatitis			25.8		30.4	4.56/0.17, P = 0.001	Increase	

Table 9. Cont.

Study	Geographic area	Age range (y)	Outcome	Time period	Baseline estimate N	Baseline estimate % (95%CI)/(SE)**	Final estimate N	Final estimate % (95%CI)/(SE)**	Summary measures	Conclusion	Quality
Southern Europe*											
Measures of symptoms of atopic eczema											
Montefort et al. (2009) [64]	Maltese Islands	5–8	ISAAC-based parental-report of:	1994–95/ 2001–02	4,465		4,761				Moderate
			lifetime prevalence of recurrent rash			7.0		6.7	P = 0.61	Stable	
			12-month prevalence of recurrent rash			5.5		5.4	P = 0.85	Stable	
Galassi et al. (2006) Italy (North) [66]		6–7	ISAAC-based parental-report of:	1994–95/ 2002	16,115		11,287		Area-adjusted absolute % Change (95% CI)		Good
			12-month prevalence of atopic eczema symptoms			8.3		14.5	6.2 (5.3–7.1)	Increase	
			12-month prevalence of atopic eczema symptoms in flexures			6.0		10.4	4.4 (3.6–5.2)	Increase	
Galassi et al. (2006) Italy (North) [66]		13–14	ISAAC-based self-report of:	1994–95/ 2002	19,723		10,267		Area-adjusted absolute % Change (95% CI)		Good
			12-month prevalence of atopic eczema symptoms			10.1		11.2	1.2 (0.1–2.4)	Increase	
			12-month prevalence of atopic eczema symptoms in flexures			6.5		8.5	2.1 (1.2–3.0)	Increase	
Anthracopoulos et al. (2009) [65]	Greece (Patras)	8–10	Parental-report of:	1991/2003	2,417		2,725				Moderate
			lifetime prevalence of atopic eczema symptoms			4.5		9.5	P trend <0.001	Increase	
			24-month prevalence of atopic eczema symptoms			2.5		5.0	P trend <0.001	Increase	
Measures of physician-diagnosed atopic eczema											
Montefort et al. (2009) [64]	Maltese Islands	5–8	ISAAC-based parental-report of:	1994–95/ 2001–02	4,465		4,761				Moderate
			lifetime prevalence of physician-diagnosed atopic eczema			4.4		11.2	P<0.0001	Increase	
Galassi et al. (2006) Italy (North) [66]		6–7	ISAAC-based parental-report of:	1994–95/ 2002	16,115		11,287		Area-adjusted absolute % Change (95% CI)		Good
			lifetime prevalence of atopic eczema			14.3		17	2.5 (1.6–3.5)	Increase	
Galassi et al. (2006) Italy (North) [66]		13–14	ISAAC-based parental-report of:	1994–95/ 2002	19,723		9,362		Area-adjusted absolute % Change (95% CI)		Good
			lifetime prevalence of atopic eczema			11.0		12.8	1.5 (0.3–2.8)	Increase	
Rosado-Pinto et al. (2006) [67]	Portugal	6–7	ISAAC-based report of:	1993–94/ 2002	5,000		5,350				Moderate

Table 9. Cont.

Study	Geographic area	Age range (y)	Outcome	Time period	Baseline estimate N	Baseline estimate % (95%CI)/(SE)**	Final estimate N	Final estimate % (95%CI)/(SE)**	Summary measures	Conclusion	Quality
			lifetime prevalence of atopic eczema			18.6		21.0	P = 0.002	Increase	
			12-month prevalence of atopic eczema			13.9		15.6	P = 0.013	Increase	
Rosado-Pinto et al. (2006) [67]	Portugal	13–14	ISAAC-based report of:	1993-94/2002	11,400		11,850				Moderate
			lifetime prevalence of atopic eczema			12.8		13.3	P = 0.22	Stable	
			12-month prevalence of atopic eczema			7.6		8.7	P = 0.002	Increase	

Northern Europe*

Measures of symptoms of atopic eczema

Study	Geographic area	Age range (y)	Outcome	Time period	Baseline estimate N	Baseline estimate % (95%CI)/(SE)**	Final estimate N	Final estimate % (95%CI)/(SE)**	Summary measures	Conclusion	Quality
Annus et al. (2005) [69]	Estonia (Tallinn)	6–7	ISAAC-based parental-report of:	1993-94/2001-02	3,070		2,383		Sex-adjusted POR (95% CI)		Good
			lifetime prevalence of itchy rash			16.9		22.0	1.40 (1.22–1.61), P<0.001	Increase	
			12-month prevalence of itchy rash			12.6		17.1	1.44 (1.24–1.67), P<0.001	Increase	
			12-month prevalence of flexural rash			12.0		13.5	1.20 (1.02–1.41), P = 0.025	Increase	
Annus et al. (2005) [69]	Estonia (Tallinn)	13–14	ISAAC-based parental-report of:	1993-94/2001-02	3,476		3,576		Sex-adjusted POR (95% CI)		Good
			lifetime prevalence of itchy rash			15.2		19.3	1.34 (1.18–1.52), P<0.001	Increase	
			12-month prevalence of itchy rash			10.4		14.9	1.51 (1.31–1.74), P<0.001	Increase	
			12-month prevalence of flexural rash			7.7		9.4	1.26 (1.07–1.50), P = 0.006	Increase	
Shamssain et al. (2007) [80]	UK (North-east England)	6–7	ISAAC-based parental-report of:	1995-96/2001-02	3,000		1,843		OR (95% CI)		Good
			lifetime prevalence of rash in boys			17.8		21.0	1.6 (1.29–1.98)	Increase	
			lifetime prevalence of rash in girls			18.7		22.5	1.8(1.35–2.30)	Increase	
			lifetime prevalence of rash with typical distribution in boys			13.2		21.1	1.9 (1.41–3.57)	Increase	
			lifetime prevalence of rash with typical distribution in girls			14.7		23.8	1.8(1.35–2.25)	Increase	
			12-month prevalence of current rash in boys			14.7		23.3	1.4 (1.31–1.61)	Increase	
			12-month prevalence of current rash in girls			16.9		25.0	1.8(1.42–2.28)	Increase	
Shamssain et al. (2007) [80]	UK (North-east England)	13–14	ISAAC-based parental-report of:	1995-96/2001-02	3,000		2,195		OR (95% CI)		Good
			lifetime prevalence of rash in boys			13.9		15.3	1.1 (0.88–1.22)	Stable	
			lifetime prevalence of rash in girls			22.8		17.5	1.6 (1.29–1.98)	Increase	
			lifetime prevalence of rash with typical distribution in boys			8.8		19.6	2.4 (1.81–3.37)	Increase	

Table 9. Cont.

Study	Geographic area	Age range (y)	Outcome	Time period	Baseline estimate N	Baseline estimate % (95%CI)/(SE)**	Final estimate N	Final estimate % (95%CI)/(SE)**	Summary measures	Conclusion	Quality
			lifetime prevalence of rash with typical distribution in girls			15.9		19.3	1.5 (1.12–1.98)	Increase	
			12-month prevalence of current rash in boys			11.3		16.8	1.6 (1.30–2.20)	Increase	
			12-month prevalence of current rash in girls			20.5		20.9	1.0 (0.89–1.32)	Stable	
Anderson et al. (2004) [68]	UK (British Isles)	12–14	ISAAC-based self-report of:	1995/2002	15,083		15,755		Absolute/Relative % Change		Moderate
			12-month prevalence of flexural rash			16.2		11.4	–4.8/–29.6	Decrease	
Bjerg et al. (2010) [70]	Sweden (Kiruna, Luleå, Piteå)	7–8	ISAAC-based parental-report of:	1996/2006	3,430		2,585				Good
			12-month prevalence of atopic eczema symptoms			27.2		25.8	P = 0.215	Stable	
Rönmark et al. (2009) [78]	Sweden (northern)	7–8	ISAAC-based parental-report of:	1996/2006	2,148		1,700				Moderate
			lifetime prevalence of atopic eczema symptoms			29.3		26.5	P = 0.048	Decrease	
Kudzytė et al. (2008) [72]	Lithuania (Kaunas)	6–7	ISAAC-based parental-report of:	1994-95/2001-02	1,879		2,772				Moderate
			12-months prevalence of itchy rash			2.6		3.9	P<0.05	Increase	
Measures of physician-diagnosed atopic eczema											
Kuehni et al. (2001) [63]	UK (Leicestershire)	1–5	Secondary analysis of:	1990/1998	1,264		2,127		Age- and sex-adjusted OR (95% CI)		Good
			lifetime prevalence of physicians' recorded atopic eczema diagnosis			29.0		44.0	1.95 (1.68–2.27), P<0.001	Increase	
Shamssain et al. (2007) [80]	UK (North-east England)	6–7	ISAAC-based parental-report of:	1995-96/2001-02					OR (95% CI)		Good
			lifetime prevalence of atopic eczema in boys		1,445	27.8	918	37.0	1.9 (1.45–3.55), P = 0.001	Increase	
			lifetime prevalence of atopic eczema in girls		1,545	27.0	925	35.5	1.8 (1.45–2.45), P = 0.001	Increase	
Shamssain et al. (2007) [80]	UK (North-east England)	13–14	ISAAC-based parental-report of:	1995-96/2001-02					OR (95% CI)		Good
			lifetime prevalence of atopic eczema in boys		1,510	13.9	1,000	27.2	6.13 (3.52–10.79), P = 0.001	Increase	
			lifetime prevalence of atopic eczema in girls		1,490	22.8	1,195	30.7	1.63 (1.48–1.81), P = 0.001	Increase	
Ng Man Kwong et al. (2001) [76]	UK (Sheffield)	8–9	ISAAC-based parental-report of:	1991/1999	4,523		4,809		Absolute % Change (95% CI)		Moderate

Table 9. Cont.

Study	Geographic area	Age range (y)	Outcome	Time period	Baseline estimate N	Baseline estimate % (95%CI)/(SE)**	Final estimate N	Final estimate % (95%CI)/(SE)**	Summary measures	Conclusion	Quality
			lifetime prevalence of atopic eczema			18.1		31.1	13.0 (11.27–14.72), P<0.001	Increase	
Anderson et al. (2004) [68]	UK (British Isles)	12–14	ISAAC-based self-report of:	1995/2002	15,083		15,755		Absolute/Relative % Change		Moderate
			lifetime prevalence of atopic eczema			21.1		24.3	3.3/15.4	Increase	
Simpson et al. (2009) [25]	UK	all	Secondary analysis of:	2001–2005	>9 million		>9 million		Relative % Change		Moderate
			age-and sex-standardised lifetime prevalence of physicians' recorded atopic eczema diagnosis			7.8 (7.8–7.8)		11.5 (11.5–11.6)	48.2, P<0.001	Increase	
McNeill et al. (2009) [75]	Scotland (Aberdeen)	7–9	ISAAC-based parental-report of:	1999/2004	2,340	24.0 (22.3–25.7)	1,070	34.6 (32.3–36.9)	No formal test	Increase	Moderate
Osman et al. (2007) [77]	Scotland (Aberdeen)	9–11	lifetime prevalence of atopic eczema	1994/2004							Moderate
			ISAAC-based parental-report of:			21.1 (19.7–22.5)		34.2 (31.8–36.6)		Increase	
			lifetime prevalence of atopic eczema in boys		2,021	17.9	935	23.6	P trend<0.0001	Increase	
			lifetime prevalence of atopic eczema in girls		2,026	17.5	980	28.9	P trend<0.0001	Increase	
McNeill et al. (2009) [75]	Scotland (Aberdeen)	9–12	ISAAC-based parental-report of:	1999/2004	3,280		1,498		No formal test		Moderate
Devenny et al. (2004) [71]	Scotland (Aberdeen)	9–12	lifetime prevalence of atopic eczema	1994/1999	4,047		3,537		RR (95% CI)	Increase	Moderate
			ISAAC-based parental-report of:			18.0		21.0	1.2 (1.10–1.33)	Increase	
Kudzyteet al. (2008) [72]	Lithuania (Kaunas)	6–7	lifetime prevalence of atopic eczema	1994–95/ 2001–02	1,879		2,772			Increase	Moderate
			ISAAC-based parental-report of:			1.4		3.5	P<0.05		
Selnes et al. (2005) [79]	Norway (subarctic)	9–11	lifetime prevalence of physician-diagnosed atopic eczema	1995/2000	1,432		3,853		RR (95% CI)	Increase	Moderate
			ISAAC-based self-report of:			21.1		20.8	0.99 (0.88–1.11)	Stable	
Bjerg et al. (2010) [70]	Sweden (Kiruna, Luleå, Piteå)	7–8	lifetime prevalence of atopic eczema	1996/2006	3,430		2,585				Moderate
			ISAAC-based parental-report of:			13.4		15.2	P=0.048	Increase	
Latvala et al. (2005) [74]	Finland	18–19	lifetime prevalence of physician-diagnosed atopic eczema	1990–2000	–		–		No formal test	Increase	Moderate
			Report of:								
			12-month prevalence of physician-diagnosed atopic eczema			1.2#		1.2#		Stable	

Table 9. Cont.

Study	Geographic area	Age range (y)	Outcome	Time period	Baseline estimate N	Baseline estimate % (95%CI)/(SE)**	Final estimate N	Final estimate % (95%CI)/(SE)**	Summary measures % (95%CI)/(SE)**	Conclusion	Quality
Eastern Europe*											
Measures of physician-diagnosed atopic eczema											
Harangi et al. (2007) [82]	Hungary (Baranya County)	7–9	Hanifin-Rajka criteria-based parental-report of:	2002/2005	587		574		No formal test		Moderate
			physician-diagnosed atopic dermatitis			17.0		17.1		Stable	
Harangi et al. (2007) [82]	Hungary (Baranya County)	7–14	Hanifin-Rajka criteria-based parental-report of:	2002/2005	1,454		1,454		No formal test		Moderate
			physician-diagnosed atopic dermatitis			15.1		16.1		Stable	
Brożek et al. (2004) [81]	Poland (Chorzów)	7–10	Parental-report of:	1993/2002	1,130		1,451				Moderate
			lifetime prevalence of physician-diagnosed atopic eczema			2.3		8.1		P<0.001	Increase	

Abbreviations – CI: confidence intervals, SE: standard error, POR: prevalence odds ratio, OR: odds ratio.
*Based on UN classification [16].
**95% CI and SE are only reported if included in original report.
#Point estimate extracted from graph or chart.

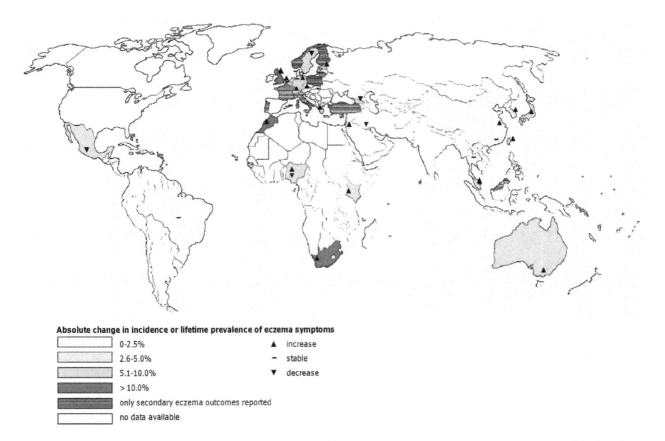

Absolute change in incidence or lifetime prevalence of eczema symptoms

- 0–2.5%
- 2.6–5.0%
- 5.1–10.0%
- >10.0%
- only secondary eczema outcomes reported
- no data available

- ▲ increase
- − stable
- ▼ decrease

Figure 2. World map of the incidence and lifetime prevalence of atopic eczema symptoms (1990–2010). Overview of absolute changes in the incidence of atopic eczema and lifetime prevalence of atopic eczema symptoms between 1990 and 2010.

different terms to describe atopic eczema [86]. In addition, not every language has disease labels, nor are they understood in the same way. This means that a diagnostic label may be influenced by region-specific guidelines for the diagnosis of atopic eczema and this may therefore render it difficult to compare estimates of physician-diagnosed atopic eczema prevalence between regions. We thus judged that the lifetime prevalence of atopic eczema symptoms was most likely to prove useful in relation to yielding comparative data on trends in atopic eczema.

Strengths and limitations. To our knowledge, no systematic review on international disease trends in the incidence and prevalence of atopic eczema has been published. We searched a large amount of potential relevant literature using seven electronic databases and included 69 papers which reported on trends in atopic eczema. These should represent a good coverage of published literature. Furthermore, we searched systematically, according to a protocol and used stipulated inclusion criteria. To ensure that included studies are above a specific quality threshold, the studies were independently quality-filtered by two reviewers. Where a consensus could not be obtained a third reviewer provided arbitration guidance. In contrast with earlier work into this field, we included all reports on atopic eczema trends, whereas previously papers have limited themselves to single estimates of atopic eczema [4,5], or to original data from the ISAAC study [2,87].

There are gaps in the literature. We could include particularly few reports from the Americas, eastern Europe and Oceania. In general, studies are available on the prevalence of atopic eczema in these regions. However, information from these studies will not be relevant until they are repeated over time. This perhaps somewhat surprising gap for North America is likely to be, at least in part, due to the fact that the ISAAC programme had difficulty identifying a regional coordinator for this region [88]. We were unable to obtain the full-text translation of one Korean paper. Nevertheless, we are reasonably confident that this report or any other additional reports would be unlikely to undermine our overall findings – that there is no clear trend in the worldwide incidence and prevalence of atopic eczema. For nearly all regions information on atopic eczema is questionnaire-based. Questionnaires are non-specific and the measured symptoms suggestive of atopic eczema may overlap with symptoms of other conditions, such as contact dermatitis. The ISAAC questionnaire stipulates the typical distribution and the onset of the itchy rash (see Table 2), which helps to enhance its specificity. At the population level and particularly for the purpose of between-population comparison, ISAAC questions are therefore likely to provide adequate symptom-derived prevalence estimates [89]. That said there is inevitably some loss of ability to differentiate between atopic eczema and other differential diagnoses such as allergic contact dermatitis. This problem may have been more pronounced had we also identified studies using the ECRHS; in the event however, no such relevant studies were found to be eligible.

Future work. Further research in this area should firstly address methodological issues to help inform the optimum design, execution and reporting of future epidemiological studies of trends in atopic eczema. In our dataset various outcome measures were reported and various assessment tools were used, data were analysed differently across studies and results were reported in

Table 10. Good and moderate quality studies reporting the prevalence of parental- or self-report of atopic eczema between 1990 and 2010 in Oceania.

Study	Geographic area	Age range (y)	Outcome	Time period	Baseline estimate N	Baseline estimate % (95%CI)/(SE)**	Final estimate N	Final estimate % (95%CI)/(SE)**	Summary measures	Conclusion	Quality
Measures of symptoms of atopic eczema											
Robertson et al. (2004)[84]	Australia (Melbourne)	6–7	ISAAC-based parental-report of:	1993/2002	2,843		2,968		No formal test		Moderate
			lifetime prevalence of atopic eczema symptoms			22.6 (20.8–24.6)		32.3 (30.4–34.2)		Increase	
			12-month prevalence of atopic eczema symptoms			11.1 (10.0–12.3)		17.2 (15.7–18.8)		Increase	
Measures of physician-diagnosed atopic eczema											
Ponsonby et al. (2008) [83]	Australia (Australian Capital Territory)	4–6	Annual school entry-based and ISAAC-based parental-report of:	2000–05	3,873		3,849		Adjusted OR (95% CI) per year		Good
			lifetime prevalence of atopic eczema			31.0#		37.0#		1.05 (1.03–1.07) P<0.001	Increase	
Toelle et al. (2004) [85]	Australia (Belmont)	8–11	ISAAC-based parental-report of:	1992/2002	908		800		% Change (95%CI)		Moderate
			lifetime prevalence of atopic eczema			24.4		24.8		0.4 (−3.7–4.5), P = not significant	Stable	

Abbreviations – CI: confidence intervals, SE: standard error, OR: odds ratio.

*Based on UN classification [16].

**95% CI and SE are only reported if included in original report.

#Point estimate extracted from graph or chart.

different formats (e.g. with and without confidence intervals (CI)), age groups did not match and studies were inconsistently stratified for sex. All of these factors enhance the incomparability of studies. In view of the above, we suggest full and elaborate reporting of the results (including CI) of all of the outcomes obtained. We recommend that the above gaps be addressed using the complete ISAAC tool (and, where possible, also include detailed clinical assessment to allow atopic eczema to be differentiated from allergic contact dermatitis) and be reported according to a standardised format, so that comparisons to other reports on trends are possible. However, even if studies are comparable the prevalence of atopic eczema may still be difficult to compare across countries, without a universal definition. Thus, we need a range of relevant measures of incidence and prevalence as well as a careful description of the diagnostic criteria used together with appropriate interpretation of these data in order to ensure that this important field of epidemiological enquiry progresses in a scientifically robust manner.

Interpretation. Although there is no consistent overall global trend in atopic eczema incidence and prevalence, there are some specific trends which are worth remarking upon further, as they may be of interest for research into the aetiology of atopic eczema. Firstly, there was a stable incidence of atopic eczema in 5–6 year olds in West Germany [12.5% (1991) and 12.8% (1997)] and a sharply increasing incidence in East Germany [from 9.6% (1991) to 23.4% (1997)] [24]. This coincides with the adoption of a "Western" lifestyle in East Germany as a result of political change. A consequence of changed lifestyle and increased socio-economic wealth may be an increased frequency of bathing and a greater availability of soaps and bubble baths, which may remove the skin's natural barrier oils and make atopic eczema more prevalent [90]. This is a biologically credible mechanism to explain an increase in incidence – in particular of mild disease. Nevertheless, Schafer et al. (2000) found that, after adjustment for potential confounders, including socio-economic status, the difference in incidence between East and West Germany remained [24]. Other factors, such as nutritional factors, allergens and irritants or infections may therefore be important in the aetiology of atopic eczema. Political changes resulting in, for example, improved access to physicians in East Germany after reunification or due to changes in disease labelling could also have impacted on measures of the incidence of atopic eczema, as has been noted in relation to asthma diagnosis and prescribing [91]. If this were the case, this would reflect an increase in reporting behaviour rather than any true change in the epidemiology of eczema.

Other trends of interest regarding aetiological hypotheses include diverging trends between neighbouring regions. For example, there are marked increases in lifetime prevalence of atopic eczema symptoms in most countries in Africa [e.g. in South Africa – from 15.5% (1995) to 26.2% (2002)] [29], whereas there is a large decrease in Nigeria [from 26.1% (1995) to 18.0% (2001–02)] [27]. This anomalous decrease is most likely a consequence of the extremely high baseline prevalence, as prevalence estimates in 2001–02 are largely comparable for all African countries. Rather than a true prevalence, this high baseline estimate may be a reflection of the presence of another skin condition, such as another rash, perhaps caused by parasites, which are common in these regions. In addition, in our dataset there were also marked baseline differences between neighbouring countries. This is indicated by the low baseline prevalence of atopic eczema symptoms in 12–15 year olds in Taiwan [2.4% (1995–96)] [32] and the much higher baseline prevalence in Korea [7.2% (1995)] [36]. In these countries too, cultural, social and diagnostic differences may potentially explain this pattern. In contrast, large changes in prevalence estimates within one country in a short space of time are of interest as such changes are likely to represent a true change. For example the doubling in lifetime prevalence of both atopic eczema diagnosis [from 13.9% (1995–96) to 27.2% (2001–02)] and atopic eczema symptoms [from 8.8% (1995–96) to 19.6% (2001–02)] in boys aged 13–14 in England [80] is likely to represent a true change and we must consider environmental explanations for this.

In conclusion, we have found no overall trend for the incidence or prevalence of atopic eczema worldwide. However, in Africa, eastern Asia, western Europe and parts of northern Europe (i.e. the UK) trends in atopic eczema prevalence were mainly increasing. There are gaps in the literature, particularly in the Americas and Oceania and for measures of atopic eczema incidence. Future research should investigate trends in what is now one of the most prevalent disorders in Europe and other regions in a scientifically robust manner. In order to do so, the careful use of key definitions, improved study design and more comprehensive reporting are essential.

Supporting Information

Appendix S1   PRISMA checklist. PRISMA checklist with 27 reporting items used for the systematic review.

Appendix S2   Search terms. Search terms and limitations used for the systematic review.

Author Contributions

Conceived and designed the experiments: ID SM MM CvS AS. Analyzed the data: ID SM SL. Wrote the paper: ID SM SL MM CvS AS.

References

1. Gupta R, Sheikh A, Strachan DP, Anderson HR (2004) Burden of allergic disease in the UK: secondary analyses of national databases. Clin Exp Allergy 34: 520–526.
2. Asher MI, Montefort S, Björkstén B, Lai CKW, Strachan DP, et al. (2006) Worldwide time trends in the prevalence of symptoms of asthma, allergic rhinoconjunctivitis, and eczema in childhood: ISAAC Phases One and Three repeat multicountry cross-sectional surveys. Lancet 368: 733–743.
3. Gupta R, Sheikh A, Strachan DP, Anderson HR (2007) Time trends in allergic disorders in the UK. Thorax 62: 91–96.
4. Odhiambo JA, Williams HC, Clayton TO, Robertson CF, Asher MI, et al. (2009) Global variations in prevalence of eczema symptoms in children from ISAAC Phase Three. J Allergy Clin Immunol 124: 1251–1258.e1223.
5. Warner JO (1999) Worldwide variations in the prevalence of atopic symptoms: what does it all mean? Thorax 54 Suppl 2: S46–51.
6. Punekar YS, Sheikh A (2009) Establishing the incidence and prevalence of clinician-diagnosed allergic conditions in children and adolescents using routinely collected data from general practices. Clin Exp Allergy: 1–8.
7. van den Oord RA, Sheikh A (2009) Filaggrin gene defects and risk of developing allergic sensitisation and allergic disorders: systematic review and meta-analysis. Bmj 339: b2433.
8. Palmer CN, Irvine AD, Terron-Kwiatkowski A, Zhao Y, Liao H, et al. (2006) Common loss-of-function variants of the epidermal barrier protein filaggrin are a major predisposing factor for atopic dermatitis. Nat Genet 38: 441–446.
9. Sandilands A, Sutherland C, Irvine AD, McLean WH (2009) Filaggrin in the frontline: role in skin barrier function and disease. J Cell Sci 122: 1285–1294.
10. Anandan C, Nurmatov U, van Schayck OC, Sheikh A (2009) Is the prevalence of asthma declining? Systematic review of epidemiological studies. Allergy 65: 152–167.
11. ISAAC steering Committee (1998) Worldwide variation in prevalence of symptoms of asthma, allergic rhinoconjunctivitis, and atopic eczema: ISAAC.

The International Study of Asthma and Allergies in Childhood (ISAAC) Steering Committee. Lancet 351: 1225–1232.

12. The European Community Respiratory Health Survey II steering committee (2002) The European Community Respiratory Health Survey II. Eur Respir J 20: 1071–1079.

13. Liberati A, Altman DG, Tetzlaff J, Mulrow C, Gotzsche PC, et al. (2009) The PRISMA statement for reporting systematic reviews and meta-analyses of studies that evaluate health care interventions: explanation and elaboration. J Clin Epidemiol 62: e1–34.

14. Public Health Resource Unit England (2006) Critical Appraisal Skills Programme (CASP) Available: http://www.sph.nhs.uk/sph-files/casp-appraisal-tools/Case%20Control%2011%20Questions.pdf. Accessed 18 July 2011.

15. Choi HS, Yun SK, Kim HU, Ihm CW (2005) A statistical study of dermatoses in the Jeonbuk Province (1979–1980, 1987–2002). Korean Journal of Dermatology 43: 606–618.

16. United Nations (2010) Composition of macro geographical (continental) regions, geographical sub-regions, and selected economic and other groupings Available: http://unstats.un.org/unsd/methods/m49/m49regin.htm.Accessed 26 Aug 2011.

17. Al Frayh AR, Shakoor Z, Fakhri SAM, Koshak EA, Al Nameem S, et al. (2004) A 17-year trend for the prevalence of asthma and allergic diseases among children in Saudi Arabia. Current Pediatric Research 8: 1–5.

18. Dorner T, Lawrence K, Rieder A, Kunze M (2007) Epidemiology of allergies in Austria. Results of the first Austrian allergy report. Wiener Medizinische Wochenschrift 157: 235–242.

19. Ellsäßer G, Diepgen TL (2002) Atopic diseases and social status of school beginners in the federal state of Brandenburg, Germany. Trend analysis 1994–2000. Monatsschrift Kinderheilkunde 150: 839–847.

20. Nishima S, Chisaka H, Fujiwara T, Furusho K, Hayashi S, et al. (2009) Surveys on the prevalence of pediatric bronchial asthma in Japan: A comparison between the 1982, 1992, and 2002 surveys conducted in the same region using the same methodology. Allergology International 58: 37–53.

21. Riikjarv MA, Annus T, Braback L, Rahu K, Bjorksten B (2000) Similar prevalence of respiratory symptoms and atopy in Estonian schoolchildren with changing lifestyle over 4 yrs. Eur Resp J 16: 86–90.

22. Saeki H, Oiso N, Honma M, Odajima H, Iizuka H, et al. (2009) Comparison of prevalence of atopic dermatitis in Japanese elementary schoolchildren between 2001/2002 and 2007/2008. The Journal of Dermatology 36: 512–514.

23. Olesen AB, Bang K, Juul S, Thestrup-Pedersen K (2005) Stable incidence of atopic dermatitis among children in Denmark during the 1990s. Acta Dermato-Venereologica 85: 244–247.

24. Schafer T, Kramer U, Vieluf D, Abeck D, Behrendt H, et al. (2000) The excess of atopic eczema in East Germany is related to the intrinsic type. Br J Dermatol 143: 992–998.

25. Simpson CR, Newton J, Hippisley-Cox J, Sheikh A (2009) Trends in the epidemiology and prescribing of medication for eczema in England. J R Soc Med 102: 108–117.

26. Bouayad Z, Aichane A, Afif A, Benouhoud N, Trombati N, et al. (2006) Prevalence and trend of self-reported asthma and other allergic disease symptoms in Morocco: ISAAC phase I and III. Int J Tuberc Lung Dis 10: 371–377.

27. Esamai F, Ayaya S, Nyandiko W (2002) Prevalence of asthma, allergic rhinitis and dermatitis in primary school children in Uasin Gishu district, Kenya. East Afr Med J 79: 514–518.

28. Falade AG, Ige OM, Yusuf BO, Onadeko MO, Onadeko BO (2009) Trends in the prevalence and severity of symptoms of asthma, allergic rhinoconjunctivitis, and atopic eczema. Journal of the National Medical Association 101: 414–418.

29. Zar HJ, Ehrlich RI, Workman L, Weinberg EG (2007) The changing prevalence of asthma, allergic rhinitis and atopic eczema in African adolescents from 1995 to 2002. Pediatr Allergy Immunol 18: 560–565.

30. Kusunoki T, Morimoto T, Nishikomori R, Yasumi T, Heike T, et al. (2009) Changing prevalence and severity of childhood allergic diseases in kyoto, Japan, from 1996 to 2006. Allergology International 58: 543–548.

31. Lee SL, Wong W, Lau YL (2004) Increasing prevalence of allergic rhinitis but not asthma among children in Hong Kong from 1995 to 2001 (Phase 3 International Study of Asthma and Allergies in Childhood). Pediatr Allergy Immunol 15: 72–78.

32. Lee YL, Li CW, Sung FC, Guo YL (2007) Increasing prevalence of atopic eczema in Taiwanese adolescents from 1995 to 2001. Clin Exp Allergy 37: 543–551.

33. Lee YL, Lin YC, Hwang BF, Guo YL (2005) Changing prevalence of asthma among Taiwanese adolescents: Two surveys 6 years apart. Pediatr Allergy Immunol 16: 157–164.

34. Liao MF, Liao MN, Lin SN, Chen JY, Huang JL (2009) Prevalence of Allergic Diseases of Schoolchildren in Central Taiwan. From ISAAC surveys 5 years apart. Journal of Asthma 46: 541–545.

35. Liao PF, Sun HL, Lu KH, Lue KH (2009) Prevalence of Childhood Allergic Diseases in Central Taiwan over the Past 15 Years. Pediatrics and Neonatology 50: 18–25.

36. Oh JW, Pyun BY, Choung JT, Ahn KM, Kim CH, et al. (2004) Epidemiological change of atopic dermatitis and food allergy in school-aged children in Korea between 1995 and 2000. Journal of Korean Medical Science 19: 716–723.

37. Wang HY, Zheng JP, Zhong NS (2006) Time trends in the prevalence of asthma and allergic diseases over 7 years among adolescents in Guangzhou city. Natl Medical J China 86: 1014–1020.

38. Yan DC, Ou LS, Tsai TL, Wu WF, Huang JL (2005) Prevalence and severity of symptoms of asthma, rhinitis, and eczema in 13- to 14-year-old children in Taipei, Taiwan. Ann Allergy Asthma Immunol 95: 579–585.

39. Yura A, Shimizu T (2001) Trends in the prevalence of atopic dermatitis in school children: longitudinal study in Osaka Prefecture, Japan, from 1985 to 1997. Br J Dermatol 145: 966–973.

40. Quah BS, Wan-Pauzi I, Ariffin N, Mazidah AR (2005) Prevalence of asthma, eczema and allergic rhinitis: two surveys, 6 years apart, in Kota Bharu, Malaysia. Respirology 10: 244–249.

41. Teeratakulpisarn J, Wiangnon S, Kosalaraksa P, Heng S (2004) Surveying the prevalence of asthma, allergic rhinitis and eczema in school-children in Khon Kaen, Northeastern Thailand using the ISAAC questionnaire: phase III. Asian Pacific Journal of Allergy & Immunology 22: 175–181.

42. Trakultivakorn M, Sangsupawanich P, Vichyanond P (2007) Time trends of the prevalence of asthma, rhinitis and eczema in Thai children-ISAAC (International Study of Asthma and Allergies in Childhood) Phase Three. Journal of Asthma 44: 609–611.

43. Wang XS, Tan TN, Shek LPC, Chng SY, Hia CPP, et al. (2004) The prevalence of asthma and allergies in Singapore; data from two ISAAC surveys seven years apart. Arch Dis Child 89: 423–426.

44. Abramidze T, Gotua M, Rukhadze M, Gamkrelidze A (2006) ISAAC I and III in Georgia: time trends in prevalence of asthma and allergies. Georgian Medical News 8: 80–82.

45. Abramidze T, Gotua M, Rukhadze M, Gamkrelidze A (2007) Prevalence of asthma and allergies among adolescents in Georgia: comparison between two surveys. Georgian Medical News 3: 38–41.

46. Demir AU, Celikel S, Karakaya G, Kalyoncu AF (2010) Asthma and allergic diseases in school children from 1992 to 2007 with incidence data. Journal of Asthma 47: 1128–1135.

47. Kalyoncu AF, Selcuk ZT, Enunlu T, Demir AU, Coplu L, et al. (1999) Prevalence of asthma and allergic diseases in primary school children in Ankara, Turkey: two cross-sectional studies, five years apart. Pediatr Allergy Immunol 10: 261–265.

48. Owayed A, Behbehani N, Al-Momen J (2008) Changing prevalence of asthma and allergic diseases among Kuwaiti children: An ISAAC study (phase III). Med Princ Pract 17: 284–289.

49. Romano-Zelekha O, Graif Y, Garty B-Z, Livne I, Green MS, et al. (2007) Trends in the prevalence of asthma symptoms and allergic diseases in Israeli adolescents: results from a national survey 2003 and comparison with 1997. Journal of Asthma 44: 365–369.

50. Barraza-Villarreal A, Hernandez-Cadena L, Moreno-Macias H, Ramirez-Aguilar M, Romieu I (2007) Trends in the prevalence of asthma and other allergic diseases in schoolchildren from Cuernavaca, Mexico. Allergy & Asthma Proceedings 28: 368–374.

51. Borges WG, Burns DAR, Guimarães FATM, Felizola MLBM, Borges VM (2008) Atopic dermatitis among adolescents from Federal District. Comparison between ISAAC phases I and III by socioeconomic status [Portugues]. Rev bras alergia imunopatol 31: 146–150.

52. Camelo-Nunes IC, Wandalsen GF, Melo KC, Naspitz CK, Solé D (2004) Prevalence of atopic eczema and associated symptoms in school children. Jornal de Pediatria (Rio J) 80: 60–64.

53. Riedi CA, Rosario NA, Ribas LFO, Backes AS, Kleiniibing GF, et al. (2005) Increase in prevalence of rhinoconjunctivitis but not asthma and atopic eczema in teenagers. J Investig Allergol Clin Immunol 15: 183–188.

54. Solé D, Melo KC, Camelo-Nunes IC, Freitas LS, Britto M, et al. (2007) Changes in the prevalence of asthma and allergic diseases among Brazilian schoolchildren (13–14 years old): Comparison between ISAAC phases one and three. Journal of Tropical Pediatrics 53: 13–21.

55. Annesi-Maesano I, Mourad C, Daures JP, Kalaboka S, Godard P (2009) Time trends in prevalence and severity of childhood asthma and allergies from 1995 to 2002 in France. Allergy 64: 798–800.

56. Grize L, Gassner M, Wuthrich B, Bringolf-Isler B, Takken-Sahli K, et al. (2006) Trends in prevalence of asthma, allergic rhinitis and atopic dermatitis in 5–7-year old Swiss children from 1992 to 2001. Allergy 61: 556–562.

57. Haidinger G, Waldhör T, Meusburger S, Süss G, Vutuc C (2008) The prevalence of childhood asthma and of allergies in 7 districts of Upper Austria - ISAAC III. [German]. Allergologie 31: 17–22.

58. Heinrich J, Hoelscher B, Frye C, Meyer I, Wjst M, et al. (2002) Trends in prevalence of atopic diseases and allergic sensitization in children in Eastern Germany. Eur Resp J 19: 1040–1046.

59. Krämer U, Oppermann H, Ranft U, Schafer T, Ring J, et al. (2009) Differences in allergy trends between East and West Germany and possible explanations. Clin Exp Allergy 40: 289–298.

60. Maziak W, Behrens T, Brasky TM, Duhme H, Rzehak P, et al. (2003) Are asthma and allergies in children and adolescents increasing? Results from ISAAC phase I and phase III surveys in Münster, Germany. Allergy 58: 572–579.

61. Schernhammer ES, Vutuc C, Waldhor T, Haidinger G (2008) Time trends of the prevalence of asthma and allergic disease in Austrian children. Pediatr Allergy Immunol 19: 125–131.

62. Vellinga A, Droste JHJ, Vermeire PA, Desager K, De Backer WA, et al. (2005) Changes in respiratory and allergic symptoms in schoolchildren from 1996 to 20029 results from the ISAAC surveys in Antwerp (Belgium). Acta Clinica Belgica 60: 219–225.

63. Weber AS, Haidinger G (2010) The prevalence of atopic dermatitis in children is influenced by their parents' education: results of two cross-sectional studies conducted in Upper Austria. Pediatr Allergy Immunol 21: 1028–1035.

64. Montefort S, Ellul P, Montefort M, Caruana S, Muscat HA (2009) Increasing prevalence of asthma, allergic rhinitis but not eczema in 5- to 8-yr-old Maltese children (ISAAC). Pediatr Allergy Immunol 20: 67–71.

65. Anthracopoulos MB, Antonogeorgos G, Liolios E, Triga M, Panagiotopoulou E, et al. (2009) Increase in chronic or recurrent rhinitis, rhinoconjunctivitis and eczema among schoolchildren in Greece: Three surveys during 1991–2003. Pediatr Allergy Immunol 20: 180–186.

66. Galassi C, De Sario M, Biggeri A, Bisanti L, Chellini E, et al. (2006) Changes in prevalence of asthma and allergies among children and adolescents in Italy: 1994–2002. Pediatrics 117: 34–42.

67. Rosado-pinto J, Gaspar A, Morais-Almeida M (2006) Epidemiology of asthma and allergic diseases in Portuguese speaking regions. Revue française d'allergologie et d'immunologie clinicque 46: 305–308.

68. Anderson HR, Ruggles R, Strachan DP, Austin JB, Burr M, et al. (2004) Trends in prevalence of symptoms of asthma, hay fever, and eczema in 12–14 year olds in the British Isles, 1995–2002: questionnaire survey. Bmj 328: 1052–1053.

69. Annus T, Riikjarv MA, Rahu K, Bjorksten B (2005) Modest increase in seasonal allergic rhinitis and eczema over 8 years among Estonian schoolchildren. Pediatr Allergy Immunol 16: 315–320.

70. Bjerg A, Sandstrom T, Lundback B, Ronmark E (2010) Time trends in asthma and wheeze in Swedish children 1996–2006: Prevalence and risk factors by sex. Allergy 65: 48–55.

71. Devenny A, Wassall H, Ninan T, Omran M, Khan SD, et al. (2004) Respiratory symptoms and atopy in children in Aberdeen: questionnaire studies of a defined school population repeated over 35 years. Bmj 329: 489–490.

72. Kudzytė J, Griška E, Bojarskas J (2008) Time trends in the prevalence of asthma and allergy among 6-7-year-old children. Results from ISAAC phase I and III studies in Kaunas, Lithuania. Medicina (Kaunas) 44: 944–952.

73. Kuehni CE, Davis A, Brooke AM, Silverman M (2001) Are all wheezing disorders in very young (preschool) children increasing in prevalence? Lancet 357: 1821–1825.

74. Latvala J, von Hertzen L, Lindholm H, Haahtela T (2005) Trends in prevalence of asthma and allergy in Finnish young men: nationwide study, 1966–2003. Bmj 330: 1186–1187.

75. McNeill G, Tagiyeva N, Aucott L, Russell G, Helms PJ (2009) Changes in the prevalence of asthma, eczema and hay fever in pre-pubertal children: A 40-year perspective. Paediatric and Perinatal Epidemiology 23: 506–512.

76. Ng Man Kwong G, Proctor A, Billings C, Duggan R, Das C, et al. (2001) Increasing prevalence of asthma diagnosis and symptoms in children is confined to mild symptoms. Thorax 56: 312–314.

77. Osman M, Tagiyeva N, Wassall HJ, Ninan TK, Devenny AM, et al. (2007) Changing trends in sex specific prevalence rates for childhood asthma, eczema, and hay fever. Pediatr Pulmonol 42: 60–65.

78. Ronmark E, Bjerg A, Perzanowski M, Platts-Mills T, Lundback B (2009) Major increase in allergic sensitization in schoolchildren from 1996 to 2006 in northern Sweden. J Allergy Clin Immunol 124: 357–363.

79. Selnes A, Nystad W, Bolle R, Lund E (2005) Diverging prevalence trends of atopic disorders in Norwegian children. Results from three cross-sectional studies. Allergy 60: 894–899.

80. Shamssain M (2007) Trends in the prevalence and severity of asthma, rhinitis and atopic eczema in 6- to 7- and 13- to 14-yr-old children from the north-east of England. Pediatr Allergy Immunol 18: 149–153.

81. Brozek GM, Zejda JE (2004) Increase in the frequency of diagnosed allergic diseases in children - Fact or artefact? [Polish]. Pediatria Polska 79: 385–392.

82. Harangi F, Fogarasy A, Muller A, Schneider I, Sebok B (2007) No significant increase within a 3-year interval in the prevalence of atopic dermatitis among schoolchildren in Baranya County, Hungary. Journal of the European Academy of Dermatology and Venereology 21: 964–968.

83. Ponsonby A-L, Glasgow N, Pezic A, Dwyer T, Ciszek K, et al. (2008) A temporal decline in asthma but not eczema prevalence from 2000 to 2005 at school entry in the Australian Capital Territory with further consideration of country of birth. Int J Epidemiol 37: 559–569.

84. Robertson CF, Roberts MF, Kappers JH (2004) Asthma prevalence in Melbourne schoolchildren: have we reached the peak? Med J Aust 180: 273–276.

85. Toelle BG, Ng K, Belousova E, Salome CM, Peat JK, et al. (2004) Prevalence of asthma and allergy in schoolchildren in Belmont, Australia: three cross sectional surveys over 20 years. Bmj 328: 386–387.

86. Galassi C, Grabenhenrich L, Hohmann C, Keil T, Thijs C, et al. (2010) Asthma and Allergy. In: Slama R, Charles M, Keil T, Kogevinas M, Sunyer J, editors. Evaluation of Health Information and Recommendations in European Birth Cohorts The ENRIECO Project: Environmental Health Risks In European Birth Cohorts, work package 3 Report to the European Commission, ENV-FP7–2008–2262852010.

87. Williams H, Stewart A, von Mutius E, Cookson W, Anderson HR, et al. (2008) Is eczema really on the increase worldwide? J Allergy Clin Immunol 121: 947–954.e915.

88. ISAAC Steering Committee (2011) The ISAAC story. Available: http://isaac.auckland.ac.nz/story/centres/regions.php?cen=North%20America. Accessed 28 Mar 2012.

89. Flohr C, Weinmayr G, Weiland SK, Addo-Yobo E, Annesi-Maesano I, et al. (2009) How well do questionnaires perform compared with physical examination in detecting flexural eczema? Findings from the International Study of Asthma and Allergies in Childhood (ISAAC) Phase Two. Br J Dermatol 161: 846–853.

90. Cork MJ, Danby S (2009) Skin barrier breakdown: a renaissance in emollient therapy. Br J Nurs 18: 872, 874, 876–877.

91. Mommers M, Swaen GM, Weishoff-Houben M, Dott W, van Schayck CP (2005) Differences in asthma diagnosis and medication use in children living in Germany and the Netherlands. Prim Care Respir J 14: 31–37.

14

Differential Effects of Peptidoglycan Recognition Proteins on Experimental Atopic and Contact Dermatitis Mediated by Treg and Th17 Cells

Shin Yong Park[1], Dipika Gupta[1]*, Chang H. Kim[2], Roman Dziarski[1]*

1 Indiana University School of Medicine–Northwest, Gary, Indiana, United States of America, **2** School of Veterinary Medicine, Purdue University, West Lafayette, Indiana, United States of America

Abstract

Skin protects the body from the environment and is an important component of the innate and adaptive immune systems. Atopic dermatitis and contact dermatitis are among the most frequent inflammatory skin diseases and are both determined by multigenic predisposition, environmental factors, and aberrant immune response. Peptidoglycan Recognition Proteins (Pglyrps) are expressed in the skin and we report here that they modulate sensitivity to experimentally-induced atopic dermatitis and contact dermatitis. $Pglyrp3^{-/-}$ and $Pglyrp4^{-/-}$ mice (but not $Pglyrp2^{-/-}$ mice) develop more severe oxazolone-induced atopic dermatitis than wild type (WT) mice. The common mechanism underlying this increased sensitivity of $Pglyrp3^{-/-}$ and $Pglyrp4^{-/-}$ mice to atopic dermatitis is reduced recruitment of Treg cells to the skin and enhanced production and activation Th17 cells in $Pglyrp3^{-/-}$ and $Pglyrp4^{-/-}$ mice, which results in more severe inflammation and keratinocyte proliferation. This mechanism is supported by decreased inflammation in $Pglyrp3^{-/-}$ mice following in vivo induction of Treg cells by vitamin D or after neutralization of IL-17. By contrast, $Pglyrp1^{-/-}$ mice develop less severe oxazolone-induced atopic dermatitis and also oxazolone-induced contact dermatitis than WT mice. Thus, Pglyrp3 and Pglyrp4 limit over-activation of Th17 cells by promoting accumulation of Treg cells at the site of chronic inflammation, which protects the skin from exaggerated inflammatory response to cell activators and allergens, whereas Pglyrp1 has an opposite pro-inflammatory effect in the skin.

Editor: Samithamby Jeyaseelan, Louisiana State University, United States of America

Funding: This work was supported by United States Public Health Services Grants AI028797 and AI073290 from the National Institutes of Health. The funders had no role in study design, data collection and analysis, decision to publish, or preparation of the manuscript.

Competing Interests: The authors have declared that no competing interests exist.

* E-mail: dgupta@iun.edu (DG); rdziar@iun.edu (RD)

Introduction

Skin protects the body from the environment and is the largest organ in mammals. Besides forming a mechanical barrier, skin is an important component of the innate and adaptive immune systems rich in anti-microbial peptides and antigen-sensing cells, and it maintains the proper homeostatic balance between pro- and anti-inflammatory responses. Atopic dermatitis and contact dermatitis are among the most frequent inflammatory skin diseases, both determined by multigenic predisposition, environmental factors, and aberrant immune response. Atopic dermatitis has a prevalence of 15–30% in children and 2–10% in adults, involves loss of barrier function of the skin and type I hypersensitivity to environmental allergens, and is manifested by pruritic erythematosus skin eruptions and increased IgE response, often with aggravating bacterial infections [1–3]. Allergic contact dermatitis (contact hypersensitivity) has a prevalence of 2–20% and involves type IV (delayed-type) hypersensitivity to environmental allergens, manifested by erythematosus skin infiltrations with inflammatory cells [2,4,5].

Peptidoglycan Recognition Proteins (PGRPs or Pglyrps) are a family of innate immunity proteins expressed in the skin. PGRPs are conserved from insects to mammals, recognize bacterial peptidoglycan, and function in antibacterial immunity. Mammals have four PGRPs, Pglyrp1, Pglyrp2, Pglyrp3, and Pglyrp4, which were initially named PGRP-S, PGRP-L, PGRP-Iα, and PGRP-Iβ, respectively [6,7]. Three PGRPs, Pglyrp1, Pglyrp3, and Pglyrp4 are directly bactericidal [8–11], whereas Pglyrp2 is an N-acetylmuramoyl-L-alanine amidase that hydrolyzes peptidoglycan [12,13]. Pglyrp1 is highly expressed in PMN's granules and to a much lower extent in other cells [7,14,15]. Pglyrp2 is constitutively expressed in the liver and secreted into blood, and its expression is induced in keratinocytes and other epithelial cells [12,13,16–20]. Pglyrp3 and Pglyrp4 have the highest expression in the skin and are also expressed in the salivary glands, throat, tongue, esophagus, stomach, intestine, and eyes [8,21,22]. Similar to Pglyrp1 and Pglyrp2, Pglyrp3 and Pglyrp4 are secreted and their expression in these tissues is both constitutive and inducible.

We hypothesized that PGRPs play a role in the development atopic dermatitis and contact dermatitis because of (a) the prominent expression of PGRPs in the skin, (b) the location of *Pglyrp3* and *Pglyrp4* genes in the epidermal differentiation gene cluster in the psoriasis sensitivity *psors4* locus, (c) coordinated expression of *Pglyrp3* and *Pglyrp4* with other genes in the *psors4* locus, (d) previous evidence of genetic association of *Pglyrp3* and *Pglyrp4* variants with psoriasis, which is another genetically- and environmentally-determined skin disease [23,24], and (e) the ability of mammalian PGRPs to protect mice against experimental colitis [22] and to modulate the development of experimental arthritis [25]. Here we tested this hypothesis using PGRP-deficient mice and mouse models of chemically-induced atopic dermatitis and contact dermatitis.

Our results show that $Pglyrp3^{-/-}$ and $Pglyrp4^{-/-}$ mice (but not $Pglyrp2^{-/-}$ mice) are more sensitive to the development of experimental atopic dermatitis than wild type (WT) mice. The common mechanism underlying this increased sensitivity of $Pglyrp3^{-/-}$ and $Pglyrp4^{-/-}$ mice is reduced recruitment of Treg cells to the skin and enhanced production and activation Th17 cells in $Pglyrp3^{-/-}$ and $Pglyrp4^{-/-}$ mice, which results in more severe inflammation and keratinocyte proliferation. By contrast, $Pglyrp1^{-/-}$ mice are less sensitive than WT mice to both experimental atopic dermatitis and contact dermatitis. Thus, Pglyrp3 and Pglyrp4 limit over-activation of Th17 cells by promoting accumulation of Treg cells at the site of chronic inflammation, which protects the skin from exaggerated inflammatory response to cell activators and allergens. By contrast, Pglyrp1 has an opposite pro-inflammatory effect in the skin.

Results

$Pglyrp3^{-/-}$ and $Pglyrp4^{-/-}$ mice have enhanced inflammatory response in the oxazolone model of atopic dermatitis

Repeated epicutaneous sensitization with oxazolone is an established mouse model of atopic dermatitis [3,26]. Initial sensitization of mice with oxazolone through abdominal skin, followed by 6-day rest and application of oxazolone to the ears every other day for 20 days induced in WT BALB/c mice progressive moderate inflammation manifested by some redness and swelling (Figure 1A). Similar application of oxazolone to $Pglyrp3^{-/-}$ or $Pglyrp4^{-/-}$ mice induced significantly enhanced inflammation, manifested first by increased redness and significantly increased swelling, accompanied by scaling (Figure 1A). This enhanced response was unique for $Pglyrp3^{-/-}$ and $Pglyrp4^{-/-}$ mice, because it was not observed in $Pglyrp1^{-/-}$, $Pglyrp2^{-/-}$, and $Pglyrp1^{-/-}$ $Pglyrp2^{-/-}$ mice, and was dominant, because it was still observed in $Pglyrp1^{-/-}Pglyrp3^{-/-}$ and $Pglyrp2^{-/-}Pglyrp3^{-/-}$ double-knock-out mice and in $Pglyrp1^{-/-}Pglyrp2^{-/-}Pglyrp3^{-/-}$ and $Pglyrp1^{-/-}$ $Pglyrp2^{-/-}Pglyrp4^{-/-}$ triple-knockout mice (Figure 1A). Deletion of $Pglyrp1$ had the opposite effect – $Pglyrp1^{-/-}$ single knockout mice showed reduced ear swelling on days 16 through 20 of oxazolone application (Figure 1A). These results indicate that in WT mice both Pglyrp3 and Pglyrp4 have a protective effect against severe atopic dermatitis-like inflammation, whereas Pglyrp1 has an enhancing proinflammatory effect and Pglyrp2 has little effect on the response to oxazolone.

To determine the pathologic basis of higher sensitivity of $Pglyrp3^{-/-}$ and $Pglyrp4^{-/-}$ mice to oxazolone, we compared the histology of oxazolone-induced skin lesions in WT and $Pglyrp$-deficient mice. Ears in untreated WT mice have one- to two-cell thick epidermis and few-cell thick subepidermal layer with blood vessels, sebaceous glands, hair follicles, muscle bundles, and central fat and connective tissue layer, with total thickness of approximately 200 μm. Histology of all untreated $Pglyrp$-deficient mice was similar to WT mice (Figure 2). Sensitization and 10 oxazolone applications to the ears (every other day) induced strong inflammatory response that was very severe in $Pglyrp3^{-/-}$ mice and $Pglyrp4^{-/-}$ mice. Cross-sections of the oxazolone-treated ears revealed severe acanthosis (thickening of the epidermis due to proliferation of keratinocytes), parakeratosis (retention of keratinocytes' nuclei in stratum corneum), and marked thickening of the sub-epidermal layer with spongiosis (intercellular edema) and

dense cellular infiltrates (composed primarily of mononuclear cells and some polymorphonuclear cells) that were all highly prominent in $Pglyrp3^{-/-}$ mice and $Pglyrp4^{-/-}$ mice (Figure 2A) and in all other double and triple knockout mice deficient in $Pglyrp3$ (not shown). All these changes are highly characteristic of atopic dermatitis lesions. These mice did not develop rete pegs (downward papillary projections of epidermis), which are characteristic of psoriasis, but not atopic dermatitis. WT mice (Figure 2A), $Pglyrp1^{-/-}$ mice, $Pglyrp2^{-/-}$ mice, and $Pglyrp1^{-/-}Pglyrp2^{-/-}$ mice (not shown) all showed much less severe acanthosis, parakeratosis, edema, and cell infiltrations, and less thickening of the subepidermal layer.

Inflammatory response to oxazolone was accompanied by a marked increase in the concentration of serum IgE, consistent with oxazolone inflammation being a model of atopic dermatitis (which is type I hypersensitivity associated with increased IgE production). The serum IgE levels in $Pglyrp3^{-/-}$ mice and $Pglyrp4^{-/-}$ mice, as well as $Pglyrp1^{-/-}Pglyrp3^{-/-}$ and $Pglyrp2^{-/-}Pglyrp3^{-/-}$ double-knockout mice and in $Pglyrp1^{-/-}Pglyrp2^{-/-}Pglyrp3^{-/-}$ and $Pglyrp1^{-/-}Pglyrp2^{-/-}Pglyrp4^{-/-}$ triple-knockout mice were all significantly higher than in WT and in $Pglyrp1^{-/-}$, $Pglyrp2^{-/-}$, and $Pglyrp1^{-/-}Pglyrp2^{-/-}$ mice (Figure 3). Pglyrp2 also played a minor role, because $Pglyrp2^{-/-}Pglyrp3^{-/-}$ double-knockout mice and $Pglyrp1^{-/-}Pglyrp2^{-/-}Pglyrp3^{-/-}$ and $Pglyrp1^{-/-}Pglyrp2^{-/-}$ $Pglyrp4^{-/-}$ triple-knockout mice had higher serum IgE levels than $Pglyrp3^{-/-}$ and $Pglyrp4^{-/-}$ single-knockout mice.

These results demonstrate that deletion of $Pglyrp3$ or $Pglyrp4$ highly predisposes mice to atopic dermatitis-like lesions in response to oxazolone, and thus in WT mice Pglyrp3 or Pglyrp4 protect the skin from excessive inflammation in the oxazolone model of atopic dermatitis.

$Pglyrp$-deficient mice have reduced response in the oxazolone model of contact dermatitis

Single epicutaneous sensitization with oxazolone followed by a single epicutaneous challenge in a different area is an established mouse model of allergic contact dermatitis (contact hypersensitivity) due to type IV hypersensitivity [27,28]. Sensitization of mice with oxazolone through abdominal skin, followed by 6-day rest and a single application of oxazolone to the ears induced on the next day a strong inflammatory response in WT BALB/c mice, manifested by redness and swelling (Figure 1B). Similar application of oxazolone to $Pglyrp$-deficient mice induced significantly lower inflammation, manifested by significantly reduced ear swelling compared to WT mice, especially in $Pglyrp1^{-/-}$ mice, and to some extent in $Pglyrp2^{-/-}$ and $Pglyrp4^{-/-}$ mice. The reduced responsiveness was dominant, because it was still observed in $Pglyrp1^{-/-}Pglyrp2^{-/-}$ (most affected), $Pglyrp1^{-/-}Pglyrp3^{-/-}$, and $Pglyrp2^{-/-}Pglyrp3^{-/-}$ double-knockout mice and in $Pglyrp1^{-/-}$ $Pglyrp2^{-/-}Pglyrp3^{-/-}$ triple-knockout mice (Figure 1B).

To determine the pathologic basis of this lower response to oxazolone in the contact dermatitis model in $Pglyrp$-deficient mice, we compared the ear histology in oxazolone-treated WT and $Pglyrp$-deficient mice. Sensitization and single oxazolone application to the ears induced strong inflammatory response in WT mice manifested by marked spongiosis of the sub-epidermal layer with cellular infiltrates of epidermal and subepidermal layers with mononuclear and polymorphonuclear cells (but no acanthosis, parakeratosis, rete pegs, or scaling, which histologically differentiates contact dermatitis from atopic dermatitis and psoriasis) (Figure 2B). $Pglyrp1^{-/-}$ and $Pglyrp1^{-/-}Pglyrp2^{-/-}$ mice still had cellular infiltrates, but had substantially reduced swelling, compared to WT mice, mostly due to reduced edema (Figure 2B). These results indicate that in

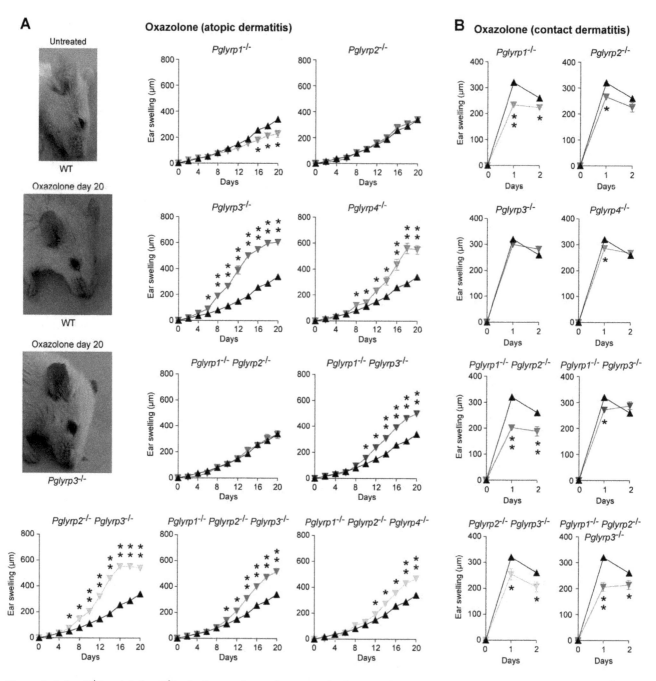

Figure 1. *Pglyrp3⁻ᐟ⁻* and *Pglyrp4⁻ᐟ⁻* mice have enhanced response in the oxazolone model of atopic dermatitis and *Pglyrp1⁻ᐟ⁻* and other *Pglyrp⁻ᐟ⁻* mice have reduced response in the oxazolone model of contact dermatitis. (**A**) Atopic dermatitis model: sensitization followed by 10 applications of oxazolone to the ears every other day induces mild inflammation (left) and mild ear swelling (right) in WT mice (black triangles) and severe inflammation with increased redness, scaling, and extensive ear swelling in *Pglyrp3⁻ᐟ⁻* and *Pglyrp4⁻ᐟ⁻* mice (color triangles). (**B**) Contact dermatitis model: sensitization followed by a single application of oxazolone to the ears induces strong ear swelling in WT mice (black triangles) and reduced ear swelling in *Pglyrp1⁻ᐟ⁻*, *Pglyrp2⁻ᐟ⁻*, and *Pglyrp4⁻ᐟ⁻* mice (color triangles). Means ± SEM (SEM were often smaller than the symbols in this and other figures); N = 9–17 mice/group; significance of differences between *Pglyrp⁻ᐟ⁻* and WT mice: *, P<0.02; **, P<0.0001.

WT mice Pglyrp1 (and also to some extent Pglyrp2 and Pglyrp4) has an enhancing proinflammatory role in this model of contact dermatitis.

Thus, altogether our results indicate that individual PGRPs have selective and distinct effects on skin inflammation. In WT mice Pglyrp3 and Pglyrp4 offer protection in the oxazolone atopic dermatitis model, Pglyrp1 has a pro-inflammatory effect both atopic and contact dermatitis models, and Pglyrp2 has little effect

on the atopic dermatitis and has a pro-inflammatory effect in the contact dermatitis model of skin inflammation.

Expression of PGRPs in inflamed ears

To gain further insight how individual PGRPs influence sensitivity to both models of skin inflammation, we compared expression of all PGRPs in the ears in untreated and oxazolone-treated mice. In both atopic and contact dermatitis models

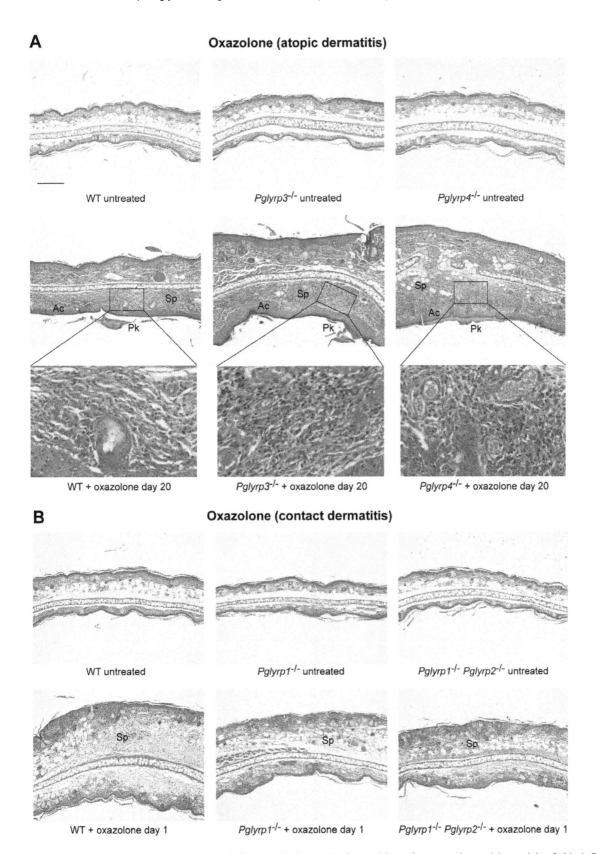

Figure 2. Ear histology in WT and *Pglyrp*-deficient mice in atopic dermatitis and contact dermatitis models of skin inflammation. (A) Oxazolone model of atopic dermatitis: sensitization and 10 applications of oxazolone to the ears every other day induced acanthosis (Ac), parakeratosis (Pk), marked thickening of the sub-epidermal layer with spongiosis (Sp) and dense cellular infiltrates of primarily mononuclear and some polymorphonuclear cells (high magnification insets), that were all highly prominent in *Pglyrp3*$^{-/-}$ mice and *Pglyrp4*$^{-/-}$ mice and much less severe in WT mice. **(B)** Oxazolone model of contact dermatitis: sensitization and a single application of oxazolone to the ears induced strong

inflammatory response in WT mice with marked spongiosis of the sub-epidermal layer (Sp) and cellular infiltrates of epidermal and sub-epidermal layers, composed of mononuclear and polymorphonuclear cells; Pglyrp1$^{-/-}$ and Pglyrp1$^{-/-}$Pglyrp2$^{-/-}$ mice still had cellular infiltrates, but had substantially reduced swelling, compared to WT mice, mostly due to reduced edema. H&E stained cross-sections; bar = 200 μm for all panels, except high magnification insets (the magnified areas are shown by rectangles).

treatment with oxazolone induced increased Pglyrp1 mRNA expression in the ears in all strains of mice (except Pglyrp1$^{-/-}$ mice, in which Pglyrp1 gene is deleted) that was significantly higher than in untreated mice (Figure 4). The expression of Pglyrp1 was significantly higher in all Pglyrp-deficient mice⁻ than in WT mice early (day 13) in the atopic dermatitis model, which correlates with their higher inflammatory response. This increase in Pglyrp1 mRNA in the ears is likely due to increased infiltration with PMNs, because PMNs highly express Pglyrp1 and expression of Pglyrp1 is not inducible in any of the cell types previously studied, including lymphocytes, monocytes, macrophages, and keratinocytes [8,14,15]. The expression of Pglyrp2 was only modestly increased early in the atopic dermatitis model and returned to the untreated level later in this model, and was not significantly changed at any time point in the contact dermatitis model, consistent with the little effect of Pglyrp2 in both atopic and contact dermatitis models (Figure 1). Pglyrp1 and Pglyrp2 were also constitutively expressed in the cervical lymph nodes at a similar level as in the ears, but following oxazolone treatment their expression in the cervical lymph nodes did not significantly change (data not shown), despite extensive stimulation and expansion of immune cells in the draining lymph nodes, which increased in diameter from <0.5 mm in untreated mice to >3 mm after 20 days of oxazolone treatment.

Pglyrp3 has high constitutive expression in untreated skin [8,21]. Pglyrp3 mRNA expression initially increased and later decreased in the atopic dermatitis model, and decreased in the contact dermatitis model. Pglyrp4 has lower constitutive expression in untreated skin than Pglyrp3. Expression of Pglyrp4 mRNA was highly increased in the atopic dermatitis model and was the highest in Pglyrp2$^{-/-}$Pglyrp3$^{-/-}$ and Pglyrp3$^{-/-}$ mice, suggesting a possibility of compensatory expression of Pglyrp4 in mice deficient in Pglyrp3 or changes in the regulation of transcription or stability

of Pglyrp4 mRNA, since Pglyrp3 and Pglyrp4 genes are tightly linked in the psoriasis sensitivity locus on chromosome 3 in mice and their expression is correlated with the expression of keratinocytes differentiation genes [21]. To further investigate which cells express Pglyrp3 and Pglyrp4 in the untreated and oxazolone-treated skin, we analyzed the expression of Pglyrp3 and Pglyrp4 proteins by immunohistochemistry. Pglyrp3 and Pglyrp4 were expressed in epidermal keratinocytes in untreated ears, and in oxazolone-treated ears they were primarily expressed in the upper layers of differentiated keratinocytes (Figure 5). Pglyrp3 and Pglyrp4 expression was not induced in other cell types, such as infiltrating inflammatory cells in oxazolone-treated ears. Moreover, Pglyrp3 and Pglyrp4 were not expressed in the cervical lymph nodes in untreated mice and their expression there was not induced following oxazolone treatment (data not shown). These results indicate that Pglyrp3 and Pglyrp4 are primarily expressed in keratinocytes, but not in immune or inflammatory cells, and thus these results raise the possibility that Pglyrp3 and Pglyrp4 exert their protective effects in the oxazolone-induced atopic dermatitis by modulating the function of keratinocytes, which are known to produce many pro-inflammatory cytokines and chemokines.

Pglyrp3$^{-/-}$ and Pglyrp4$^{-/-}$ mice have increased Th17 cells and Th17 responses in the skin

To determine the cellular basis for the differences in the inflammatory responses in Pglyrp-deficient mice, we next determined the types of inflammatory cells in the ears in both models of skin inflammation, and then we determined which cell types significantly differed in Pglyrp-deficient mice compared to WT mice. This was first accomplished by measuring the amounts of mRNA for several marker genes characteristic of various immune and inflammatory cell types in the untreated and the affected ears. To determine which marker genes (and thus cell types) are increased or decreased in Pglyrp-deficient mice compared to WT mice, we calculated how many times higher or lower they were induced in Pglyrp-deficient mice than in WT mice (fold induction in Pglyrp-deficient mice/fold induction in WT mice).

Prolonged treatment with oxazolone in the atopic dermatitis model induced increases in mRNA of several cell types in WT mice, and especially mature B cells, CD8$^+$ T cells, monocytes, PMNs, and mast cells, as well as changes associated with de-differentiation, proliferation, and activation of keratinocytes, which are all expected changes consistent with the atopic dermatitis model (Figure 6A and Figure S1). Atopic dermatitis-sensitive mice (Pglyrp3$^{-/-}$, Pglyrp4$^{-/-}$, and Pglyrp2$^{-/-}$Pglyrp3$^{-/-}$ mice) had increased expression of genes characteristic of B cells and T cells. Also increased was Rorγt mRNA, which is preferentially expressed in Th17 cells [29] (Figure 6A and Figure S1).

Short-term treatment with oxazolone in the contact dermatitis model in WT mice induced increases primarily in monocytes and PMNs at 6 hrs after challenge (Figure 6B and Figure S2) and later in T cells (18 hrs, not shown). Contact dermatitis-resistant mice (Pglyrp1$^{-/-}$, Pglyrp2$^{-/-}$, and Pglyrp1$^{-/-}$Pglyrp2$^{-/-}$ mice) had initially (6 hrs after challenge) increased B cells and Treg cells and decreased other cell-types, compared to WT mice (Figure 6B and Figure S2). Later (18 hrs after challenge) the cell markers in

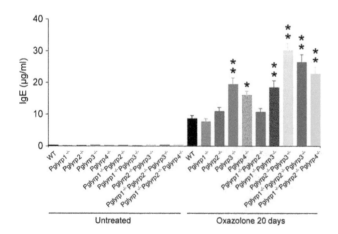

Figure 3. Pglyrp3$^{-/-}$ and Pglyrp4$^{-/-}$ mice have higher serum IgE levels than WT mice in the oxazolone model of atopic dermatitis. Sensitization followed by 10 applications of oxazolone to the ears every other day induced higher level of serum IgE in Pglyrp3$^{-/-}$ and Pglyrp4$^{-/-}$ mice than in WT, Pglyrp1$^{-/-}$ or Pglyrp2$^{-/-}$ mice; means ± SEM of 8–20 mice/group; *, P<0.002; **, P<0.0001, Pglyrp$^{-/-}$ versus WT.

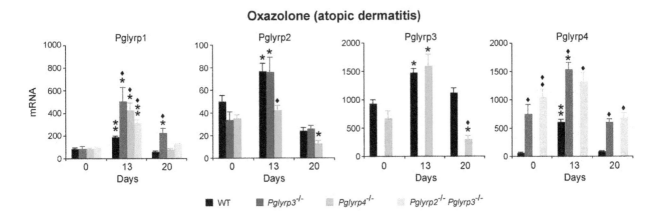

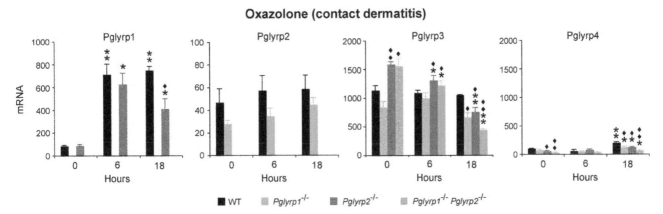

Figure 4. Pglyrp1, Pglyrp2, Pglyrp3, and Pglyrp4 expression is increased in the affected skin in the atopic dermatitis and contact dermatitis models of inflammation. The amounts of each PGRP mRNA in WT mice and in the indicated *Pglyrp*-deficient mice sensitized and treated with oxazolone every other day (atopic dermatitis model) or sensitized and treated with oxazolone at 0 hrs only (contact dermatitis model) were measured by qRT-PCR. The results are means of 3–4 mice ± SEM; *, P<0.04; **, P<0.001, treated versus untreated; ♦, P<0.04; ♦♦, P<0.001, *Pglyrp*$^{-/-}$ versus WT.

Pglyrp2$^{-/-}$ and *Pglyrp1*$^{-/-}$*Pglyrp2*$^{-/-}$ mice were similar (most cells) or increased (monocytes), compared to WT mice (not shown), consistent with comparable cell infiltrates seen in all mice on tissue sections on day 1 (Figure 2B).

To further define the cell types responsible for differential sensitivity of *Pglyrp*-deficient mice to atopic dermatitis and contact dermatitis, we measured the expression of an extended panel of cytokines, chemokines, and other marker genes characteristic of Th1, Th2, Th17, Treg, NK, and other cell types to determine which of these genes were differentially induced in the affected skin in *Pglyrp*-deficient mice, compared to WT mice. We included these cell types, because in addition to Th1 and Th2 cells, Th17 cells and other cell types may also be involved in these skin diseases.

Prolonged epicutaneous sensitization with oxazolone (20 days), which induced atopic dermatitis-like skin inflammation, was accompanied in WT mice by high activation (more than 15-fold) of 14 out of 44 studied genes in the affected skin. These genes were Ifng (Th1), Il4 and Il10 (Th2), Cxcl2, Cxcl5, and Il21 (Th17), Cxcl9 and Cxcl10 (NK cells), and Ccl3, Ccl4, Ccr5, Fasl, Il1b, and Il6 (several cell types) (Figure 7A and Figures S3 and S4). Atopic dermatitis-sensitive mice initially (day 13) had several genes activated higher than in WT mice, characteristic of several cell types, including Th2 and Th17 (Figure 7A and Figure S3). Later (day 20), atopic dermatitis-sensitive mice (*Pglyrp3*$^{-/-}$, *Pglyrp4*$^{-/-}$, and *Pglyrp2*$^{-/-}$*Pglyrp3*$^{-/-}$ mice) had four genes characteristic of

Th17 cells (Cxcl1, Cxcl5, IL17a, IL22) and one gene characteristic of several cell types (Ccl2) activated more than three-fold higher in *Pglyrp*-deficient than in WT mice (Figure 7A and Figure S4).

A single oxazolone challenge in sensitized WT mice (in the contact dermatitis model) also induced many genes characteristic of several cell types, and the early (6 hrs) activation of these genes in *Pglyrp*-deficient mice was mostly reduced, compared to WT mice (Figure 7B and Figure S5). These results are consistent with lower clinical responses of *Pglyrp*-deficient mice to a single oxazolone challenge in the contact dermatitis model (Figures 1B and 2B).

The above results indicate that the atopic dermatitis-sensitive *Pglyrp*-deficient mice have increased activity of Th17 cells in the affected skin, compared to WT mice. To further investigate the role Th17 cells (and other Th cell types) in increased sensitivity of *Pglyrp*-deficient mice in atopic dermatitis model, we used flow cytometry to directly measure Th cell types in the ears, draining lymph nodes, and the spleen.

Untreated ears in WT and *Pglyrp*$^{-/-}$ mice had <400 CD4$^+$ cells/ear, whereas after sensitization and 20 days of oxazolone treatment the numbers of CD4$^+$ cells/ear increased >50 times to ~18,000–19,000/ear in WT and *Pglyrp3*$^{-/-}$ mice (Figure 8A). Regarding Th cell subpopulations, oxazolone treatment for 13 days induced significantly higher numbers of Th2 cells (CD4$^+$IL-4$^+$) in the affected ears in *Pglyrp3*$^{-/-}$ mice compared to WT mice, whereas oxazolone treatment for 20 days induced significantly

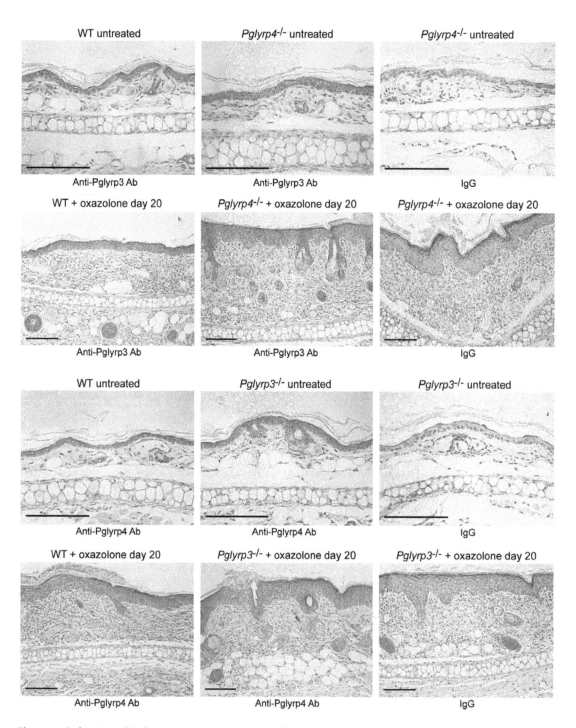

Figure 5. Pglyrp3 and Pglyrp4 are expressed primarily in the differentiated epidermal cells in both untreated and oxazolone-treated skin in the atopic dermatitis model. Transverse sections of the ears from either untreated or oxazolone-treated mice (sensitization followed by 10 applications of oxazolone to the ears every other day) were stained by an immunoperoxidase method with either anti-Pglyrp3 or anti-Pglyrp4 antibodies or IgG (negative control); bar = 50 μm.

higher numbers of Th17 cells (CD4$^+$IL-17$^+$) in the affected ears in $Pglyrp3^{-/-}$ mice compared to WT mice (Figure 8A, B and C). Thus, on day 20 in $Pglyrp3^{-/-}$ mice the numbers of Th17 cells in the ears increased from undetectable (<10/ear) to ~650 Th17 cells/ear, 3.5 times higher than in WT mice (Figure 8A). Virtually all detectable IL-17$^+$ cells in the oxazolone-treated ears were CD4$^+$ (Th17 cells) and there were very few (<50/ear, not shown) other IL-17$^+$ cells in the inflamed skin (such as CD8$^+$, γ/δ T cells, or

NKT cells), and therefore the observed increases in the numbers IL-17$^+$ cells mostly represent increases in Th17 cells (CD4$^+$IL-17$^+$). There was no significant difference in the numbers of Th1 (CD4$^+$IFN-γ$^+$) and Th2 (CD4$^+$IL-4$^+$) cells in the ears of WT and $Pglyrp3^{-/-}$ mice on day 20 (Figure 8C). Oxazolone-treated mice had substantially swollen cervical lymph nodes (>3 mm in diameter, compared to <0.5 mm in untreated mice), where on day 13 the numbers of Th2 cells and on day 20 the numbers of all

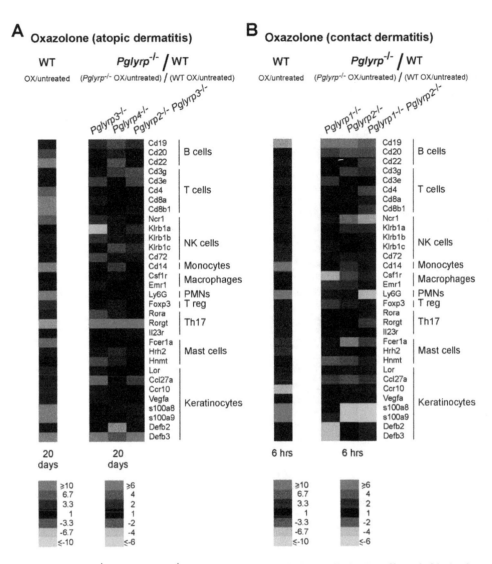

Figure 6. *Pglyrp3⁻/⁻* **and** *Pglyrp4⁻/⁻* **mice have increased Th17 cells in the affected skin in the atopic dermatitis model, whereas** *Pglyrp1⁻/⁻* **and** *Pglyrp2⁻/⁻* **mice have most cell types decreased (except B cells and Treg cells) in the contact dermatitis model.** Expression of a panel of marker genes characteristic of various inflammatory cell types in the ears of mice after (**A**) sensitization and 10 applications of oxazolone to the ears every other day, or (**B**) after sensitization and 6 hrs after a single application of oxazolone to the ears, measured by qRT-PCR is shown. For WT mice (left panels in A and B), the ratio of the amount of mRNA in oxazolone-treated to untreated mice for each gene (fold induction by oxazolone) is shown; for *Pglyrp⁻/⁻* mice (right panels in A and B), the results are the ratios of fold induction of each gene by oxazolone in *Pglyrp⁻/⁻* mice to fold induction of each gene by oxazolone in WT mice (which represents the fold difference in the response to oxazolone in *Pglyrp⁻/⁻* versus WT mice). The results are means of 3 arrays from 4–5 mice/group in heat map format. The means ± SEM bar graphs for these results are shown in Figures S1 and S2.

Th cell types were significantly higher in *Pglyrp3⁻/⁻* mice compared to WT mice (Figure 8B and C).

These results indicate initial (day 13) preferential activation of Th2 cells in the affected ears and draining lymph nodes in *Pglyrp3⁻/⁻* mice compared to WT mice, consistent with B-cell-dependence of atopic dermatitis model. However, continued treatment with oxazolone (20 days) showed a switch to preferential infiltration of the affected ears with Th17 cells in *Pglyrp3⁻/⁻* mice compared to WT mice (Figure 8), consistent with our mRNA gene expression data (Figures 6 and 7 and Figures S1, S3, and S4).

IL-17 is required for enhanced response to oxazolone in *Pglyrp3⁻/⁻* mice

To further study the role of IL-17 (Th17 cytokine) in high sensitivity of *Pglyrp3⁻/⁻* mice to oxazolone-induced atopic

dermatitis, we determined the protein levels of an IL-17-induced chemokine, CXCL-1, in the ears of WT and *Pglyrp3⁻/⁻* mice. CXCL-1 was undetectable (<7 pg/ear) in the ears of untreated mice, and after sensitization and 20 days of skin treatment with oxazolone, the amount of CXCL-1 increased to >350 pg/ear in *Pglyrp3⁻/⁻* mice, the level that was significantly higher than in WT mice (Figure 9A).

To determine whether IL-17 is required for the high sensitivity of *Pglyrp3⁻/⁻* mice to atopic dermatitis, we compared the severity of ear inflammation in oxazolone-treated *Pglyrp3⁻/⁻* mice in which IL-17 activity was inhibited with neutralizing anti-IL-17 mAb. In vivo neutralization of IL-17 activity in *Pglyrp3⁻/⁻* mice in the oxazolone-induced atopic dermatitis significantly reduced ear inflammation, compared to mice treated with an isotype control IgG (Figure 9B). These results demonstrate that IL-17 is required

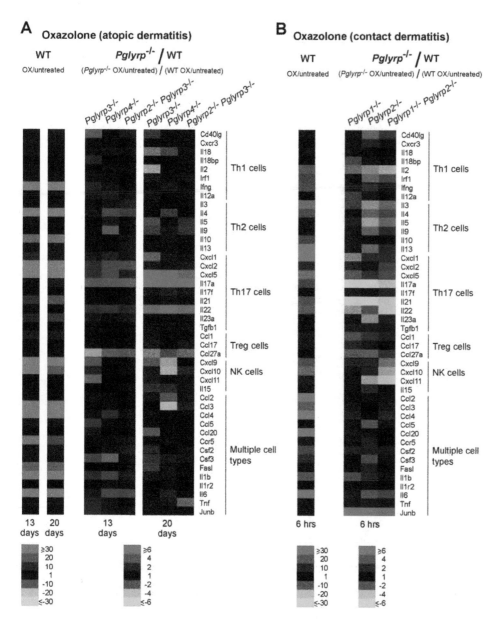

Figure 7. Th17 gene expression profile is preferentially induced in the atopic dermatitis model in *Pglyrp3*[−/−] and *Pglyrp4*[−/−] mice, whereas expression of most immune genes is reduced in the contact dermatitis model in *Pglyrp*[−/−] mice. Expression of a panel of cytokines, chemokines, and other marker genes characteristic of Th1, Th2, Th17, Treg, NK, and other cell types in the ears of mice was measured by qRT-PCR. (**A**) After sensitization and 10 applications of oxazolone to the ears every other day the expression of several Th17 marker genes was higher in *Pglyrp3*[−/−] and *Pglyrp4*[−/−] mice than in WT mice. (**B**) After sensitization and a single application of oxazolone to the ears the expression of most of immune marker genes was lower in *Pglyrp*[−/−] mice than in WT mice. For WT mice (left panels in A and B), the ratio of the amount of mRNA in oxazolone-treated to untreated mice for each gene (fold induction by oxazolone) is shown; for *Pglyrp*[−/−] mice (right panels in A and B), the results are the ratios of fold induction of each gene by oxazolone in *Pglyrp*[−/−] mice to fold induction of each gene by oxazolone in WT mice (which represents the fold difference in the response to oxazolone in *Pglyrp*[−/−] versus WT mice). The results are means of 3 arrays from 4–5 mice/group in heat map format. The means ± SEM bar graphs for these results are shown in Figures S3, S4, and S5.

for full manifestation of severe skin inflammation in *Pglyrp3*[−/−] mice in the atopic dermatitis model.

Pglyrp3[−/−] and *Pglyrp4*[−/−] mice have decreased numbers of Treg cells in the skin

Because WT mice were able to limit skin inflammation in the atopic dermatitis model more effectively than *Pglyrp3*[−/−] and *Pglyrp4*[−/−] mice, we then tested whether this difference is due to impaired generation or function of regulatory T cells (CD4+FoxP3+ Treg) in *Pglyrp*-deficient mice.

In the atopic dermatitis model WT mice efficiently recruited Treg cells into the affected skin, as evidenced by an increase in FoxP3-expressing Treg cells in the affected skin shown both by the qRT-PCR (Figure 6A and Figure S1) and by flow cytometry, in which high numbers of CD4+FoxP3+ Treg cells were found in the affected skin in WT mice (Figure 8B–D). By contrast, atopic dermatitis-sensitive *Pglyrp*-deficient mice (*Pglyrp3*[−/−], *Pglyrp4*[−/−] and *Pglyrp2*[−/−]*Pglyrp3*[−/−] mice) all had lower expression of FoxP3 mRNA in the affected ears compared to WT mice (Figure 6A and Figure S1). *Pglyrp3*[−/−] mice in the atopic dermatitis model also

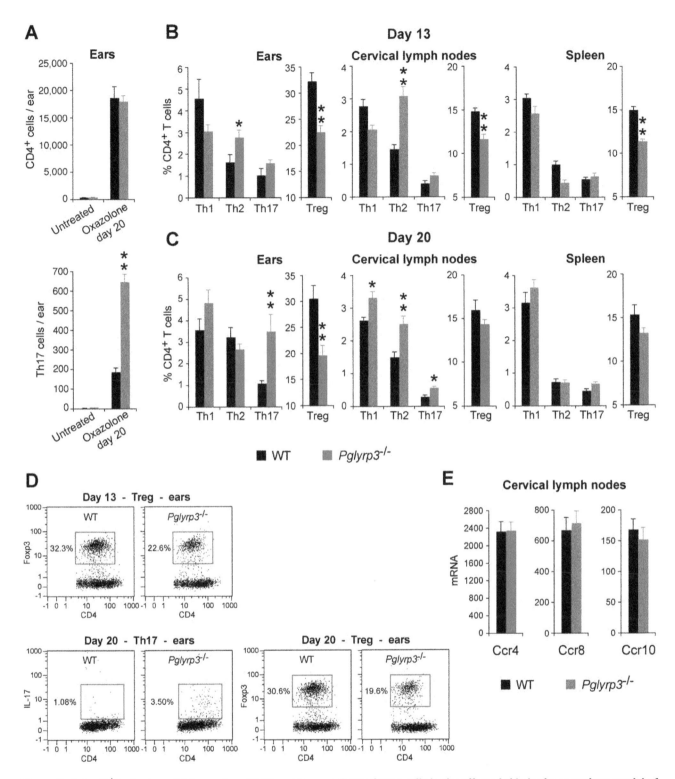

Figure 8. *Pglyrp3*$^{-/-}$ **mice have high numbers Th17 and low numbers of Treg cells in the affected skin in the oxazolone model of atopic dermatitis.** (**A**) Numbers of CD4$^+$ cells and Th17 cells in the ears or (**B–D**) percentages of Th1, Th2, Th17, and Treg cells in the ears, cervical lymph nodes, and spleen in sensitized WT and *Pglyrp3*$^{-/-}$ mice on days 13 or 20 of ear treatment with oxazolone, measured by flow cytometry; means ± SEM of 5–9 mice/group (*, P<0.05; **, P<0.005; *Pglyrp3*$^{-/-}$ versus WT) or representative dot plots are shown. (**E**) Expression of receptors for chemokines that attract Treg cells in cervical lymph nodes of sensitized WT and *Pglyrp3*$^{-/-}$ mice on day 20 of ear treatment with oxazolone measured by qRT-PCR; amounts of mRNA are shown as means ± SEM of 3 arrays from 5 mice/group.

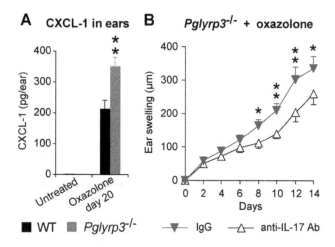

Figure 9. IL-17 is required for enhanced response to oxazolone in *Pglyrp3*^{−/−} mice. (A) The level of IL-17-induced chemokine, CXCL-1, is higher in the ears of *Pglyrp3*$^{-/-}$ mice than WT mice after sensitization and application of oxazolone for 20 days. **(B)** Ear swelling in *Pglyrp3*$^{-/-}$ mice sensitized and treated 7 times with oxazolone every other day and also treated with neutralizing anti-IL-17 mAbs is lower than in *Pglyrp3*$^{-/-}$ mice similarly treated with oxazolone and isotype control IgG. Means ± SEM; N = 6 mice/group; significance of differences between *Pglyrp3*$^{-/-}$ and WT mice (A) or IgG control and anti-IL-17 mAbs-treated mice (B): *, P<0.05; **, P<0.005.

had significantly lower numbers of CD4$^+$FoxP3$^+$ Treg cells in the affected skin compared to WT mice measured by flow cytometry (Figure 8B–D). These results suggest impaired recruitment and/or maintenance of Treg cells in the inflamed skin in *Pglyrp3*$^{-/-}$ and *Pglyrp4*$^{-/-}$ mice.

To further investigate whether *Pglyrp3*$^{-/-}$ mice have less efficient generation of induced Treg cells in lymphoid tissues in general or less efficient recruitment and/or maintenance of these cells in the inflamed skin, we compared the numbers of Treg cells in the draining cervical lymph nodes and in the spleen of WT and *Pglyrp3*$^{-/-}$ mice treated with oxazolone. Oxazolone-treated *Pglyrp3*$^{-/-}$ mice on day 13 had lower numbers of Treg cells than WT mice in cervical lymph nodes and spleen (Figure 8B). However, at the peak of inflammation (day 20) *Pglyrp3*$^{-/-}$ mice had similar numbers of Treg cells in the draining lymph nodes and spleen compared to WT mice (Figure 8C). These results indicate that *Pglyrp3*$^{-/-}$ mice can eventually generate sufficient numbers of induced Treg cells in lymphoid organs and suggest a possible reduced migration and retention of Treg cells in the affected skin.

There could be at least two reasons for this less efficient recruitment of Treg cells to the skin in *Pglyrp3*$^{-/-}$ mice: insufficient production of Treg-attracting chemokines in the skin, and/or insufficient expression of receptors for these chemokines in Treg cells in *Pglyrp3*$^{-/-}$ mice. Our results show lower expression of mRNA for Treg-attracting chemokines, CCL-27 (both on days 13 and 20) and CCL-17 (on day 20), in the ears of oxazolone-treated *Pglyrp3*$^{-/-}$ mice compared to WT mice (Figure 7A and Figures S3 and S5), indicating insufficient production of Treg-attracting chemokines in the skin in *Pglyrp3*$^{-/-}$ mice. To investigate the second of the above-mentioned possibilities, we determined whether Treg cells in the draining cervical lymph nodes in *Pglyrp3*$^{-/-}$ mice had sufficient expression of receptors for Treg-attracting chemokines (Ccr4, Ccr8, and Ccr10). The expression of mRNA for Ccr4, Ccr8, and Ccr10 in the draining cervical lymph nodes in oxazolone-treated *Pglyrp3*$^{-/-}$ mice and WT mice was similar (Figure 8E). These results support the

conclusion that Treg cells in the draining lymph nodes in oxazolone-treated *Pglyrp3*$^{-/-}$ mice have sufficient expression of receptors for Treg-attracting chemokines, but that these Treg cells are not recruited to the inflamed skin, likely because of the insufficient production of Treg-attracting chemokines in the skin (Figure 7A and Figures S3 and S4). Our results thus indicate that Pglyrp3 promotes efficient population of the skin with Treg cells in oxazolone-induced atopic dermatitis.

Induction of Treg cells in *Pglyrp3*$^{-/-}$ mice reduces Th17 cells and sensitivity to atopic dermatitis

To further investigate the role of Treg cells in high sensitivity of *Pglyrp3*$^{-/-}$ mice to atopic dermatitis, we induced generation of Treg cells by application of vitamin D to the skin (which is known to induce Treg cells [30,31]) together with the sensitizing allergen, oxazolone. Vitamin D applied to the ears of *Pglyrp3*$^{-/-}$ mice together with oxazolone significantly reduced ear swelling compared to *Pglyrp3*$^{-/-}$ mice similarly treated with oxazolone alone (Figure 10A). Vitamin D applied to the ears (together with oxazolone) also significantly increased the percentages of Treg cells both in the ears and cervical lymph nodes (as expected [30,31]), and, moreover, it significantly reduced the percentages of Th17 cells in the ears compared to the ears treated with oxazolone alone, measured on day 20 by flow cytometry (Figure 10B–D). Thus, increasing the numbers of Treg cells in the affected skin in *Pglyrp3*$^{-/-}$ mice to the numbers found in WT mice could revert the inflammatory phenotype of *Pglyrp3*$^{-/-}$ mice to the less inflammatory phenotype characteristic of WT mice. These results further demonstrate the critical role of Treg cells in preventing high levels of Th17 cells in the skin and excessive inflammation in the oxazolone model of atopic dermatitis. In summary, our results indicate that in WT mice Pglyrp3 and Pglyrp4 promote efficient population of the skin with Treg cells in the experimental model of atopic dermatitis.

Discussion

Skin diseases such as atopic dermatitis and contact dermatitis involve complex interactions of many cell types. Atopic dermatitis is thought to have Th2 bias [2,26], but recent findings also show involvement of Th17 cells [32,33]. The initially identified in vivo role of Th17 cells was promoting some autoimmune diseases and recruitment of PMNs to the sites of inflammation [34–37]. However, Th17 cells have many other functions – they play a role in inflammatory bowel diseases, skin diseases, asthma, graft rejection, atherosclerosis, periodontal disease, and arthritis [32,33,38–40]. We extend these findings by showing that Th17 cells exacerbate skin inflammation in experimental model of atopic dermatitis in a PGRP-dependent manner.

We demonstrate here that *Pglyrp3*$^{-/-}$ and *Pglyrp4*$^{-/-}$ mice develop more severe oxazolone-induced atopic dermatitis than WT mice. By contrast, *Pglyrp1*$^{-/-}$ mice develop less severe oxazolone-induced atopic dermatitis and also less severe contact dermatitis than WT mice. Thus, individual PGRPs play distinct roles in these two models of skin diseases: in WT mice Pglyrp3 and Pglyrp4 protect mice from the development of experimental atopic dermatitis, whereas Pglyrp1 enhances the development of both atopic and contact dermatitis and Pglyrp2 has less effect on both disease models.

The common mechanism underlying these protective effects of PGRPs is decreased recruitment and activity of Treg cells and enhanced production and activation of Th17 cells in the affected skin in *Pglyrp3*$^{-/-}$ and *Pglyrp4*$^{-/-}$ mice, which results in more severe inflammation and keratinocyte proliferation. Thus, in WT

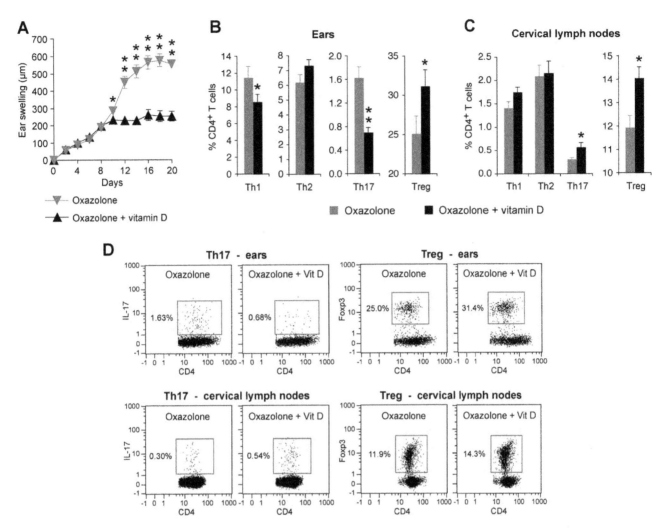

Figure 10. Induction of Treg cells by vitamin D reduces the inflammatory response to oxazolone and decreases the numbers of Th17 cells in the skin of _Pglyrp3_ _^{−/−}_ mice. (A) Vitamin D applied to the skin of _Pglyrp3_ _^{−/−}_ mice together with oxazolone reduces ear swelling compared to _Pglyrp3_ _^{−/−}_ mice similarly treated with oxazolone alone. (**B–D**) Vitamin D applied to the skin of _Pglyrp3_ _^{−/−}_ mice together with oxazolone increases the percentages of Treg cells in the ears and cervical lymph nodes and reduces the percentages of Th17 cells in the ears compared to the application of oxazolone alone, measured on day 20 by flow cytometry. Means ± SEM of 8 mice/group (A–C; *, P<0.05; **, P<0.005; oxazolone versus oxazolone + vitamin D) or representative dot plots (D) are shown.

mice Pglyrp3 and Pglyrp4 promote recruitment and retention of Treg cells in the inflamed skin, which limits over-activation of Th17 cells and protects the skin from exaggerated inflammatory response to allergens.

Our results do show prominent activation of Th2 cells in the oxazolone model of atopic dermatitis and prominent production of IgE, characteristic of Th2 bias in atopic diseases. In our model, however, the main difference at the peak of inflammation between WT and atopic dermatitis-sensitive _Pglyrp_-deficient mice, which determines the enhanced inflammatory responses and higher IgE production in _Pglyrp_-deficient mice, is the over-activation of Th17 cells and reduced numbers of Treg cells in the atopic dermatitis-sensitive mice. Our results indicate that initial Th2 response changes with time to Th17 response and that Th17 cells play an important role in enhancing inflammation and production of IgE in atopic dermatitis. Our results thus further extend recent findings of the enhancing role of Th17 cells in B cell maturation and differentiation [41–43]. Therefore, our results indicate that Pglyrp3 and Pglyrp4 are involved in

controlling multiple functions of Treg and Th17 cells in the skin in atopic dermatitis.

Contact dermatitis, which is a skin model of type IV hypersensitivity, is usually considered to be mediated by Th1 cells. However, this is an oversimplification, because recent findings show involvement of multiple cell types [2,4,5,44]. Our results show that Pglyrp1 (and other Pglyrps to a lesser extent) promotes Th1 responses, because _Pglyrp1_ _^{−/−}_ mice (and also _Pglyrp2_ _^{−/−}_ and _Pglyrp4_ _^{−/−}_ mice) have reduced inflammation in oxazolone-induced contact dermatitis. This shift of balance to Th1 cells is likely beneficial for the desirable anti-microbial responses and may taper exaggerated inflammatory responses in the skin to allergens. Note that Pglyrp1 is mainly delivered to the sites of inflammation by PMNs, which are usually recruited to fight infections.

Our results show that PGRPs, a family of innate immunity proteins, influence the functions of both innate and adaptive immune cells with an outcome of enhancing the activity of Treg cells and inhibiting the activity of Th17 cells. _Pglyrp3_ _^{−/−}_ and

Pglyrp4$^{-/-}$ mice have decreased numbers of Treg cells and increased numbers of Th17 cells in the inflamed skin, compared to WT mice. Allergens and proinflammatory stimuli (such as oxazolone) in WT mice initially induce vigorous cytokine and chemokine production. However, upon chronic exposure, WT mice recruit and maintain large numbers of Treg cells in the inflamed skin and are able to limit the proinflammatory response by reducing the number of proinflammatory genes that are activated and reducing the level of their activation. By contrast, *Pglyrp3*$^{-/-}$ and *Pglyrp4*$^{-/-}$ mice have fewer Treg cells and higher numbers of Th17 cells in the affected skin and are unable to limit inflammatory responses. This T cell imbalance in Treg/Th17 cells in *Pglyrp3*$^{-/-}$ and *Pglyrp4*$^{-/-}$ mice could come from reduced recruitment of Treg cells and increased recruitment of Th17 cells to the affected skin, and/or from enhanced local differentiation of T cells into Th17 cells (including conversion of Treg cells into Th17 cells) under the influence of locally produced chemokines and cytokines. T cell populations are dynamic and have considerable plasticity based on local cytokine milieu, as, for example, Treg cells can differentiate into Th17 under the influence of locally-produced proinflammatory cytokines [45,46].

The enhanced recruitment and differentiation of Th17 cells is supported by higher production of Th17 cell promoting cytokines (IL-17, IL-22, IL-23) in the inflamed skin in *Pglyrp3*$^{-/-}$ and *Pglyrp4*$^{-/-}$ mice. Decreased recruitment of Treg cells to the inflamed skin is supported by the presence of adequate numbers of Treg cells and adequate expression of receptors for Treg-attracting chemokines on these Treg cells in the draining lymph nodes and spleen in oxazolone-treated *Pglyrp3*$^{-/-}$ mice, but lower numbers in the skin than in WT mice. These results suggest efficient generation of induced Treg cells in lymphoid organs but defective recruitment to the inflamed skin. This mechanism is further supported by decreased production of Treg cell-attracting chemokines (CCL1, CCL17, CCL27) in the skin of *Pglyrp3*$^{-/-}$ and *Pglyrp4*$^{-/-}$ mice. Thus both increased recruitment and generation of Th17 cells and decreased recruitment and retention of Treg cells in the skin are likely responsible for increased inflammation in *Pglyrp3*$^{-/-}$ and *Pglyrp4*$^{-/-}$ mice.

Pglyrp3 and Pglyrp4 are primarily expressed in keratinocytes and other epithelial cells, but not in immune cells and stimulation of immune cells does not induce expression of Pglyrp3 and Pglyrp4 [7,8,18,20,21]. Our results extend these findings by showing expression of Pglyrp3 and Pglyrp4 in differentiated keratinocytes in untreated and oxazolone-treated skin, and no expression of Pglyrp3 and Pglyrp4 in the inflammatory cells infiltrating the skin and in the draining lymph nodes, which primarily contain resting and activated lymphocytes and antigen-presenting cells that migrated from the inflamed skin. Thus, Pglyrp3 and Pglyrp4 most likely exert their anti-inflammatory effect in the skin through their expression in keratinocytes. Keratinocytes are an important local source of chemokines and cytokines, and activation of keratinocytes by proinflammatory stimuli also leads to increased expression of Pglyrp3 and Pglyrp4 in the skin, which correlates with the ability of WT mice to reduce chronic inflammation in the skin. By contrast, increased Pglyrp1 expression in the inflamed skin likely comes from the influx of PMNs, because PMNs express high amounts of Pglyrp1 in their granules and, unlike other PGRPs, Pglyrp1 expression is not increased by proinflammatory stimuli in epithelial cells, including keratinocytes [7,8,14,15]. Thus, the effects of PGRPs in the inflamed skin are likely exerted through a change in the local production of chemokines and cytokines in the skin, which modulates the recruitment and activity of these Treg and Th17 cells. In *Pglyrp3*$^{-/-}$ and *Pglyrp4*$^{-/-}$ mice reduced numbers of Treg cells allow dominating expansion of Th17 cells,

which can increase inflammatory responses in the atopic dermatitis model, but may reduce Th1-mediated response in the contact dermatitis model by shifting T cell differentiation into Th17 cells instead of Th1 cells. Thus in WT mice, compared to *Pglyrp3*$^{-/-}$ and *Pglyrp4*$^{-/-}$ mice, the immune balance is shifted towards Th1 cells, which are protective against microbial infections (rather than Th17 cells) and towards Treg cells that control detrimental inflammation induced by proinflammatory chemicals and allergens. Our results suggest that defects in *Pglyrp3* and *Pglyrp4* genes could be predisposing to atopic dermatitis through the aforementioned shifts in immune homeostasis.

Materials and Methods

Ethics statement

All experiments on mice were performed according to the guidelines and approved by the Indiana University School of Medicine–Northwest Institutional Animal Care and Use Committee (approval number IUSM-NW-16).

Mice

We generated *Pglyrp1*$^{-/-}$, *Pglyrp2*$^{-/-}$, *Pglyrp3*$^{-/-}$, and *Pglyrp4*$^{-/-}$ mice as described previously [15,22,25]. We generated *Pglyrp1*$^{-/-}$*Pglyrp2*$^{-/-}$, *Pglyrp1*$^{-/-}$*Pglyrp3*$^{-/-}$, and *Pglyrp2*$^{-/-}$*Pglyrp3*$^{-/-}$ double knockout mice and *Pglyrp1*$^{-/-}$*Pglyrp2*$^{-/-}$*Pglyrp3*$^{-/-}$ and *Pglyrp1*$^{-/-}$*Pglyrp2*$^{-/-}$*Pglyrp4*$^{-/-}$ triple knockout mice by breeding single and double knockout mice (all on BALB/c background) and screening for homozygous deletion of each *Pglyrp* gene by PCR analysis of genomic DNA as previously described [15,22,25]. The lack of expression of the *Pglyrp* genes was confirmed by qRT-PCR in mRNA from the ears. Double and triple homozygous *Pglyrp* knockout mice were viable and fertile, bred normally, and yielded the expected male:female ratios and similar litter size as the wild type and heterozygous mice. They had similar weight as the WT and single *Pglyrp* knockout mice and developed normally with no obvious defects. Their major internal organs had normal macroscopic appearance, and normal histological appearance on hematoxylin/eosin-stained sections.

All mice used in experiments were 8–10 week-old and on BALB/c background. The original colony founder WT BALB/c breeder mice were obtained from Harlan-Sprague-Dawley. All knockout mice were backcrossed to the same WT BALB/c mice from our breeding colony, and all WT and knockout mice were bred and kept under conventional pathogen-free conditions in the same room in our facility to minimize the influence of differences in the environment. For each experiment, mice from several different cages and breeder pairs were used. The BALB/c background of *Pglyrp*-deficient mice and their negative status for all common viral and bacterial pathogens and parasites were confirmed as previously described [22].

Oxazolone atopic dermatitis and contact dermatitis models

To induce atopic dermatitis female mice were first sensitized with 10 µl of 5% oxazolone (in 80% acetone, 20% olive oil) applied to the abdomen (after removing hair with Nair cream); 6 days later applications of 30 µl of 0.1% oxazolone (in 80% acetone, 20% olive oil) to each ear (15 µl to each side) were started (day 0) and continued every other day through day 18 [26]. In some experiments to induce Treg cells [30,31] 3 µM vitamin D (1α,25-dihydroxyvitamin D$_3$ from Sigma) was added to the oxazolone solution and used for the initial sensitization and applications to the ears. Ear thickness was measured each time before oxazolone application with Digimatic Micrometer (Mitutoyo, Japan) under constant pressure at the lowest setting. Ear swelling was determined by subtracting the untreated ear thickness. The significance of differences in ear swelling was determined using t-test.

To induce contact dermatitis female mice were first sensitized with 50 µl of 2% oxazolone (Sigma, in 80% acetone, 20% olive oil) applied to the abdomen (after removing hair with Nair cream) and 5 µl applied to each paw. The contact dermatitis reaction was then elicited 6 days later with a single application of 20 µl of 1% oxazolone (in 80% acetone, 20% olive oil) to each ear (10 µl to each side) [27,28]. Ear thickness was measured as described above before and 24 and 48 hrs after oxazolone application, and ear swelling was determined by subtracting the untreated ear thickness. The significance of differences in ear swelling was determined using t-test.

Histology and immunohistochemistry

For histological analysis ears were fixed in Bouin's fixative, postfixed in 70% ethanol, and embedded in paraffin, and 5 µm cross-sections were stained with hematoxylin/eosin, and evaluated microscopically. For immunohistochemistry, antibodies to mouse Pglyrp3 and Pglyrp4 were obtained by immunizing rabbits with peptides corresponding to the following amino acids: CLVPQHSEIPKKA for Pglyrp3 (exon 5), and CWENPQTDQV-SEG for Pglyrp4 (exon 2), coupled to KLH, followed by affinity purification on SulfoLink gel (Pierce) with corresponding peptides linked through the N-terminal Cys, elution with Tris-glycine buffer, pH 2.5, and dialysis against PBS, pH 7.2. A rabbit IgG antibody to a different peptide, which did not react with mouse Pglyrp3 and Pglyrp4, prepared and purified by the same method, was used as a negative control. Paraffin 5 µm cross-sections of were stained by the immunoperoxidase method as previously described [8], including standard deparaffinization, re-hydration, quenching of endogenous peroxidase by 30 min incubation in 0.3% H_2O_2, and incubation with 0.5 µg/ml of anti-Pglyrp3 or Pglyrp4 antibodies or control IgG overnight, followed by biotinylated second Ab and Vectastain Elite ABC kit (Vector) with DAB as a substrate (which generates brown reaction product) and counterstaining with hematoxylin (blue).

RNA and quantitative real-time reverse transcription PCR (qRT-PCR)

RNA was isolated from either the entire untreated or treated ears or lymph nodes using the TRIZOL method (InVitrogen), followed by digestion with RNase-free DNase (Qiagen) and purification on RNeasy spin columns using RNeasy Minikit (Qiagen). Quantitative reverse transcription real-time PCR (qRT-PCR) was used to quantify the amounts of mRNA in the ears or lymph nodes using custom RT^2 Profiler PCR Arrays designed by us and manufactured by Qiagen/SA Biosciences, as previously described [22,25]. The arrays typically included 30 to 44 assay genes, 5 housekeeping genes and reverse transcription efficiency and DNA contamination controls. All primer sets were from Qiagen/SA Biosciences, except the following primers designed by us: Pglyrp1, exons 1 and 2 primers, GTGGTGATCTCACACA-CAGC and GTGTGGTCACCCTTGATGTT; Pglyrp2, exons 3 and 4 primers, ACCAGGATGTGCGCAAGTGGGAT and AGTGACCCAGTGTAGTTGCCCA; and Pglyrp4, exons 4 and 5 primers, CGACCAGGGCTACAAGAA and CCAGG-CAGTCTTCACTTTTC. cDNA was synthesized from 2 µg of RNA using RT^2 PCR Array First Strand Kit (Qiagen/SA Biosciences) and the arrays were performed according to the manufacturer instructions using Qiagen/SA Biosciences Master

Mix. The lists of genes are provided in the figures. The experiments were performed on RNA pooled from 4–5 mice/group and repeated 3 times usually with another set of 4–5 mice/group (usually total of 8–10 mice per treatment).

For each gene, ΔCt was calculated using the same threshold (0.2) for all genes and $Ct \leq 35$ considered as no expression, followed by normalization to 5 housekeeping genes (Hsp90ab1, Gusb, Hprt1, Gapdh, and Actb) included in each array, followed by calculation of $\Delta\Delta Ct$ for each gene from two arrays: $\Delta\Delta Ct = \Delta Ct1 - \Delta Ct2$, where $\Delta Ct1$ is the oxazolone treated mice and $\Delta CT2$ is the untreated mice, using the program provided by Qiagen/SA Biosciences. This calculation gives the fold increase in expression of each gene in the treated mice versus untreated mice per µg RNA. The genomic DNA contamination controls, reverse transcription controls, and positive PCR controls were included in each array and were all passed. Additional control to assure amplification from RNA, but not from possible contaminating DNA included parallel reaction sets from which reverse transcriptase was omitted, and which showed no amplification. To compare baseline gene expression in untreated mice, $\Delta CT1$ was from untreated PGRP-deficient mice and $\Delta CT2$ was from untreated WT mice.

The results were reported as mean fold increases after oxazolone treatment (treated/untreated) for WT mice, or ratios of fold increases in $Pglyrp$-deficient to WT mice, calculated as follows: $[(Pglyrp^{-/-}\ \text{treated})/(Pglyrp^{-/-}\ \text{untreated})]/[(\text{WT treated})/(\text{WT untreated})]$ and presented as heat maps or bar graphs. The latter fold differences (ratios) of >1 or <1 reflect higher or lower expression levels of the genes (respectively) in $Pglyrp$-deficient than in WT mice. Heat maps were generated using Java TreeView after converting <1 ratios to negative fold difference using the formula: $(-1)/\text{ratio}$. In some bar graph figures, <1 ratios were also converted to negative fold difference using the formula: $(-1)/\text{ratio}$. The significance of differences in gene activation between groups of mice was determined using the two-sample one-tailed t-test, and typically the differences of >2 fold were significant at $P<0.05$.

Expression of mRNA for PGRPs and some chemokine receptors was similarly measured by qRT-PCR using Qiagen/SA Biosciences First Strand Kit (with random primers) and amplification for 40 cycles with Qiagen/SA Biosciences SYBR Green Master Mix, and calculated using comparative cycle threshold method with 5 housekeeping genes (Hsp90ab1, Gusb, Hprt1, Gapdh, and Actb) as controls.

Isolation of cells and flow cytometry

Mouse ears were placed in RPMI-1640 with 3 mg/ml of Dispase II (Roche), separated into dorsal and ventral halves and scored on the dermal side with a scalpel. The tissue was digested for 8 hrs at 37°C in 5% CO_2. Dermis was then separated from the epidermis and epidermis was further digested with 0.25% trypsin in RPMI-1640 for 10 min at 37°C. Cells were washed twice with RPMI-1640 with 5% fetal bovine serum (FBS) and incubated for 20 hrs in the same medium at 37°C in 5% CO_2. Cells were then strained through a 40 µm filter and resuspended at 2.0×10^7 cells/ml in RPMI-1640 with 5% FBS. Single cells from cervical lymph nodes and spleen were obtained by passing the tissue through a 40 µm filter, red blood cells were removed from the spleen cells with a lysis buffer (Biolegend), and cells were suspended at 2.0×10^7 cells/ml in RPMI-1640 with 5% FBS.

1×10^6 cells were stained with CD4-APC (clone RM4-5, Biolegend) antibody for 20 min at 4°C. CD4-stained cells were then stained for Foxp3-PE (clone FJK-16s, eBioscience) or for cytokines IFN-γ-PE (clone XMG1.2), IL4-PE (clone 11B11) and

IL-17-PE (clone TC11-18H10.1) with antibodies from Biolegend, used at 0.2 mg/1×10^6 cells according to Biolegend protocols using Biolegend buffers. Prior to staining for cytokines, CD4-APC stained cells were activated with TPA (12-O-Tetradecanoylphorbol 13-acetate, 25 ng/ml) and ionomycin (250 ng/ml) in the presence of the Golgi inhibitor, monensin, for 4 hrs at 37°C in 5% CO_2. Cells were analyzed by flow cytometry using MACSQuant (Miltenyi) cytometer. Foxp3, IFN-γ, IL-4 and IL-17 positive cells were measured within the CD4$^+$ gate.

Neutralization of IL-17 and ELISA

IL-17 was neutralized by intravenous injections of anti-IL-17 mAb (specific for IL-17A and not reactive with IL-1F, rat clone 50104, endotoxin-free from R&D Systems) 100 μg at sensitization and 50 μg on days 0, 3, 6, 9, 12, and 15 of oxazolone treatment. Control mice were similarly treated with isotype control rat IgG2aκ mAb (clone 16-4321, endotoxin-free from eBioscience). The amount of CXCL-1 in ears was measured by ELISA as previously described [25], after each ear was homogenized with Polytron in 0.5 ml of PBS (without Ca/Mg) with 1 mM EDTA, 1 mM PMSF, 1:100 dilution of protease inhibitors (Sigma P1860), and 0.5% Triton X-100, followed by sonication and centrifugation.

Supporting Information

Figure S1 *Pglyrp3$^{-/-}$* and *Pglyrp4$^{-/-}$* mice have increased Th17 cells in the affected skin in the oxazolone atopic dermatitis model. Expression of a panel of marker genes characteristic of various inflammatory cell types in the ears of mice after sensitization and 10 applications of oxazolone to the ears every other day measured by qRT-PCR (day 20) is shown. For WT mice (top panel), the ratio of the amount of mRNA in oxazolone-treated to untreated mice for each gene (fold induction by oxazolone) is shown; for *Pglyrp$^{-/-}$* mice, the results are the ratios of fold induction of each gene by oxazolone in *Pglyrp$^{-/-}$* mice to fold induction of each gene by oxazolone in WT mice (which represents the fold difference in the response to oxazolone in *Pglyrp$^{-/-}$* versus WT mice). The results are means ± SEM of 3 arrays from 4–5 mice/group and are shown as heat maps in Figure 6A in the main article.

Figure S2 In the oxazolone contact dermatitis model in *Pglyrp1$^{-/-}$* and *Pglyrp2$^{-/-}$* mice most cell types are decreased in the affected skin, but Treg cells and B cells are increased. Expression of a panel of marker genes characteristic of various inflammatory cell types in the ears of mice after sensitization and 6 hrs after single application of oxazolone to the ears measured by qRT-PCR is shown. For WT mice (top panel), the ratio of the amount of mRNA in oxazolone-treated to untreated mice for each gene (fold induction by oxazolone) is shown; for *Pglyrp$^{-/-}$* mice, the results are the ratios of fold induction of each gene by oxazolone in *Pglyrp$^{-/-}$* mice to fold induction of each gene by oxazolone in WT mice (which represents the fold difference in the response to oxazolone in *Pglyrp$^{-/-}$* versus WT mice). The results are means ± SEM of 3 arrays from 4–5 mice/group and are shown as heat maps in Figure 6B in the main article.

Figure S3 Multiple inflammatory and immune genes are induced at an early stage of oxazolone model of atopic dermatitis. Expression of a panel of cytokines, chemokines, and other marker genes characteristic of Th1, Th2, Th17, Treg, NK, and other cell types in the ears of mice after sensitization and 7 applications of oxazolone to the ears every other day measured by qRT-PCR (day 13). For WT mice (top panel), the ratio of the amount of mRNA in oxazolone-treated to untreated mice for each gene (fold induction by oxazolone) is shown; for *Pglyrp3$^{-/-}$* or *Pglyrp4$^{-/-}$* mice, the results are the ratios of fold induction of each gene by oxazolone in *Pglyrp$^{-/-}$* mice to fold induction of each gene by oxazolone in WT mice (which represents the fold difference in the response to oxazolone in *Pglyrp$^{-/-}$* versus WT mice). The results are means ± SEM of 3 arrays from 4–5 mice/group and are shown as heat maps in Figure 7A in the main article.

Figure S4 Th17 gene expression profile is preferentially induced in the oxazolone model of atopic dermatitis in *Pglyrp3$^{-/-}$* and *Pglyrp4$^{-/-}$* mice. Expression of a panel of cytokines, chemokines, and other marker genes characteristic of Th1, Th2, Th17, Treg, NK, and other cell types in the ears of mice after sensitization and 10 applications of oxazolone to the ears every other day shows higher induction of several Th17 marker genes in *Pglyrp3$^{-/-}$* and *Pglyrp4$^{-/-}$* compared to WT mice measured by qRT-PCR. For WT mice (top panel), the ratio of the amount of mRNA in oxazolone-treated to untreated mice for each gene (fold induction by oxazolone) is shown; for *Pglyrp$^{-/-}$* mice, the results are the ratios of fold induction of each gene by oxazolone in *Pglyrp$^{-/-}$* mice to fold induction of each gene by oxazolone in WT mice (which represents the fold difference in the response to oxazolone in *Pglyrp$^{-/-}$* versus WT mice). The results are means ± SEM of 3–4 arrays from 4–5 mice/group and are shown as heat maps in Figure 7A in the main article.

Figure S5 Expression of most immune genes is reduced in the oxazolone model of contact dermatitis in *Pglyrp$^{-/-}$* mice. Expression of a panel of cytokines, chemokines, and other marker genes characteristic of Th1, Th2, Th17, Treg, NK, and other cell types in the ears of mice after sensitization and a single application of oxazolone to the ears shows lower induction of immune marker genes in *Pglyrp$^{-/-}$* mice compared to WT mice measured by qRT-PCR. For WT mice (top panel), the ratio of the amount of mRNA in oxazolone-treated to untreated mice for each gene (fold induction by oxazolone) is shown; for *Pglyrp$^{-/-}$* mice, the results are the ratios of fold induction of each gene by oxazolone in *Pglyrp$^{-/-}$* mice to fold induction of each gene by oxazolone in WT mice (which represents the fold difference in the response to oxazolone in *Pglyrp$^{-/-}$* versus WT mice, negative numbers show lower gene induction in *Pglyrp$^{-/-}$* than in WT mice). The results are means ± SEM of 3–4 arrays from 4–5 mice/group and are shown as heat maps in Figure 7B in the main article.

Acknowledgments

We are grateful to Patrick Bankston for help in interpreting histology slides, and Robert Rukavina, Julie Cook, Panida Girddonfag, and Tiffany Caluag for maintaining and breeding our mice.

Author Contributions

Conceived and designed the experiments: SYP DG CHK RD. Performed the experiments: SYP DG RD. Analyzed the data: SYP DG CHK RD. Wrote the paper: RD.

References

1. De Benedetto A, Agnihothri R, McGirt LY, Bankova LG, Beck LA (2009) Atopic dermatitis: a disease caused by innate immune defects? J Invest Dermatol 129: 14–30.

2. Fonacier LS, Dreskin SC, Leung DY (2010) Allergic skin diseases. J Allergy Clin Immunol 125(Suppl 2): S138–149.

3. Jin H, He R, Oyoshi M, Geha RS (2009) Animal models of atopic dermatitis. J Invest Dermatol 129: 31–40.

4. Wang B, Feliciani C, Freed I, Cai Q, Sauder DN (2001) Insights into molecular mechanisms of contact hypersensitivity gained from gene knockout studies. J Leukoc Biol 70: 185–191.

5. Martin SF, Jakob T (2008) From innate to adaptive immune responses in contact hypersensitivity. Curr Opin Allergy Clin Immunol 8: 289–293.

6. Kang D, Liu G, Lundstrom A, Gelius E, Steiner H (1998) A peptidoglycan recognition protein in innate immunity conserved from insects to humans. Proc Natl Acad Sci USA 95: 10078–10082.

7. Liu C, Xu Z, Gupta D, Dziarski R (2001) Peptidoglycan recognition proteins: a novel family of four human innate immunity pattern recognition molecules. J Biol Chem 276: 34686–34694.

8. Lu X, Wang M, Qi J, Wang H, Li X, et al. (2006) Peptidoglycan recognition proteins are a new class of human bactericidal proteins. J Biol Chem 281: 5895–5907.

9. Tydell CC, Yuan J, Tran P, Selsted ME (2006) Bovine peptidoglycan recognition protein-S: antimicrobial activity, localization, secretion, and binding properties. J Immunol 176: 1154–1162.

10. Wang M, Liu L-H, Wang S, Li X, Lu X, et al. (2007) Human peptidoglycan recognition proteins require zinc to kill both Gram-positive and Gram-negative bacteria and are synergistic with antibacterial peptides. J Immunol 178: 3116–3125.

11. Kashyap DR, Wang M, Liu L-H, Boons G-J, Gupta D, Dziarski R (2011) Peptidoglycan recognition proteins kill bacteria by activating protein-sensing two-component systems. Nature Med 17: 676–683.

12. Gelius E, Persson C, Karlsson J, Steiner H (2003) A mammalian peptidoglycan recognition protein with N-acetylmuramoyl-L-alanine amidase activity. Biochem Biophys Res Commun 306: 988–994.

13. Wang Z-M, Li X, Cocklin RR, Wang M, Wang M, et al. (2003) Human peptidoglycan recognition protein-L is an N-acetylmuramoyl-L-alanine amidase. J Biol Chem 278: 49044–49052.

14. Liu C, Gelius E, Liu G, Steiner H, Dziarski R (2000) Mammalian peptidoglycan recognition protein binds peptidoglycan with high affinity, is expressed in neutrophils, and inhibits bacterial growth. J Biol Chem 275: 24490–24499.

15. Dziarski R, Platt KA, Gelius E, Steiner H, Gupta D (2003) Defect in neutrophil killing and increased susceptibility to infection with non-pathogenic Gram-positive bacteria in peptidoglycan recognition protein-S (PGRP-S)-deficient mice. Blood 102: 689–697.

16. Lo D, Tynan W, Dickerson J, Mendy J, Chang HW, et al. (2003) Peptidoglycan recognition protein expression in mouse Peyer's Patch follicle associated epithelium suggests functional specialization. Cell Immunol 224: 8–16.

17. Xu M, Wang Z, Locksley RM (2004) Innate immune responses in peptidoglycan recognition protein L-deficient mice. Mol Cell Biol 24: 7949–7957.

18. Wang H, Gupta D, Li X, Dziarski R (2005) Peptidoglycan recognition protein 2 (N-acetylmuramoyl-L-Ala amidase) is induced in keratinocytes by bacteria through the p38 kinase pathway. Infect Immun 73: 7216–7225.

19. Zhang Y, van der Fits L, Voerman JS, Melief M-J, Laman JD, et al. (2005) Identification of serum N-acetylmuramoyl-L-alanine amidase as liver peptidoglycan recognition protein 2. Biochim Biophys Acta 1752: 34–46.

20. Li X, Wang S, Wang H, Gupta D (2006) Differential expression of peptidoglycan recognition protein 2 in the skin and liver requires different transcription factors. J Biol Chem 281: 20738–20748.

21. Mathur P, Murray B, Crowell T, Gardner H, Allaire N, et al. (2004) Murine peptidoglycan recognition proteins PglyrpIα and PglyrpIβ are encoded in the epidermal differentiation complex and are expressed in epidermal and hematopoietic tissues. Genomics 83: 1151–1163.

22. Saha S, Jing X, Park SY, Wang S, Li X, et al. (2010) Peptidoglycan recognition proteins protect mice from experimental colitis by promoting normal gut flora and preventing induction of interferon-γ. Cell Host Microbe 8: 147–162.

23. Sun C, Mathur P, Dupuis J, Tizard R, Ticho B, et al. (2006) Peptidoglycan recognition proteins Pglyrp3 and Pglyrp4 are encoded from the epidermal differentiation complex and are candidate genes for the Psors4 locus on chromosome 1q21. Hum Genet 119: 113–125.

24. Kainu K, Kivinen K, Zucchelli M, Suomela S, Kere J, et al. (2009) Association of psoriasis to PGLYRP and SPRR genes at PSORS4 locus on 1q shows heterogeneity between Finnish, Swedish and Irish families. Exp Dermatol 18: 109–115.

25. Saha S, Qi J, Wang S, Wang M, Li X, et al. (2009) PGLYRP-2 and Nod2 are both required for peptidoglycan-induced arthritis and local inflammation. Cell Host Microbe 5: 137–150.

26. Man MQ, Hatano Y, Lee SH, Man M, Chang S, et al. (2008) Characterization of a hapten-induced, murine model with multiple features of atopic dermatitis: structural, immunologic, and biochemical changes following single versus multiple oxazolone challenges. J Invest Dermatol 128: 79–86.

27. Lange-Asschenfeldt B, Weninger W, Velasco P, Kyriakides TR, von Andrian UH, et al. (2002) Increased and prolonged inflammation and angiogenesis in delayed-type hypersensitivity reactions elicited in the skin of thrombospondin-2-deficient mice. Blood 99: 538–545.

28. Kunstfeld R, Hirakawa S, Hong YK, Schacht V, Lange-Asschenfeldt B, et al. (2004) Induction of cutaneous delayed-type hypersensitivity reactions in VEGF-A transgenic mice results in chronic skin inflammation associated with persistent lymphatic hyperplasia. Blood 104: 1048–1057.

29. Ivanov II, McKenzie BS, Zhou L, Tadokoro CE, Lepelley A, et al. (2006) The orphan nuclear receptor RORγt directs the differentiation program of proinflammatory IL-17+ T helper cells. Cell 126: 1121–1133.

30. Gorman S, Kuritzky LA, Judge MA, Dixon KM, McGlade JP, et al. (2007) Topically applied 1,25-dihydroxyvitamin D3 enhances the suppressive activity of CD4+CD25+ cells in the draining lymph nodes. J Immunol 179: 6273–6283.

31. Ghoreishi M, Bach P, Obst J, Komba M, Fleet JC, et al. (2009) Expansion of antigen-specific regulatory T cells with the topical vitamin D analog calcipotriol. J Immunol 182: 6071–6078.

32. Koga C, Kabashima K, Shiraishi N, Kobayashi M, Tokura Y (2008) Possible pathogenic role of Th17 cells for atopic dermatitis. J Invest Dermatol 128: 2625–2630.

33. Oyoshi MK, Murphy GF, Geha RS (2009) Filaggrin-deficient mice exhibit TH17-dominated skin inflammation and permissiveness to epicutaneous sensitization with protein antigen. J Allergy Clin Immunol 124: 485–493.

34. Ye P, Rodriguez FH, Kanaly S, Stocking KL, Schurr J, et al. (2001) Requirement of interleukin 17 receptor signaling for lung CXC chemokine and granulocyte colony-stimulating factor expression, neutrophil recruitment, and host defense. J Exp Med 194: 519–527.

35. Cua DJ, Sherlock J, Chen Y, Murphy CA, Joyce B, et al. (2003) Interleukin-23 rather than interleukin-12 is the critical cytokine for autoimmune inflammation of the brain. Nature 421: 744–748.

36. Murphy CA, Langrish CL, Chen Y, Blumenschein W, McClanahan T, et al. (2003) Divergent pro- and antiinflammatory roles for IL-23 and IL-12 in joint autoimmune inflammation. J Exp Med 198: 1951–1957.

37. Langrish CL, Chen Y, Blumenschein WM, Mattson J, Basham B, et al. (2005) IL-23 drives a pathogenic T cell population that induces autoimmune inflammation. J Exp Med 201: 233–240.

38. Korn T, Bettelli E, Oukka M, Kuchroo VK (2009) IL-17 and Th17 cells. Annu Rev Immunol 27: 485–517.

39. Miossec P, Korn T, Kuchroo VK (2009) Interleukin-17 and type 17 helper T cells. N Engl J Med 361: 888–898.

40. Alcorn JF, Crowe CR, Kolls JK (2010) TH17 cells in asthma and COPD. Annu Rev Physiol 72: 495–516.

41. Hsu HC, Yang P, Wang J, Wu Q, Myers R, et al. (2008) Interleukin 17-producing T helper cells and interleukin 17 orchestrate autoreactive germinal center development in autoimmune BXD2 mice. Nat Immunol 9: 166–175.

42. Mitsdoerffer M, Lee Y, Jäger A, Kim HJ, Korn T, et al. (2010) Proinflammatory T helper type 17 cells are effective B-cell helpers. Proc Natl Acad Sci USA 107: 14292–14297.

43. Wu HJ, Ivanov II, Darce J, Hattori K, Shima T, et al. (2010) Gut-residing segmented filamentous bacteria drive autoimmune arthritis via T helper 17 cells. Immunity 32: 815–827.

44. O'Leary JG, Goodarzi M, Drayton DL, von Andrian UH (2006) T cell- and B cell-independent adaptive immunity mediated by natural killer cells. Nat Immunol 7: 507–516.

45. Zhou L, Chong MM, Littman DR (2009) Plasticity of CD4+ T cell lineage differentiation. Immunity 30: 646–655.

46. Campbell DJ, Koch MA (2011) Phenotypical and functional specialization of FOXP3+ regulatory T cells. Nat Rev Immunol 11: 119–130.

15

Childhood Atopic Diseases and Early Life Circumstances: An Ecological Study in Cuba

Suzanne D. van der Werff[1,2]*, Katja Polman[1,2], Maiza Campos Ponce[1], Jos W. R. Twisk[1,3], Raquel Junco Díaz[4], Mariano Bonet Gorbea[4], Patrick Van der Stuyft[5,6]

1 Department of Health Sciences, VU University Amsterdam, Amsterdam, The Netherlands, 2 Department of Biomedical Sciences, Prince Leopold Institute of Tropical Medicine, Antwerp, Belgium, 3 Department of Epidemiology and Biostatistics, EMGO Institute of Health and Care Research, VU University Medical Center, Amsterdam, The Netherlands, 4 National Institute of Hygiene, Epidemiology and Microbiology, Havana, Cuba, 5 Department of Public Health, Prince Leopold Institute of Tropical Medicine, Antwerp, Belgium, 6 Department of Public Health, Ghent University, Ghent, Belgium

Abstract

Background: Children are especially vulnerable during periods of resource shortage such as economic embargoes. They are likely to suffer most from poor nutrition, infectious diseases, and other ensuing short-term threats. Moreover, early life circumstances can have important consequences for long-term health. We examined the relationship between early childhood exposure to the Cuban economic situation in the nineties and the occurrence of atopic diseases later in childhood.

Methodology/Principal Findings: A cross-sectional study of 1321 primary schoolchildren aged 4–14 was conducted in two Cuban municipalities. Asthma, allergic rhinoconjunctivitis and atopic dermatitis were diagnosed using the International Study of Asthma and Allergies in Childhood questionnaire. Children were divided into three groups of exposure to the economic situation in the nineties according to birth date: (1) unexposed; (2) exposed during infancy; (3) exposed during infancy and early childhood. Associations were assessed using multiple logistic regression models. Exposure during infancy had a significant inverse association with the occurrence of asthma (OR 0.56, 95%CI 0.33–0.94) and allergic rhinoconjunctivitis (OR 0.46, 95%CI 0.25–0.85). The associations were stronger after longer exposure, i.e. during infancy and early childhood, for asthma (OR 0.40, 95% CI 0.17–0.95) and allergic rhinoconjunctivitis (OR 0.29, 95%CI 0.11–0.77). No significant associations were found for atopic dermatitis.

Conclusions/Significance: Exposure to the economic situation in the nineties during infancy and early childhood was inversely associated with asthma and allergic rhinoconjunctivitis occurrence later in childhood. We hypothesize that factors related to this period, such as infectious diseases and undernutrition, may have an attenuating effect on atopic disease development. The exact cause and underlying mechanisms need to be further elucidated.

Editor: Vincent W V. Jaddoe, Erasmus Medical Center, The Netherlands

Funding: This work was supported by a grant of the Directorate-General for Development Cooperation (DGDC) within the Framework Agreement 2 (2003–2007) DGDC-ITM 'IPK/INHEM/CUBA' project [ITM-DGD FA2 920501]. The funder had no role in study design, data collection and analysis, decision to publish, or preparation of the manuscript.

Competing Interests: The authors have declared that no competing interests exist.

* E-mail: suzanne.vander.werff@vu.nl

Introduction

Economic crises can have a negative impact on health [1,2]. In Cuba a period of great economic difficulty, known as the "Special Period", affected the country in the early 1990 s. The United States instated an economic blockade against the island in 1961. This embargo, along with the collapse of the Soviet Union and the Eastern European socialist block in the late 1980 s, reduced Cuban foreign trade by 80%. Multiple economic constraints evolved which further deteriorated when the U.S. intensified their sanctions in the early 1990 s. The situation improved during 1995–1996 and especially from 1996 on, but complete economic recovery was not reached until after 2000 [3–6].

The economic problems affected the health of the Cuban population in various ways, due to a sudden shortage of essential products such as food, energy, drugs and medical equipment [3–

5]. Approximately half of the food needed to meet caloric and protein needs was imported. Therefore, the decline in food imports combined with an already low food production within Cuba resulted in a 40% reduction in the availability of nutritional energy per capita [3–6]. Furthermore, diet quality, composition and patterns were affected [5]. Vitamin deficiencies led to an increase of anaemia in pregnant women and infants and an epidemic of optic neuropathy predominantly among males [3,7,8]. The incidence of tuberculosis increased as did the mortality rates from infectious and parasitic disorders, and influenza and pneumonia [3]. Although the economic crisis in Cuba was severe, the harmful effects on general public health were reduced to a minimum due to appropriate economic and social measures taken by the government to counter the crisis [9]. For example, vulnerable groups like children, women, and the elderly were prioritized for protection against nutritional deficiencies [3].

Children under the age of five are especially vulnerable during economic embargoes. They are likely to suffer most from poor nutrition, increased infectious disease risk, and other ensuing short-term threats [2,10]. Moreover, early life circumstances may have serious consequences for long-term health, such as cardiovascular and other chronic diseases [11,12]. Previous research on the health impact of economic crises mostly focused on morbidity, mortality, impact on health care, and nutritional status during and shortly after a crisis [13–16]. Longer term consequences, like altered chronic disease occurrence, have been studied less and mostly in adults [11].

In this ecological study, we examined the relationship between early childhood exposure to the Cuban economic situation in the nineties and the occurrence of atopic diseases later in childhood. Possible contributing factors and underlying mechanisms for this association will be discussed.

Methods

Study Design

A cross-sectional study was conducted in 1321 primary schoolchildren of two municipalities in Cuba: San Juan y Martínez (SJM) in Pinar del Rio (December 2003), a province in the west of Cuba, and Fomento in Sancti Spiritus (May 2004), a province in the centre of Cuba. Rural and urban primary schools were randomly selected from SJM (N = 5) and Fomento (N = 14). All children were included in the study, i.e. 398 children from SJM and 923 children from Fomento. Data on atopic diseases, other relevant health and environmental factors, and demographic characteristics were collected. Further details have been described elsewhere [17,18].

Ethics Statement

Informed written consent was obtained from the parents or guardians of each participating child. This study is part of a larger investigation on atopic diseases and helminth infections in Cuban children, for which approval was obtained from the Ethical Committees of the Prince Leopold Institute of Tropical Medicine in Antwerp, Belgium, the Pedro Kourí Institute (IPK) of Tropical Medicine and the National Institute for Hygiene, Epidemiology and Microbiology (INHEM) in Havana, Cuba.

Atopic Diseases

Atopic disease occurrence, i.e. asthma, allergic rhinoconjunctivitis and atopic dermatitis, was determined by means of the standard Spanish version of the International Study of Asthma and Allergies in Childhood (ISAAC) questionnaire [19], whereby a parent or guardian of each child was interviewed by a trained local team member. ISAAC definitions of atopic diseases were used in this study: current asthma, shortened to 'asthma' throughout the text, was defined as an affirmative answer to the second ISAAC core asthma question on current wheeze [20]; allergic rhinoconjunctivitis was defined as an affirmative answer to the second and third core questions of the ISAAC modules on rhinitis [21]; and atopic dermatitis was defined as an affirmative answer to the second and third core questions of the ISAAC modules on eczema [22].

Exposure to Economic Situation

Exposure to the Cuban economic situation in the nineties was determined using the child's date of birth. None of the children in our study group were born before 1990. The gross domestic product (GDP) dropped dramatically starting in 1990 [4]. As the situation improved during 1995–1996 [5,6], the exposure period

was set from January 1st 1990 until January 1st, 1996. Children were divided into three groups: (1) exposed during infancy (<24 months) and early childhood (2–6 year), i.e. born before January 1st, 1994; (2) exposed only during infancy, i.e. born from January 1st, 1994 till January 1st, 1996; and (3) unexposed, i.e. born from January 1st, 1996 and later.

Covariates

Demographic variables considered were sex, age (in years), municipality (SJM vs. Fomento) and area of residence (rural vs. urban). Socio-economic variables were monthly household income (250 pesos (≈ 7 euro)/month or less vs. more than 250 pesos/month) and education level of the parents (less than grade 12 vs. grade 12 or higher). Perinatal variables considered were low birth weight (LBW), i.e. a birth weight less than 2500 gram (yes or no), and premature birth, i.e. a gestational age of less than 37 weeks (yes or no). The variables included regarding the first year of life were breastfeeding for more than six months (yes or no) and antibiotics use (yes or no). All these variables were collected by means of a structured parental questionnaire.

Statistical Analysis

Statistical analyses were conducted using SPSS (SPSS Inc., Chicago, IL, USA) version 17.0 for Windows. A P-value of 0.05 or less was regarded as statistically significant.

Characteristics of the study population are given as numbers and percentages, except age which is given as median and its interquartile range (IQR). Differences in the covariates between the three exposure groups were tested using the Chi-square test, except age for which the Kruskal-Wallis test was used. Univariate logistic regression models were performed to assess crude associations between exposure to the economic situation in the nineties and atopic disease outcomes with the unexposed group as the reference. Subsequently, the covariates were entered using a stepwise forward approach to examine possible confounding or effect modification. Only relevant confounders, i.e. which satisfied a change-in-estimate criterion of ≥10% [23], and significant effect modifiers were included in the final multiple logistic regression models.

To test the robustness of the results, sensitivity analyses were performed: the two cut-off dates that distinguished the three groups were shifted forward for three and six months, and the 'transition groups' with a range of six months before and after both cut-off dates were removed, and associations were re-assessed.

Results

All 1321 children were included in the analysis. The participating children were aged 4 till 14 (median 8 years) and consisted of 678 boys (51%) and 643 girls (49%). The response rate to the questionnaires was 100%. Characteristics of the study population according to their exposure to the economic situation in the nineties are shown in Table 1. The three groups significantly differed from each other on age, municipality, and education level of the mother.

Based on the parental ISAAC questionnaire 279 of the 1321 children (21.1%) were diagnosed with asthma, 180 (13.6%) with allergic rhinoconjunctivitis, and 110 (8.3%) with atopic dermatitis. The percentages of positives for the different atopic diseases according to exposure status (Figure 1) show that (longer) exposure to the economic situation in the nineties corresponds with decreased atopic disease occurrence.

Table 2 shows the crude and adjusted ORs of the two groups exposed to the economic situation in the nineties for the different

Table 1. Characteristics of study population according to exposure to the Cuban economic situation in the nineties.

	Unexposed		Exposed during infancy		Exposed during infancy and early childhood		N	P-value[*]
Number of children	541		400		380		1321	
Sex (male)	265	(49.0%)	202	(50.5%)	211	(55.5%)	1321	0.14
Age (years)	6	(1)	9	(1)	11	(1)	1321	**<0.001**
Municipality (Fomento)	375	(69.3%)	259	(64.8%)	289	(76.1%)	1321	**0.003**
Area of residence (urban)	280	(51.8%)	210	(52.5%)	200	(52.6%)	1321	0.96
Family income (>250 peso/month)	249	(46.2%)	182	(45.8%)	162	(43.1%)	1312	0.62
Education level father (≥12 grades)	239	(44.8%)	181	(46.5%)	159	(42.4%)	1297	0.51
Education level mother (≥12 grades)	261	(48.6%)	204	(51.1%)	151	(39.9%)	1314	**0.004**
LBW (<2500 g)	51	(9.5%)	51	(13.0%)	31	(8.3%)	1304	*0.07*
Premature birth (<37 weeks)	37	(6.8%)	29	(7.3%)	23	(6.1%)	1321	0.80
Breastfeeding (>6 months)	284	(52.7%)	198	(49.7%)	181	(47.9%)	1315	0.34

Data are given as numbers and percentage, except age which is given as median (IQR).
Statistically significant differences are given in bold and borderline significant differences in italic.
*Chi-square test for difference between the three exposure groups, expect for age which was done by Kruskal-Wallis test.

atopic diseases compared to the unexposed group. The adjusted ORs confirmed the observations of Figure 1, with significant associations between exposure and asthma and allergic rhinoconjunctivitis. These associations tended to be stronger for longer exposure, i.e. during both infancy and early childhood. However, the differences between the two exposure groups were not significant. No significant association was found between exposure and atopic dermatitis.

The sensitivity analysis by shifting forward the cut-off dates confirmed the general trend found for asthma and allergic rhinoconjunctivitis (Table S1). As expected, removing the transition groups slightly strengthened most associations (Table S2). Only for atopic dermatitis the results were altered after sensitivity analysis, confirming the instability of the original results for atopic dermatitis due to the small group sizes (Table S1 and S2).

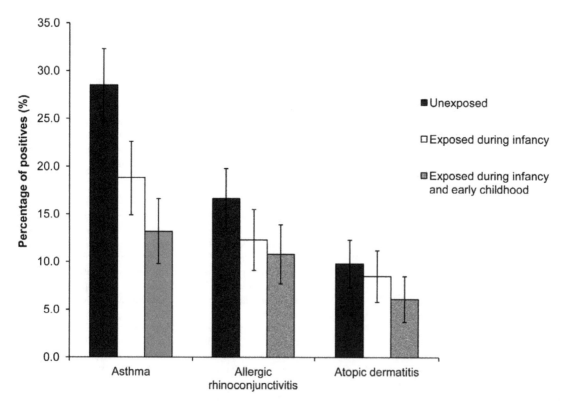

Figure 1. Atopic diseases according to exposure status to the Cuban economic situation in the nineties. (asthma resp. 28.5%, 18.8% and 13.2%; allergic rhinoconjunctivitis resp. 16.6%, 12.3% and 10.8%; atopic dermatitis resp. 9.8%, 8.5% and 6.1%).

Table 2. Crude and adjusted odds ratio's (OR) with 95% confidence intervals (CI) of exposure to the Cuban economic situation in the nineties for the different atopic diseases.

	Crude OR (95% CI)	P-value	Adjusted OR (95% CI)*	P-value
Asthma				
Unexposed	1.0		1.0	
Exposed during infancy	0.58 (0.42–0.79)	**0.001**	0.56 (0.33–0.94)	**0.03**
Exposed during infancy and early childhood	0.38 (0.27–0.54)	**<0.001**	0.40 (0.17–0.95)	**0.04**
Allergic rhinoconjunctivitis				
Unexposed	1.0		1.0	
Exposed during infancy	0.70 (0.48–1.02)	*0.06*	0.46 (0.25–0.85)	**0.01**
Exposed during infancy and early childhood	0.61 (0.41–0.90)	**0.01**	0.29 (0.11–0.77)	**0.01**
Atopic dermatitis				
Unexposed	1.0		1.0	
Exposed during infancy	0.86 (0.55–1.35)	0.51	1.58 (0.72–3.44)	0.25
Exposed during infancy and early childhood	0.59 (0.36–0.99)	**0.04**	1.86 (0.52–6.65)	0.34

Statistically significant associations are given in bold and borderline significant associations in italic.
*Adjusted for age & municipality.

Discussion

So far most studies on the impact of economic crises on health have focussed on immediate health consequences during or shortly after the crisis [4,5,13–16]. Longer term health consequences like chronic diseases have been investigated to a lesser extent. Here, we studied the effects of the Cuban economic situation in the nineties on the occurrence of atopic diseases in Cuban children 10 years later. We observed that exposure to the economic circumstances during infancy and early childhood had an attenuating effect on atopic disease development later in childhood.

A few limitations of this study should be noted. Firstly, all ecological studies are potentially prone to the so-called 'ecological fallacy', and our study findings should thus be interpreted cautiously. Although we checked for potential confounders, we cannot exclude that unknown or unmeasured contemporary factors not related to the economic situation may have influenced the study results. Our atopic disease data are based on the ISAAC questionnaire, which has become the standard diagnostic method in childhood epidemiology of atopic diseases worldwide [19]. Nevertheless, questionnaires have important inherent limitations, such as information and recall bias, which should be kept in mind when interpreting the data. Also, an independent trend of increasing atopic diseases prevalence over time, like in the Western world, cannot be ruled out [24]. Moreover, we used GDP to define the period of exposure, as this seems to be the most objective and well-documented proxy for exposure to the Cuban economic situation in the nineties. However, we do realize that GDP is an indirect measure of exposure. Thus, the possibility remains that our conclusions are based on an inadequate assumption of how GDP translates into exposure to the economic circumstances. Also, we did not take severity of the economic situation into account, e.g. the first years of the exposure period may have been less severe than the following years, resulting in differences in impacts on health in infancy and childhood. However, such data are scarce, and usually report on one aspect, such as per capita calorie consumption or low birth weight prevalence [3,5], so we could not to take this aspect into account.

Although we corrected for age, we are aware that this cannot completely adjust for age-related trends in the prevalence of atopic diseases. However, the adjusted effects we found show that older children are less likely to have asthma and allergic rhinoconjunctivitis and more likely to have atopic dermatitis. Therefore, these effects are different or even opposite of the normal age trends, suggesting that the effect of the economic circumstances is genuine. Finally, since it is difficult to determine an exact end point for the exposure period, the chosen cut-off date (January 1st, 1996) is somewhat arbitrary and therefore possible misclassification cannot be ruled out. Nevertheless, we believe that our results are robust, as demonstrated by the sensitivity analyses, and do indicate an inverse association between atopic diseases in today's Cuban schoolchildren and exposure to the economic circumstances in the nineties.

The associations found suggest an attenuating effect of factors related to the economic situation on atopic disease development. Below we speculate on potential factors and mechanisms underlying the observed associations.

During Cuba's Special Period there were two important health trends. One was a small and temporary rising in mortality rates from infectious and parasitic disorders and increased incidence of tuberculosis [3,25]. Even though we do not have exact data on other infectious disease incidences, it is very likely that these were elevated as well, since infectious pathogens normally thrive during natural disasters, civil unrest or economic upheaval [26–28]. The relationship between infection and atopic diseases has been subject of many studies and originates from the so-called hygiene hypothesis which could explain our results. According to this hypothesis, early childhood infections can down-regulate inflammatory immune responses, thereby suppressing allergic disorders [29]. The rise in infectious disease rates during the 1990 s may thus as such have had an attenuating effect on the development of atopic diseases as observed in our study.

The other major health trend during Cuba's special period was the declining nutritional status of the population with caloric restrictions, marginal vitamin deficiencies in children and high anemia rates in infants and pregnant women [3,5]. Several studies have been carried out and different hypotheses have been put forward on the relationship between nutritional status and atopic diseases. According to the Barker hypothesis, undernutrition in early-life, by altering the body's metabolism, is positively associated with (risk factors for) chronic diseases in adulthood in general [10,30,31] and with asthma specifically by impairing lung development [32,33]. Furthermore, several dietary hypotheses postulate that diet changes, e.g. reduced antioxidant intake, increases the risk for asthma and other atopic diseases, but the available evidence is inconclusive [34,35]. Neither of these hypotheses are in line with our study results, possibly due to differences in study groups, i.e. schoolchildren from a resource poor country versus adults and populations from resource rich countries, respectively. A number of studies have been devoted to the relationship between obesity and the occurrence of asthma, suggesting that obesity increases the risk of asthma, although the underlying mechanisms are still unresolved [36,37]. In Cuba obesity decreased during the 1990 s [6] and thus may have been accompanied by a decrease in asthma, but this does not necessarily explain our findings that children that were possibly exposed to a period of undernutrition had lower odds of developing atopic diseases than those unexposed.

The hygiene hypothesis and the relationship between nutrition and atopic diseases are usually considered separately. However, infection and undernutrition are closely related and share a similar geographical distribution, with the same individuals often experiencing both disease states simultaneously [38]. Their co-existence has been explained by two causal pathways: infection leads to undernutrition and alternatively undernutrition increases susceptibility to infection [38,39], with a strong involvement of the immune system [38,40], which in turn underlies atopic disease pathology [41,42]. The observed inverse relationship between atopic diseases and exposure to the economic situation in the nineties of our study group may thus well be the result of some immuno-regulated effect of a synergistic interplay between infection and undernutrition on the development of atopic disease. To our knowledge no studies have been carried out so far about the effect of concurrent undernutrition and infection on atopic disease.

Within the limitations of an ecological analysis, our findings indicate an inverse relationship between exposure to the Cuban economic situation in the nineties during infancy and early childhood and asthma and allergic rhinoconjunctivitis occurrence later in childhood. These results suggest that factors related to this period may have an attenuating effect on atopic disease development. We hypothesized that increased levels of infectious disease incidence and undernutrition during this special period may have been influential factors, either separately or concurrently. However, the exact cause and underlying mechanisms for the observed relationship need to be further elucidated.

Supporting Information

Table S1 Adjusted odds ratio's (OR) with 95% confidence intervals (CI) of exposure to the Cuban economic situation in the nineties for the different atopic diseases if cut-off date is shifted three or six months forward.

Table S2 Adjusted odds ratio's (OR) with 95% confidence intervals (CI) of exposure to the Cuban economic situation in the nineties for the different atopic diseases if transition groups around the cut-off dates are removed.

Acknowledgments

We especially thank Meike Wördemann, Lenina Menocal Heredia, and Ana María Collado Madurga for their valuable help during the study. We also like to thank Colleen Doak for her useful suggestions to improve the text. Furthermore, we thank all children, parents, teachers, school staff as well as the staff in the policlinics, the health authorities and all field workers in SJM and Fomento who participated in this study.

Author Contributions

Conceived and designed the experiments: KP MBG PS SDW. Performed the experiments: SDW RJD. Analyzed the data: SDW JWRT. Wrote the paper: SDW MCP MBG PS. Interpreted the data: SDW JWRT MCP PS KP Drafted the manuscript: SDW contributed to the critical revision of the manuscript: SDW KP MCP JWRT RJD MBG PS Approved the final version of the published manuscript:SDW KP MCP JWRT RJD MBG PS.

References

1. Abel-Smith B (1986) The world economic crisis. Part 1: Repercussions on health. Health Policy Plan 1: 202–213.
2. Garfield R, Devin J, Fausey J (1995) The health impact of economic sanctions. Bull N Y Acad Med 72: 454–469.
3. Garfield R, Santana S (1997) The impact of the economic crisis and the US embargo on health in Cuba. Am J Public Health 87: 15–20.
4. Nayeri K, Lopez-Pardo CM (2005) Economic crisis and access to care: Cuba's health care system since the collapse of the Soviet Union. Int J Health Serv 35: 797–816.
5. Rodriguez-Ojea A, Jimenez S, Berdasco A, Esquivel M (2002) The nutrition transition in Cuba in the nineties: an overview. Public Health Nutr 5: 129–133.
6. Franco M, Ordunez P, Caballero B, Tapia Granados JA, Lazo M, et al. (2007) Impact of energy intake, physical activity, and population-wide weight loss on cardiovascular disease and diabetes mortality in Cuba, 1980–2005. Am J Epidemiol 166: 1374–1380.
7. Hedges TR, Hirano M, Tucker K, Caballero B (1997) Epidemic optic and peripheral neuropathy in Cuba: a unique geopolitical public health problem. Surv Ophthalmol 41: 341–353.
8. Centers for Disease Control and Prevention (1994) Epidemic neuropathy–Cuba, 1991–1994. MMWR Morb Mortal Wkly Rep 43: 183, 189–192.
9. De Vos P (2005) "No one left abandoned": Cuba's national health system since the 1959 revolution. Int J Health Serv 35: 189–207.
10. Garfield R (1997) The impact of economic embargoes on the health of women and children. J Am Med Womens Assoc 52: 181–184, 198.
11. Painter RC, Roseboom TJ, Bleker OP (2005) Prenatal exposure to the Dutch famine and disease in later life: an overview. Reprod Toxicol 20: 345–352.

12. Galobardes B, Smith GD, Lynch JW (2006) Systematic review of the influence of childhood socioeconomic circumstances on risk for cardiovascular disease in adulthood. Ann Epidemiol 16: 91–104.
13. Waters H, Saadah F, Pradhan M (2003) The impact of the 1997–98 East Asian economic crisis on health and health care in Indonesia. Health Policy Plan 18: 172–181.
14. Khang YH, Lynch JW, Kaplan GA (2005) Impact of economic crisis on cause-specific mortality in South Korea. Int J Epidemiol 34: 1291–1301.
15. Hopkins S (2006) Economic stability and health status: evidence from East Asia before and after the 1990 s economic crisis. Health Policy 75: 347–357.
16. Waters H, Saadah F, Surbakti S, Heywood P (2004) Weight-for-age malnutrition in Indonesian children, 1992–1999. Int J Epidemiol 33: 589–595.
17. Wordemann M, Polman K, Junco Diaz R, Menocal Heredia LT, Collado Madurga AM, et al. (2006) The challenge of diagnosing atopic diseases: outcomes in Cuban children depend on definition and methodology. Allergy 61: 1125–1131.
18. Wordemann M, Polman K, Menocal Heredia LT, Junco Diaz R, Collado Madurga AM, et al. (2006) Prevalence and risk factors of intestinal parasites in Cuban children. Trop Med Int Health 11: 1813–1820.
19. Asher MI, Keil U, Anderson HR, Beasley R, Crane J, et al. (1995) International Study of Asthma and Allergies in Childhood (ISAAC): rationale and methods. Eur Respir J 8: 483–491.
20. The International Study of Asthma and Allergies in Childhood (ISAAC) Steering Committee (1998) Worldwide variation in prevalence of symptoms of asthma, allergic rhinoconjunctivitis, and atopic eczema: ISAAC. Lancet 351: 1225–1232.

21. Strachan D, Sibbald B, Weiland S, Ait-Khaled N, Anabwani G, et al. (1997) Worldwide variations in prevalence of symptoms of allergic rhinoconjunctivitis in children: the International Study of Asthma and Allergies in Childhood (ISAAC). Pediatr Allergy Immunol 8: 161–176.

22. Williams H, Robertson C, Stewart A, Ait-Khaled N, Anabwani G, et al. (1999) Worldwide variations in the prevalence of symptoms of atopic eczema in the International Study of Asthma and Allergies in Childhood. J Allergy Clin Immunol 103: 125–138.

23. Sonis J (1998) A closer look at confounding. Fam Med 30: 584–588.

24. von Mutius E (1998) The rising trends in asthma and allergic disease. Clin Exp Allergy 28 Suppl 5: 45–49.

25. Ministerio de Salud Publica (2000) Anuario Estadistico de Salud en Cuba 2000. Havana. Available at: http://www.infomed.sld.cu/servicios/estadisticas/.

26. Ligon BL (2006) Infectious diseases that pose specific challenges after natural disasters: a review. Semin Pediatr Infect Dis 17: 36–45.

27. Morens DM, Folkers GK, Fauci AS (2004) The challenge of emerging and re-emerging infectious diseases. Nature 430: 242–249.

28. Suhrcke M, Stuckler D, Suk JE, Desai M, Senek M, et al. (2011) The impact of economic crises on communicable disease transmission and control: a systematic review of the evidence. PLoS One 6: e20724.

29. Wills-Karp M, Santeliz J, Karp CL (2001) The germless theory of allergic disease: revisiting the hygiene hypothesis. Nat Rev Immunol 1: 69–75.

30. Barker DJP, Godfrey KM (2004) Maternal Nutrition, Fetal Programming and Adult Chronic Disease. In: Gibney MJ, Margetts BM, Kearney JM, Arab L, editors. Public Health Nutrition. 1st ed. Oxford: Blackwell Publishing Ltd.

31. Roseboom T, de Rooij S, Painter R (2006) The Dutch famine and its long-term consequences for adult health. Early Hum Dev 82: 485–491.

32. Lopuhaa CE, Roseboom TJ, Osmond C, Barker DJ, Ravelli AC, et al. (2000) Atopy, lung function, and obstructive airways disease after prenatal exposure to famine. Thorax 55: 555–561.

33. Shaheen SO, Sterne JA, Montgomery SM, Azima H (1999) Birth weight, body mass index and asthma in young adults. Thorax 54: 396–402.

34. Devereux G, Seaton A (2005) Diet as a risk factor for atopy and asthma. J Allergy Clin Immunol 115: 1109–1117.

35. Devereux G (2006) The increase in the prevalence of asthma and allergy: food for thought. Nat Rev Immunol 6: 869–874.

36. Shore SA, Johnston RA (2006) Obesity and asthma. Pharmacol Ther 110: 83–102.

37. Weiss ST (2005) Obesity: insight into the origins of asthma. Nat Immunol 6: 537–539.

38. Koski KG, Scott ME (2001) Gastrointestinal nematodes, nutrition and immunity: breaking the negative spiral. Annu Rev Nutr 21: 297–321.

39. Scrimshaw NS (2003) Historical concepts of interactions, synergism and antagonism between nutrition and infection. J Nutr 133: 316S-321S.

40. Bhaskaram P (2002) Micronutrient malnutrition, infection, and immunity: an overview. Nutr Rev 60: S40–45.

41. Ngoc PL, Gold DR, Tzianabos AO, Weiss ST, Celedon JC (2005) Cytokines, allergy, and asthma. Curr Opin Allergy Clin Immunol 5: 161–166.

42. Eisenbarth SC, Cassel S, Bottomly K (2004) Understanding asthma pathogenesis: linking innate and adaptive immunity. Curr Opin Pediatr 16: 659–666.

16

Filaggrin Gene Mutation c.3321delA Is Associated with Various Clinical Features of Atopic Dermatitis in the Chinese Han Population

Li Meng[1,2,3⑨], Li Wang[1,2,3⑨], Huayang Tang[1,2,3⑨], Xianfa Tang[1,2,3], Xiaoyun Jiang[1,2,3], Jinhua Zhao[1,2,3], Jing Gao[1,2,3], Bing Li[1,2,3], Xuhui Fu[1,2,3], Yan Chen[1,2,3], Weiyi Yao[1,2,3], Wenying Zhan[1,2,3], Bo Wu[1,2,3], Dawei Duan[1,2,3], Changbing Shen[1,2,3], Hui Cheng[1,2,3], Xianbo Zuo[1,2,3], Sen Yang[1,2,3], Liangdan Sun[1,2,3*], Xuejun Zhang[1,2,3,4,5*]

1 Institute of Dermatology and Department of Dermatology, No.1 Hospital, Anhui Medical University, Hefei, Anhui, China, 2 Key Laboratory of Dermatology, Anhui Medical University, Ministry of Education, China, Hefei, Anhui, China, 3 State Key Laboratory Incubation Base of Dermatology, Anhui Medical University, Hefei, Anhui, China, 4 Department of Dermatology at No.2 Hospital, Anhui Medical University, Hefei, Anhui, China, 5 Department of Dermatology, Huashan Hospital of Fudan University, Shanghai, China

Abstract

Background: We confirmed that the filaggrin gene mutation c.3321delA is associated with atopic dermatitis in our previous genome wide association study of the Chinese Han population. c.3321delA is the most common filaggrin gene mutation in Chinese atopic dermatitis patients but is not present in European populations.

Objective: To investigate the genetic model for the c.3321delA mutation and to determine the correlation between c.3321delA and atopic dermatitis clinical phenotypes in the Chinese Han population.

Method: The filaggrin gene mutation c.3321delA was sequenced in 1,080 atopic dermatitis patients and 908 controls from the Chinese population. The χ^2 test, ANOVA, nonparametric tests and logistic regression were used to investigate the relationship between the c.3321delA genotype and atopic dermatitis clinical phenotypes in the Chinese Han population.

Results: Analyses of the genetic model revealed that the additive model best described the c.3321delA mutation ($P = 3.09E-11$, OR = 3.43, 95%CI = 2.38–4.96). Stratified analyses showed that the c.3321delA allele frequency distribution is significantly associated with concomitant skin xerosis ($P = 1.68E-03$, OR = 2.13, 95%CI = 1.32–3.46), palmar hyperlinearity ($P = 3.64E-17$, OR = 4.0, 95%CI = 2.86–5.70), white dermatographism ($P = 4.25E-03$, OR = 1.82, 95%CI = 1.22–2.71), food intolerance ($P = 1.51E-03$, OR = 1.76, 95%CI = 1.23–2.50) and disease severity ($P = 9.67E-05$).

Conclusion: Our study indicates that the filaggrin gene mutation c.3321delA is associated with clinical phenotypes of atopic dermatitis in the Chinese Han population, which might help us gain a better understanding on the pathogenesis of atopic dermatitis.

Editor: Yong-Gang Yao, Kunming Institute of Zoology, Chinese Academy of Sciences, China

Funding: This study was funded by General Program of National Natural Science Foundation of China (31171224, 31000528), Program for New Century Excellent Talents in University (NCET-11-0889), Science and Technological Foundation of Anhui Province for Outstanding Youth (1108085J10), Pre-project of State Key Basic Research Program 973 of China (No. 2012CB722404), and Hospital incubation program (3101005002354). The funders had no role in study design, data collection and analysis, decision to publish, or preparation of the manuscript.

* E-mail: ayzxj@vip.sina.com (X. Zhang); ahmusld@163.com (LS)

⑨ These authors contributed equally to this work.

Introduction

Atopic dermatitis (AD) has long been recognized as a complex trait, wherein multiple genes and environmental stimuli contribute to disease manifestation. To date, 81 genes have been implicated in over 100 published reports on AD genetic association studies, and 46 of these genes have demonstrated at least one positive association with AD. Of these genes, filaggrin gene (*FLG*) is the most consistently replicated gene, appearing in 20 reports [1].

Filaggrin, also known as filament-aggregating protein, plays a major role in the epidermal barrier function. To date, approximately 60 loss-of-function *FLG* mutations have been identified in European and Asian populations [2]. All of the mutations that are predicted to cause loss of function, including nonsense mutations as well as out-of-frame insertions or deletions, are specific to certain ethnic groups, with distinct profiles observed in the European and Asian populations that have been well studied [3].

AD, with a prevalence of 1.4 to 22.3% worldwide [4], has a complex clinical phenotype strongly associated with food allergies, asthma, and allergic rhinitis (AR) in a patient's life (i.e., the atopic march) [5]. Over the last decade, numerous association studies on *FLG* mutations and AD-associated phenotypes have been conducted. The majority of the studies focused on combined *FLG* mutations, and only a few studies referred to single mutation. c.3321delA is an Asian-specific *FLG* mutation that has been described in Chinese, Japanese, Korean and Singaporean populations [6]. c.3321delA is the most common *FLG* mutation in the Chinese population; however, it is not found in European populations. In our previous Genome Wide Association Study (GWAS) of AD, we identified the *FLG* variant rs3126085 that correlates with c.3321delA. In this study, we investigated the genetic model for c.3321delA, the genotype–phenotype correlation between c.3321delA and AD in the Chinese population. This study employs the largest sample size of all of the genotype-phenotype correlation studies of AD to date.

Materials and Methods

Patients and controls

A total of 1,080 AD patients and 908 controls were enrolled in this study (**Table 1**). All samples were from the Chinese Han population and were used in our previous GWAS. AD patients meeting the Hanifin-Rajka diagnostic criteria [7] were recruited from the No. 1 Hospital of Anhui Medical University and the Xinhua Hospital affiliated with the Shanghai Jiaotong University School of Medicine in China. Physician specialists collected clinical data from the affected individuals through a full clinical checkup. Additional demographic information was collected from the cases and controls through a structured questionnaire. The disease severity was evaluated using the objective SCORing Atopic Dermatitis (SCORAD) index [8], which categorizes patients as mild ($\leq$15 points), moderate (15–40 points) and severe ($>$40 points). Patients were considered to have food intolerance either evaluated by allergen test of venous blood samples or patients' self-reports. All controls were clinically assessed to be without AD or other atopic diseases, a family history of atopic diseases (including first-, second- and third-degree relatives) or ichthyosis vulgaris (IV). All participants provided written informed consent. The study was approved by the Institutional Ethics Committee of Anhui Medical University and was conducted according to the Declaration of Helsinki principles.

Statistical analyses

c.3321delA genotyping adhered to quality control standards, with a call rate $>$95% and meeting Hardy–Weinberg equilibrium ($P>0.01$) in the controls. The c.3321delA allelic and genotypic frequencies were compared between the AD patients and controls using the χ^2 test with 2$\times$2 and 2$\times$3 contingency tables (SPSS 10.0, Statistical Program for Social Sciences, Illinois). The Fisher's exact test was used to compare the variable frequencies when the expected count was less than 5. Stratified analyses were performed to examine the relation between c.3321delA and the AD phenotypes. $P<0.05$ (two-tailed) was considered significant. The genetic models (dominant, recessive and additive models) were calculated for c.3321delA using logistic regression. To assess the effect of c.3321delA on the age of onset and disease severity, quantitative trait locus(QTL)analyses were performed in cases using ANOVA and nonparametric tests.

Results

Characteristics of the study subjects

The clinical characteristics of 1,080 patients (629 male and 451 female with a mean age of 5.14$\pm$6.42 years), including age of onset, AD with asthma, AD with AR, total IgE and AD severity, are summarized in Table 1. The 908 controls (629 male and 451 female) have a mean age of 16.35$\pm$9.32 years.

The association of AD with c.3321delA

The c.3321delA *FLG* mutation was significantly associated with AD ($P=3.09$ E-12,OR = 3.43, 95%CI = 2.38–4.96; $P_{genotype}$ = 1.75E-11, OR = 2.93, 95%CI = 2.00–4.28). We further evaluated the homozygous and heterozygous odds ratio (OR_{hom}/OR_{het}) for c.3321delA in the cases and controls. Using allele A as the reference allele, the OR_{het} estimate of c.3321delA was 2.93 (95% CI = 2.00–4.28); however, the OR_{hom} estimates could not be calculated because no controls were homozygous for c.3321delA (**Table 2**). Overall, the genetic model analysis revealed that the additive model best described the association of c.3321delA with AD ($P=3.09$E-11, OR = 3.43, 95%CI = 2.38–4.96).

Clinical phenotype stratification analyses

We also assessed the association between c.3321delA and AD phenotypes (**Table 3**) using stratified analyses in the cases. Significant associations were observed between c.3321delA and concomitant skin xerosis ($P=1.68$E-03, OR = 2.13, 95%CI = 1.32–3.46), IV ($P=2.17$E-02, OR = 1.63, 95%CI = 1.07–2.49), palmar hyperlinearity ($P=3.64$E-17, OR = 4.03, 95%CI = 2.86–5.70), keratosis pilaris ($P=1.72$E-02, OR = 1.70, 95%CI = 1.09–2.64), white dermatographism ($P=4.25$E-03, OR = 1.82, 95%CI = 1.22–2.71) and food intolerance ($P=1.51$E-03, OR = 1.76, 95%CI = 1.23–2.50) (**Table 3**). In the QTL analysis, we found that c.3321delA was associated with disease severity ($P=9.67$E-05). The c.3321delA homozygous and heterozygous patients displayed a significantly increased average SCORAD score (32.87 and 30.79, respectively) compared with the patients with a wild-type genotype (25.73) (**Table 4**). The patients harboring c.3321delA (homozygous and heterozygous) displayed a trend of earlier age of onset (0.16 and 0.81 years, respectively) compared with the wild-type genotype (1.07 years), which although displayed no statistical significance but showed a trend among three groups ($P=0.056$) (**Table 4**). We observed that the c.3321delA allele frequencies in AD patients without asthma or AR were slightly higher than in patients with asthma or AR, but the differences were not statistically significant (all $P>0.05$) (**Table 3**). In stratified analyses, c.3321delA was not associated with other phenotypes of AD, including early age of onset, elevated total serum IgE levels and orbital darkening ($P>0.05$) (**Table 3**).

The relationship between age of onset and c.3321delA-associated phenotypes of AD

In order to explore whether patients with earlier onset tend to present the phenotypes associated with c.3321delA or whether patients with mutation related phenotypes display a trend of earlier onset, we divided the patients into two groups (early age of onset and late age of onset), calculated these phenotypes' prevalence of the two groups, and compared the phenotype-distribution difference using the χ^2 test. We observed that the prevalence of AD concomitant with IV in the early age of onset group was significant lower than late age of onset group (13.37% vs 27.27%, $P=0.004$). On the other hand, AD concomitant with IV displayed a trend of later onset than without IV (1.56 years vs 0.91 years, $P=0.026$), as well as AD concomitant with keratosis

Table 1. The clinical characteristics of 1,080 cases.

Phenotype	Patients
Male (%)	629(58.24%)
Female (%)	451(41.76%)
Age (years), mean±SD (range)	5.14±6.42(0.5–58)
Age of onset (years), mean±SD (range)	1.03±3.00(0.02–37)
Early age of onset (≤2 years) (%) (n*)	999(92.59%)(1,079)
AD with asthma (%) (n*)	246(22.82%)(1,078)
AD with allergic rhinitis (%) (n*)	344(32.12%)(1,071)
AD with xerosis (%) (n*)	812(75.19%)(1,080)
AD with IV (%) (n*)	155(14.35%)(1,080)
AD with palmar hyperlinearity (%) (n*)	237(22.11%)(1,072)
AD with keratosis pilaris (%) (n*)	134(12.51%)(1,071)
AD with orbital darkening (%) (n*)	89(8.27%)(1,076)
AD with food intolerance (%) (n*)	407(42.66%)(954)
AD with white dermatographism (%) (n*)	158(14.65%)(1,080)
Elevated total IgE (>100 IU/ml) (%) (n*)	575(66.45%)(816)
Mild AD (objective SCORAD≤15) (%) (n*)	179(16.57%)(1,080)
Moderate AD (15< objective SCORAD≤40) (%) (n*)	764(70.74%)(1,080)
Severe AD (objective SCORAD>40) (%) (n*)	137(12.69%)(1,080)

pilaris also had a trend of later onset than without keratosis pilaris (1.69 years vs 0.91 years, $P=0.034$) (**Table 5**). There was no significant difference between age of onset and phenotypes (xerosis, palmar hyperlinearity, food intolerance and white dermatographism) (**Table 5**).

Discussion

In our previous GWAS, we confirmed that the *FLG* mutation c.3321delA is associated with AD in the Chinese Han population [9]. In the current study, our genotype–phenotype analyses of AD may aid in the investigation of various disease phenotypes and the identification of phenotype-specific genetic factors, thereby providing new insights into the pathogenesis of AD. Our findings indicate that c.3321delA significantly associates with various AD clinical phenotypes, including skin xerosis, IV, palmar hyperli-

nearity, keratosis pilaris, white dermatographism, food intolerance and disease severity.

The association of c.3321delA in our group was best described with an additive model that displayed a clear trend for increased disease risk in heterozygous and homozygous c.3321delA patients. Our analysis comparing AD severity (measured by the objective SCORAD score) between the genotype groups in the QTL analysis showed that homozygous and heterozygous c.3321delA patients were more likely to have a more severe form of the disease, and this finding is consistent with the Singaporean study that showed that the combined null *FLG* genotype of 17 mutations detected in cases and controls were strongly associated with increased AD severity (permutation test $P=0.0063$) [6]. However, the association was inconsistent in other studies [2,10,11] in the Chinese Han population, all of which were assessing compound genotypes of *FLG* including c.3321delA with smaller samples. *FLG*

Table 2. Genotype of c.3321delA in 1,080 cases and 908 control.

	Cases (n=1080)	Controls (n=908)	OR (95% CI)	P
Genotype				
AA	949(87.87%)	871(95.93%)	Reference	
Aa	118(10.93%)	37(4.07%)	2.93(2.00–4.28)	1.75E-11
aa	13(1.20%)	0(0%)	NA	
Recessive model				
aa/(Aa+AA)	13/1067	0/908	NA	9.10E-04
Dominant model				
(aa+Aa)/AA	131/949	37/871	3.25(2.23–4.73)	1.26E-10
Additive model				
aa/Aa/AA	13/118/949	0/37/871	3.43(2.38–4.96)	3.09E-11

Table 3. The association between c.3321delA and clinical phenotypes in AD.

Clinical phenotypes	Allele frequencies		P	OR	95%CI
	3321delA	A			
Early age of onset (≤2 years)	0.0691	0.9309	1.24E-01	1.90	0.83–4.38
Late age of onset (>2 years)	0.0375	0.9625			
AD with asthma	0.0650	0.9350	8.60E-01	0.96	0.64–1.45
AD without asthma	0.0673	0.9327			
AD with AR	0.0581	0.9419	2.97E-01	0.82	0.56–1.19
AD without AR	0.0702	0.9299			
AD with elevated IgE	0.0740	0.9260	6.59E-01	1.10	0.77–1.56
AD with normal IgE	0.0685	0.9315			
AD with Xerosis	0.0764	0.9237	1.68E-03	2.13	1.32–3.46
AD without Xerosis	0.0373	0.9627			
AD with IV	0.0968	0.9032	2.17E-02	1.63	1.07–2.49
AD without IV	0.0616	0.9384			
AD with Palmar hyperlinearity	0.1519	0.8481	3.64E-17	4.03	2.86–5.70
AD without Palmar hyperlinearity	0.0425	0.9575			
AD with Keratosis pilaris	0.1007	0.8993	1.72E-02	1.70	1.09–2.64
AD without Keratosis pilaris	0.0619	0.9381			
AD with Orbital darkening	0.0506	0.9494	3.62E-01	0.73	0.36–1.45
AD without Orbital darkening	0.0684	0.9316			
AD with food intolerance	0.0842	0.9158	1.51E-03	1.76	1.23–2.50
AD with food tolerance	0.0496	0.9504			
AD with White dermatographism	0.1107	0.8893	4.25E-03	1.82	1.22–2.71
AD without White dermatographism	0.0642	0.9358			

mutations predict dose-dependent alterations in epidermal permeability barrier function [12], and our results confirmed that the *FLG* null mutations might serve as an indicator of severe disease phenotypes.

Several studies indicate that *FLG* mutations have an effect on the age of onset of AD such that individuals carrying *FLG* mutations (R501X, 2282del4, R2447X or S3247x) can lead to early-onset (age of onset ≤2 years) AD that persisits well into adulthood [13–16]. Moreover, Ma et al. reported that c.3321delA was associated with early-onset of AD in Northern Chinese patients (*P*= 0.020) [17]. However, in our study, no statistical significance was observed for the association between early-onset at AD and *FLG* mutation c.3321delA in stratified analysis (*P*= 1.24E-01), which may be attributed to the fact that the majority of AD cases begin early in life (age of onset ≤2 years). It's reported that *FLG* mutations were associated with much earlier age at onset for AD [11,18], AD patients carrying *FLG* mutations were younger than those without *FLG* mutations. However, one

study in China did not observe the association (*P*= 0.307) [2]. In our study, we observed that the average/median age of onset in AD tended to decrease among the three groups (wide-type, homozygous and heterozygous genotype) in the QTL analysis, but there were no statistical differences (*P*= 0.056), which may be due to the low proportion of AD cases with homozygous c.3321delA. Further analysis using larger sample sizes will be helpful for determining the effect of c.3321delA on age of onset.

Our data provide evidence for the association between c.3321delA and various AD phenotypes, including concomitant IV, palmar hyperlinearity, and keratosis pilaris (**Table 3**), consistent with previous studies [6,10] regarding *FLG* compound mutations. A recent study in Northern China indicated that combined *FLG* variants were significantly associated with IV and palmar hyperlinearity; however, no association with keratosis pilaris was observed [2]. These results are attributed to the fact that AD has a well-recognized association with IV [19,20] and that *FLG* is the pathogenic gene of IV; thus, AD patients from non-IV

Table 4. Association between genotype of c.3321delA and SCORAD and age of onset in AD.

Genotypes	AA	Aa	aa	P
Patients (n)	927	118	13	
Objective SCORAD (median)	25.73(24.00)	30.79(29.30)	32.87(32.00)	9.67E-05
Age of onset (years) (median)	1.07 (0.17)	0.81 (0.17)	0.16 (0.083)	0.056

Table 5. The relationship between age of onset and c.3321delA related phenotypes in AD.

c.3321delA related phenotypes of AD	Early age of onset	Late age of onset	P*	OR(95%CI)	Cases(n)	Mean onset age(SD)	P#
With xerosis	750(75.53%)	56(72.73%)	0.953	0.99(0.69-1.42)	812	0.95(3.10)	0.256
Without xerosis	243(24.47%)	21(27.27%)			266	1.19(2.59)	
With IV	132(13.37%)	21(27.27%)	0.004	2.09(1.25-3.50)	154	1.56(3.35)	0.026
Without IV	855(86.63%)	56(72.73%)			917	0.91(2.91)	
With palmar hyperlinearity	221(22.39%)	16(20.78%)	0.872	0.96(0.55-1.67)	237	1.13(2.86)	0.468
Without palmar hyperlinearity	766(77.61%)	61(79.22%)			834	0.97(3.02)	
With keratosis pilaris	118(11.96%)	15(20.00%)	0.084	1.67(0.93-3.00)	134	1.69(4.12)	0.034
Without keratosis pilaris	869(88.04%)	60(30.00%)			937	0.91(2.77)	
With food intolerance	379(43.22%)	22(30.14%)	0.163	0.70(0.43-1.14)	404	0.97(2.90)	0.322
Without food intolerance	498(56.78%)	51(69.86%)			552	1.18(3.31)	
With white dermatographism	119(14.39%)	10(15.87%)	0.718	1.14(0.57-2.28)	131	1.38(3.43)	0.109
Without white dermatographism	708(85.61%)	53(84.13%)			763	0.93(2.94)	

P* value: calculated by χ^2 test; P# value:calculated by T test;

family trios have a low probability of carrying *FLG* mutations [10]. Hyperlinear palms and keratosis pilaris, the phenotypic characteristics of IV, have been previously reported to be strong clinical markers of *FLG*-null mutations [21]. Greater than 60% of patients carrying *FLG* mutations develop palmar hyperlinearity manifested as criss-cross hyperlinearity of the thenar eminence [22]. Hyperlinear palms,keratosis pilaris and IV were all skin barrer dysfunction disorders, and they have common pathogenesis with AD, thus they could represent good phenotypic indicators of *FLG*-null mutations and AD.

In this study, we first reported that c.3321delA was associated with AD coexistent skin xerosis in Asian populations. A similar study using a smaller sample in Northern China did not find this association [2]. But the German study has reported a strong association between combined *FLG* mutations and dry skin [21]. *FLG* gene number polymorphisms has been associated with the dry skin phenotype [23]. The loss or reduction of filaggrin expression disrupts barrier formation making filaggrin-deficient skin susceptible to increased transepidermal water loss and easy penetrated by environmental allergens, which can manifest as varying degrees of dry skin. The filaggrin degradation products, namely several amino acids (alanine, pyrrolidone carboxylic acid, and urocanoic acid) act as natural moisturizing factors (NMFs) in the stratum corneum. The hygroscopic NMFs are important for the maintenance of epidermal barrier hydration. NMFs are less abundant in dry skin [24], which becomes more pronounced with age [25] and changing seasons. Biochemical and immunological evidence indicate that profilaggrin and processed filaggrin are completely absent in patients carrying *FLG* mutations [26]. *FLG* deficiency or absence results in reduced NMFs and impaired epidermal barrier function, which likely contribute to the etiopathogenesis of AD and AD-associated skin xerosis. Therefore, our results are the first to suggest that *FLG* mutations may be associated with an individual's predisposition to skin xerosis in the context of AD.

We also were the first to report that c.3321delA was associated with AD coexistent white dermatographism using a large sample study of an Asian population, whereas a similar study using a smaller sample from Northern China did not observe the association [2]. White dermatographism expresses as local erythema followed by edema and a surrounding flare reaction caused by a stroke with a dull object. Dermatographism is likely considered to be caused by mechanicoimmunological stimulation of mast cells that release histamine. Mechanical trauma is thought to release an antigen that interacts with IgE-sensitized mast cells, which further release inflammatory mediators like histamine into the tissues. Filaggrin degradation can release histidine acting as putative ultraviolet photoprotector [27]. Our result indicated that *FLG* mutation c.3321delA might involve in the development of white dermatographism.

In addition, we found that c.3321delA was associated with food intolerance, consistent with the Southern China study [11] assessing compound genotypes for combined *FLG* variants and the study by Linneberg et al [28] assessing *FLG* mutations R501X or 2282del4. *FLG* mutations predispose individuals to AD with allergic sensitization [29]. Studies have indicated that the absorption of allergens through the skin of patients with *FLG* mutations may be a predisposing factor for the development of other allergic disorders [30]. The destruction of normal epidermal barrier function is considered a key event in allergic sensitization [31]. A damaged epidermal barrier allows allergens to penetrate into the skin easily and exposes the allergens to antigen-presenting cells, causing allergic sensitization. Except skin keratinizing epithelial tissue, filaggrin is also expressed in other keratinizing epithelia, such as the oral and nasal mucosa, and is also presumed to contribute to the oral epithelial barrier function. Since, allergen through oral can also cause allergy. Our results confirm that skin barrier defects due to *FLG* mutations play a crucial role in the pathogenesis of other allergic disorders, such as food sensitization.

The relationship among AD, asthma, AR and *FLG* mutations is complex. Common and varying genetic factors for AD and asthma have been reported in the Chinese Han population [32]. A large European cohort study demonstrated that *FLG* null mutations predispose to allergic phenotypes, such as asthma and AR involved in the atopic march only in the presence of eczema [33]. Several studies have shown that *FLG* mutations predispose to asthma but only in the context of prior eczema or AD and their families, which indicating that *FLG* mutations did not have an independent effect on asthma [34–36]. A study [17] in Northern China reported that c.3321delA was associated with AD-associated AR or asthma in stratified analysis ($P = 0.035$). However, a Polish study also found evidence for the association between combined *FLG* variants with asthma and AR, and an association between *FLG*-null variants and atopic asthma was also observed in individuals without AD or a history thereof [37]. In one study in Northern China, no association was observed between the combined *FLG* mutations and AD-associated asthma or AR; however, an association between the mutation K4671X and AD-associated AR was found [2]. An additional study in Southern China did not find an association between the combined *FLG* mutations and AD-associated asthma or AR. However, c.3321delA was found more frequently in AD patients without asthma than patients with asthma. In addition, a significant association between c.3321delA and AD patients with asthma was observed ($P = 0.016$) [11], implying that c.3321delA may serve as a protective factor for asthma that occurs in the context of AD. In this larger sample study, we observed that the c.3321delA allele frequencies in AD patients without asthma or AR were slightly increased compared with AD patients with asthma or AR, but the findings were not statistically significant ($P = 0.86$, OR = 0.96, 95%CI = 0.64–1.45 and $P = 0.297$, OR = 0.82, 95%CI = 0.56–1.19, respectively) **(Table 3)**. The negative association between *FLG* mutations and atopies found in our study may be attributed to sample bias, environmental factors and ethnic differences. The majority of our patients displayed an age of onset for asthma and AR well below the median age at onset. However, we confirmed the previous hypothesis that c.3321delA might be a protective factor for asthma. Additional studies are needed to clarify the relationship between *FLG* mutations and AD-associated respiratory allergic disorders.

We also performed an analysis regarding orbital darkening, but no significant difference was found, consistent with the Northern China study [2]. AD patients tend to have increased IgE levels. A study from Japan reported that c.3321delA is associated with elevated IgE levels [38], but we were unable to replicate that association in this study, which is consistent with the south China [11] and Polish [37] studies.Above all, according to our results, mutation c.3321delA was associated with several AD phenotypes, and AD patients with c.3321delA tended to have earlier age of onset, though the association is not significant. Since this, we performed further stratified analysis to explore the possible relationship between age of onset and these six AD phenotypes associated with c.3321delA. And we found that AD patients with late age of onset were more likely to accompany with IV, and AD patients with IV or keratosis pilaris tended to have later age of onset in AD. This may be due to the later predilection ages of IV and keratosis pilaris than that of AD.

Of course, there are some limitations in our study. Our study is limited by all cases and controls being of Chinese Han and it is possible that the *FLG* mutations may not exert the same effect in other races of China and other Asian countries. Our sample size was not large enough, so that most (92.59%) of our patients were early age of onset (≤2 years), and only 13 patients were homozygous, which may lead to minor bias. In addition, the phenotypes-genotypes association analysis in current study was just focused on AD patients, and all the results about phenotypes-genotypes relationship were in the presence of AD. In future study, we will perform the associated analyses of c.3321delA in the non-AD group, such as groups of IV, asthma and AR, et al.

In conclusion, our study confirmed that the *FLG* mutation c.3321delA was associated with AD under an additive genetic model in a large Chinese cohort. In addition, we observed a correlation between c.3321delA and various clinical features of AD, and we demonstrated that c.3321delA has an effect on these phenotypes in the context of AD. These findings may help to further define the role of *FLG* in AD susceptibility, thereby assisting in the categorization of various subtypes of the disease and building the foundation for genetic diagnosis and personalized treatment for patients with AD in the near future.

Acknowledgments

We thank all study participants and all the volunteers who have so willingly participated in this study, thus make this study possible.

Author Contributions

Conceived and designed the experiments: LS X. Zhang SY. Performed the experiments: LM LW XJ JZ JG BL XF YC WY WZ BW DD CS HC. Analyzed the data: X. Zuo HT. Wrote the paper: LM. Rectified the manuscript: LM HT LS XT.

References

1. Barnes KC (2010) An update on the genetics of atopic dermatitis: scratching the surface in 2009. J Allergy Clin Immunol 125: 16-29 e11-11; quiz 30–11.
2. Li M, Liu Q, Liu J, Cheng R, Zhang H, et al. (2013) Mutations analysis in filaggrin gene in northern China patients with atopic dermatitis. J Eur Acad Dermatol Venereol 27: 169–174.
3. Irvine AD, McLean WH, Leung DY (2011) Filaggrin mutations associated with skin and allergic diseases. N Engl J Med 365: 1315–1327.
4. Williams H, Stewart A, von Mutius E, Cookson W, Anderson HR (2008) Is eczema really on the increase worldwide? J Allergy Clin Immunol 121: 947–954 e915..
5. Spergel JM, Paller AS (2003) Atopic dermatitis and the atopic march. J Allergy Clin Immunol 112: S118–127.
6. Chen H, Common JE, Haines RL, Balakrishnan A, Brown SJ, et al. (2011) Wide spectrum of filaggrin-null mutations in atopic dermatitis highlights differences between Singaporean Chinese and European populations. Br J Dermatol 165: 106–114.
7. Hanifin JM RG (1980) Diagnostic features of atopic dermatitis. Acta Derm 92(Suppl.): 44–47.
8. (1993) Severity scoring of atopic dermatitis: the SCORAD index. Consensus Report of the European Task Force on Atopic Dermatitis. Dermatology 186: 23–31.
9. Sun LD, Xiao FL, Li Y, Zhou WM, Tang HY, et al. (2011) Genome-wide association study identifies two new susceptibility loci for atopic dermatitis in the Chinese Han population. Nat Genet 43: 690–694.
10. Cheng R, Li M, Zhang H, Guo Y, Chen X, et al. (2012) Common FLG mutation K4671X not associated with atopic dermatitis in Han Chinese in a family association study. PLoS One 7: e49158.
11. Zhang H, Guo Y, Wang W, Shi M, Chen X, et al. (2011) Mutations in the filaggrin gene in Han Chinese patients with atopic dermatitis. Allergy 66: 420–427.
12. Gruber R, Elias PM, Crumrine D, Lin TK, Brandner JM, et al. (2011) Filaggrin genotype in ichthyosis vulgaris predicts abnormalities in epidermal structure and function. Am J Pathol 178: 2252–2263.
13. Weidinger S, Rodriguez E, Stahl C, Wagenpfeil S, Klopp N, et al. (2007) Filaggrin mutations strongly predispose to early-onset and extrinsic atopic dermatitis. J Invest Dermatol 127: 724–726.

14. Barker JN, Palmer CN, Zhao Y, Liao H, Hull PR, et al. (2007) Null mutations in the filaggrin gene (FLG) determine major susceptibility to early-onset atopic dermatitis that persists into adulthood. J Invest Dermatol 127: 564–567.

15. Greisenegger E, Novak N, Maintz L, Bieber T, Zimprich F, et al. (2010) Analysis of four prevalent filaggrin mutations (R501X, 2282del4, R2447X and S3247X) in Austrian and German patients with atopic dermatitis. J Eur Acad Dermatol Venereol 24: 607–610.

16. Brown SJ, Sandilands A, Zhao Y, Liao H, Relton CL, et al. (2008) Prevalent and low-frequency null mutations in the filaggrin gene are associated with early-onset and persistent atopic eczema. J Invest Dermatol 128: 1591–1594.

17. Ma L, Zhang L, Di ZH, Zhao LP, Lu YN, et al. (2010) Association analysis of filaggrin gene mutations and atopic dermatitis in Northern China. Br J Dermatol 162: 225–227.

18. Carson CG, Rasmussen MA, Thyssen JP, Menne T, Bisgaard H (2012) Clinical presentation of atopic dermatitis by filaggrin gene mutation status during the first 7 years of life in a prospective cohort study. PLoS One 7: e48678.

19. Mevorah B, Marazzi A, Frenk E (1985) The prevalence of accentuated palmoplantar markings and keratosis pilaris in atopic dermatitis, autosomal dominant ichthyosis and control dermatological patients. Br J Dermatol 112: 679–685.

20. Sandilands A, O'Regan GM, Liao H, Zhao Y, Terron-Kwiatkowski A, et al. (2006) Prevalent and rare mutations in the gene encoding filaggrin cause ichthyosis vulgaris and predispose individuals to atopic dermatitis. J Invest Dermatol 126: 1770–1775.

21. Novak N, Baurecht H, Schafer T, Rodriguez E, Wagenpfeil S, et al. (2008) Loss-of-function mutations in the filaggrin gene and allergic contact sensitization to nickel. J Invest Dermatol 128: 1430–1435.

22. Brown SJ, Relton CL, Liao H, Zhao Y, Sandilands A, et al. (2009) Filaggrin haploinsufficiency is highly penetrant and is associated with increased severity of eczema: further delineation of the skin phenotype in a prospective epidemiological study of 792 school children. Br J Dermatol 161: 884–889.

23. Ginger RS, Blachford S, Rowland J, Rowson M, Harding CR (2005) Filaggrin repeat number polymorphism is associated with a dry skin phenotype. Arch Dermatol Res 297: 235–241.

24. Horii I, Nakayama Y, Obata M, Tagami H (1989) Stratum corneum hydration and amino acid content in xerotic skin. Br J Dermatol 121: 587–592.

25. Jacobson TM, Yuksel KU, Geesin JC, Gordon JS, Lane AT, et al. (1990) Effects of aging and xerosis on the amino acid composition of human skin. J Invest Dermatol 95: 296–300.

26. Smith FJ, Irvine AD, Terron-Kwiatkowski A, Sandilands A, Campbell LE, et al. (2006) Loss-of-function mutations in the gene encoding filaggrin cause ichthyosis vulgaris. Nat Genet 38: 337–342.

27. McLoone P, Simics E, Barton A, Norval M, Gibbs NK (2005) An action spectrum for the production of cis-urocanic acid in human skin in vivo. J Invest Dermatol 124: 1071–1074.

28. Linneberg A, Fenger RV, Husemoen LL, Thuesen BH, Skaaby T, et al. (2013) Association between loss-of-function mutations in the filaggrin gene and self-reported food allergy and alcohol sensitivity. Int Arch Allergy Immunol 161: 234–242.

29. Weidinger S, Illig T, Baurecht H, Irvine AD, Rodriguez E, et al. (2006) Loss-of-function variations within the filaggrin gene predispose for atopic dermatitis with allergic sensitizations. J Allergy Clin Immunol 118: 214–219.

30. Scharschmidt TC, Man MQ, Hatano Y, Crumrine D, Gunathilake R, et al. (2009) Filaggrin deficiency confers a paracellular barrier abnormality that reduces inflammatory thresholds to irritants and haptens. J Allergy Clin Immunol 124: 496–506, 506 e491–496.

31. Schuttelaar ML, Kerkhof M, Jonkman MF, Koppelman GH, Brunekreef B, et al. (2009) Filaggrin mutations in the onset of eczema, sensitization, asthma, hay fever and the interaction with cat exposure. Allergy 64: 1758–1765.

32. Tang HY, Tang XF, Zuo XB, Gao JP, Sheng YJ, et al. (2012) Association analysis of single nucleotide polymorphisms at five loci: comparison between atopic dermatitis and asthma in the Chinese Han population. PLoS One 7: e35334.

33. Marenholz I, Nickel R, Ruschendorf F, Schulz F, Esparza-Gordillo J, et al. (2006) Filaggrin loss-of-function mutations predispose to phenotypes involved in the atopic march. J Allergy Clin Immunol 118: 866–871.

34. Morar N, Cookson WO, Harper JI, Moffatt MF (2007) Filaggrin mutations in children with severe atopic dermatitis. J Invest Dermatol 127: 1667–1672.

35. Henderson J, Northstone K, Lee SP, Liao H, Zhao Y, et al. (2008) The burden of disease associated with filaggrin mutations: a population-based, longitudinal birth cohort study. J Allergy Clin Immunol 121: 872–877 e879.

36. Weidinger S, O'Sullivan M, Illig T, Baurecht H, Depner M, et al. (2008) Filaggrin mutations, atopic eczema, hay fever, and asthma in children. J Allergy Clin Immunol 121: 1203–1209 e1201.

37. Poninska J, Samolinski B, Tomaszewska A, Raciborski F, Samel-Kowalik P, et al. (2011) Filaggrin gene defects are independent risk factors for atopic asthma in a Polish population: a study in ECAP cohort. PLoS One 6: e16933.

38. Enomoto H, Hirata K, Otsuka K, Kawai T, Takahashi T, et al. (2008) Filaggrin null mutations are associated with atopic dermatitis and elevated levels of IgE in the Japanese population: a family and case-control study. J Hum Genet 53: 615–621.

17

Clinical Presentation of Atopic Dermatitis by Filaggrin Gene Mutation Status during the First 7 Years of Life in a Prospective Cohort Study

Charlotte Giwercman Carson[1], Morten Arendt Rasmussen[2], Jacob P. Thyssen[3], Torkil Menné[3], Hans Bisgaard[1]*

1 Copenhagen Prospective Studies on Asthma in Childhood; COPSAC, Health Sciences, University of Copenhagen, Copenhagen University Hospital, Gentofte, Copenhagen, Denmark, **2** Faculty of Life Sciences, University of Copenhagen, Frederiksberg, Denmark, **3** National Allergy Research Centre, Department of Dermato-Allergology, Copenhagen University Hospital Gentofte, Hellerup, Denmark

Abstract

Background: Filaggrin null mutations result in impaired skin barrier functions, increase the risk of early onset atopic dermatitis and lead to a more severe and chronic disease. We aimed to characterize the clinical presentation and course of atopic dermatitis associated with filaggrin mutations within the first 7 years of life.

Method: The COPSAC cohort is a prospective, clinical birth cohort study of 411 children born to mothers with a history of asthma followed during their first 7 years of life with scheduled visits every 6 months, as well as visits for acute exacerbations of dermatitis. Atopic dermatitis was defined in accordance with international guidelines and described at every visit using 35 predefined localizations and 10 different characteristics.

Results: A total of 170 (43%) of 397 Caucasian children developed atopic dermatitis. The R501X and/or 2282del4 filaggrin null mutations were present in 26 (15%) of children with atopic dermatitis and were primarily associated with predilection to exposed skin areas (especially the cheeks and back of the hands) and an up-regulation of both acute and chronic dermatitis. Furthermore, we found the filaggrin mutations to be associated with a higher number of unscheduled visits (3.6 vs. 2.7; p = 0.04) and more severe (moderate-severe SCORAD 44% vs. 31%; p = 0.14), and widespread dermatitis (10% vs. 6% of the body area, p<0.001) with an earlier age at onset (246 vs. 473 days, p<0.0001) compared to wild-type.

Conclusion: In children, filaggrin mutations seem to define a specific endotype of atopic dermatitis primarily characterized by predilection to exposed areas of the body, in particular hands and cheeks, and an up-regulation in both acute and chronic morphological markers. Secondary, this endotype is characterized by an early onset of dermatitis and a more severe course, with more generalized dermatitis resulting in more frequent medical consultations.

Editor: Michel Simon, CNRS-University of Toulouse, France

Funding: COPSAC is funded by private and public research funds. Grants above 100.000 Euro were donated by the Lundbeck Foundation, the Pharmacy Foundation of 1991, Augustinus Foundation, the Danish Medical Research Council and the Danish Pediatric Asthma Centre. The funders had no role in study design, data collection and analysis, decision to publish, or preparation of the manuscript.

Competing Interests: The authors have declared that no competing interests exist.

* E-mail: bisgaard@copsac.dk

Introduction

Approximately 10% of the general population carry at least one null mutation in the filaggrin gene (*FLG*) [1]. Normal gene expression results in intracellular filaggrin proteins which aggregate keratin filaments, leading to keratinocyte compaction and formation of the stratum corneum. Also, filaggrin expression is crucial for loading of lamellar body contents, uniform extracellular distribution of secreted organelle contents, and correct lamellar bilayer architecture; key features in upholding the function of the two compartment cornified envelope that prevents transepidermal water loss and penetration of micro-organisms, chemicals and allergens [2,3]. Heterozygous, and in particular homozygous or compound heterozygous carriers of *FLG* null variants, experience dry, scaly and fissured skin more often that non-mutation carriers

[4,5] and recent *in vivo* measurements of the stratum corneum in patients with AD also found lower levels of natural moisturizing factor among *FLG* deficient patients [6,7]. Furthermore, *FLG* mutations are major predisposing factors for atopic dermatitis (AD) [1,8–11] and are associated with early onset of AD, persistence of AD into adulthood and asthma and allergic sensitization [8,9,12–14]. Mutations seem to predict dose-dependent alterations in epidermal permeability barrier function and in accordance with this, homozygous carriers typically develop ichtyoisis vulgaris and/or AD very early in life, whereas heterozygous carriers may experience a milder course or no symptoms at all [3,15,16].

Phenotyping based on *FLG* null mutations might represent a novel endotype with known underlying molecular causes and, presumably, distinct clinical features. Endotyping of AD is important for segmentation of patients and future investigations of individualized treatment possibilities. Phenotypical characterization based on prospective data collection has not yet been reported for the *FLG* mutations. We meticulously characterized the pattern of AD in the Copenhagen Prospective Birth Cohort during the first 7 years of life and performed stratification by *FLG* mutation status.

Materials and Methods

Ethics Statement

The Copenhagen Study on Asthma in Childhood (COPSAC) was conducted in accordance with the guiding principles of the Declaration of Helsinki, approved by the Ethics Committee for Copenhagen (KF 01-289/96) and The Danish Data Protection Agency (2002-41-2434). Data validity was assured by compliance with "Good Clinical Practice" (GCP) guidelines and quality control procedures. Data were collected on-line and locked after external monitoring and an audit trail was run routinely. Informed written consent was obtained from all parents.

Participants

The Copenhagen Study on Asthma in Childhood (COPSAC) is a prospective, clinical, birth cohort study including 411 children born to mothers with asthma. The children were enrolled at one month of age and visited the clinical research unit at scheduled visits every six months as well as for any acute skin symptoms. The main recruiting area of the cohort was greater Copenhagen, Denmark and all children were born between August 1998 and December 2001. The study was previously detailed [17–19]. In this study, we included data from Caucasians only, i.e. 397 of 411 enrolled children. Among these, 172 (43%) were diagnosed with AD before age 7 years. In two cases, information about *FLG* mutation status and registration of dermatitis were missing, leaving 170 children for analysis. Two homozygous/compound heterozygous children were grouped with the heterozygous children. Skin examinations, diagnoses and treatment of dermatitis were handled by medical doctors employed for this purpose in the clinical research unit.

Risk Assessments

AD was stratified by *FLG* mutation status and the groups were analyzed for differences during the first 7 years of life. AD was defined based on the criteria of Hanifin and Rajka [20]. *FLG* genotyping was performed for R501X and 2282del4 mutations using TaqMan-based allelic discrimination assay and fluorescently labelled PCR (Applied Biosystems 3100, 3730 and 7700 sequence detection system, Foster City, CA, USA) [8]. Individuals designated as "wild type" were therefore patients not carrying these two common mutations, but carrier status of other, rare *FLG* mutations, cannot be excluded for this group.

At each visit, the following observations were registered:

- **Anatomical localization** of dermatitis lesions were divided into 35 predefined areas: abdomen, ankle (back), ankle (front), back (lower), back (upper), cheek, chest, chin, ear, elbow (back), elbow (front), eye area, foot (back), foot (sole), forearm (back), forearm (front), forehead, hand (back), hand (palm), knee (back), knee (front), lower leg (back), lower leg (front), nappy region, neck (back), neck (front), nose, perioral, scalp, upper arm (back), upper arm (front), upper leg (back), upper leg (front), wrist (back) and wrist (front).
- **Morphology** of the single dermatitis lesion was based on the following characteristics: area (in percent of the total body surface area), erythema, lichenification, crusts, dryness, vesicles, squamation, fissures, edema and excoriations (graduated from 0 (none) to 3 (severe)).
- **Severity** of the dermatitis episode was assessed using the Scoring Atopic Dermatitis index (SCORAD) [21].

Statistical Analyses

Associations between *FLG* mutation status (null vs. wild type) and different variables were investigated using the following analyses: Cox proportional-hazards regression (PROC PHREG) (AD diagnosis), chi-square test (PROC FREQ) (frequency of localizations), log-rank test (PROC LIFETEST) (age at onset of AD), the non-parametric Wilcoxon Rank-Sum Test (PROC NPAR1WAY) (number of visits in the clinical research unit), and GEE-model (PROC GENMOD) (SCORAD, total area of the body involved pr visit). All analyses were done in SAS version 9.1 (SAS Institute Inc, Cary, NC). The overall significance level used was 0.05.

A multivariate approach was employed to detect clinical patterns related to *FLG* null mutation status. We applied Partial Least Squares Discriminant Analysis (PLSDA) [22] to describe the anatomical location of dermatitis and Principal Component Analysis (PCA) to describe dermatitis morphology, in both cases with the aim of exploring differences in relation to *FLG* mutation status.

1) Anatomical location. The number of registrations (continuous) was used as predictors. The pattern of the 35 different regions was visualized including how they were associated with the *FLG* genotype both individually and compared to the other regions. The component consists of a *score matrix* with samples distribution and a *loading matrix* where the relation between the predictors (regions) was created and displayed.

2) Dermatitis morphology. For each region (n = 35) and each *FLG* mutation type (wild type and null), the morphology parameters (erythema, lichenification, crusts, dryness, vesicles, squamation, fissures, edema and excoriations) were represented by a weighted average across all registrations taking the different registration frequencies into account. This resulted in a 70 by 9 matrix. PCA with two components and varimax rotation was then conducted on this matrix. Here the *score plot* displays the similarity between regions in connection with *FLG* mutation status. The *loading plot* unravels the correlation structure between the morphology parameters [23].

PLSDA and PCA were conducted using the PLStoolbox ver. 6.0.1 (Eigenvector Inc, Manson, Washington, USA.). In addition in-house algorithms were used for visualization. All analysis where conducted in Matlab® R2010b version 7.11.0.584.

Additional methodological details are given in "Supporting Information S1: Materials and methods".

Results

Twenty six (15.3%) of 170 AD children and 15 (7.1%) of 212 non-AD children were *FLG* null mutation carriers (HR 2.23, 95% CI 1.47–3.39, p = 0.0002). The lifetime prevalence of AD was 63% in children with the *FLG* null genotype and 43% in children with the wild type.

Anatomical Dermatitis Localizations

The anatomical localization of dermatitis stratified by *FLG* mutation status (affected per visit) is presented in figure 1. Here, the 35 predefined areas were grouped into 11 areas (for details, please see Table S1). The analysis showed that involvement of the palm and back of the hands, the flexor and extensor extremities, the feet and the cheeks was statistically significant associated with the *FLG* null genotype (p values between <0.0001 and 0.002). PLSDA analysis of the original 35 regions confirmed this positive association, with a tendency towards higher number of different localizations for the *FLG* null children, as all loading values were positive in the first component, mainly driven by affection of the cheeks and the back of the hands, No differences were seen for the flexural area (p<0.01) (Figure S1). Figure 2 summarizes the localizations that were more often affected in *FLG* null children (red and blue areas), with the red areas illustrating the localizations significantly selected by the PLSDA (cheeks and back of the hand). To investigate whether the anatomical localizations associated with the *FLG* null genotype were age dependent, further stratification was performed (0–3 and 3–7 years). However, we found no change in predilection of dermatitis (data not shown).

Morphology

Firstly, three regions were excluded from the analyses due to a low number of registrations (eye area, plantar part of the foot, and the nose). Secondly, two components, describing 58% of the total variation, were extracted by PCA (component 1 and 2). The PCA loading plot separated chronic signs of dermatitis such as fissures, lichenification and crusting (x-axis) from acute signs of dermatitis such as oedema and erythema (y-axis). Characteristics closely positioned are correlated and therefore exhibited similar pattern, e.g. high loadings for erythema track with high loadings for edema and vesicles etc. (Figure 3a). It is important to notice that the PCA does not aim at separating different markers (unsupervised), and that the chronic and acute components simply

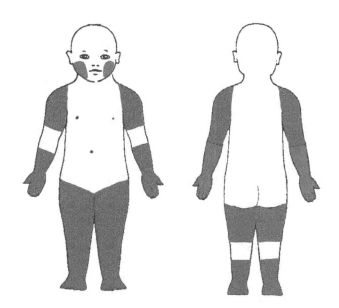

Figure 2. Summary of skin localizations in respect to filaggrin status. The figure summarizes the localizations more often affected in children with *FLG* null mutations compared to wild type children (red and blue areas), with red areas illustrating the localizations specifically selected by PLSDA as driving sites.

appear, because the main variation turns out to be reflected by these two patterns. Thirdly, the information obtained in the PCA loading plot, was combined with information about the morphol-

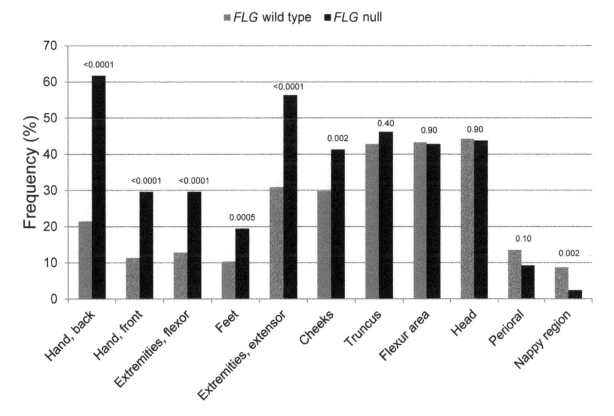

Figure 1. Frequency of skin localizations in respect to filaggrin status. Frequency of localizations in relation to the number of visits at the clinical research unit, 0–7 years, grouped and stratified by *FLG* status. Numbers above the bars indicate the p values.

ogy at the separate skin localizations via a score plot (figure 3b). At the score plot, the positions in truncated principal component space of the dermatitis lesions are shown. The figure describes the distribution of the skin regions, so that closely positioned points exhibit a similar pattern with respect to the morphology parameters reflected in the loading plot (figure 3a). Each region is shown as two points (blue and red circles representing *FLG* wild type and *FLG* null, respectively) connected with an arrow from the *FLG* wild genotype to the *FLG* null genotype. To get an idea of how these two plots are interpreted, consider the skin region *Extremities flex* as an example. The location of *FLG* null is high in component 2 compared to *FLG* wild type (figure 3b). This means that this skin region exhibits a more severe dermatitis for *FLG* null with respect to the acute inflammatory markers, that span this component (component 2– figure 3a). On the other hand, there seems to be no difference between the severities of the chronic inflammatory markers between the two genotypes reflected by the position on component 1. Likewise, it is registered that *Wrist back,* in terms of chronic inflammatory markers, is one of the skin regions with the most severe dermatitis with slightly higher severity for the *FLG* null type compared to the *FLG* wild type, but with no difference between the severities of acute markers (component 2). Figure 3b showed that the majority of arrows pointed up or towards the right, i.e. pointing in the same directions as the acute and chronic markers at the loading plot, which means that a general up-regulation of both acute and chronic markers was observed in *FLG* null children when compared to wild type children. Interpretation of single region differences between the two groups, revealed a pattern with certain regions up-regulated in acute markers (extensor areas, extremities flex areas, truncus, hand (palm/back)) and in chronic markers (feet area, wrist (front/back), hand back). These two figures (3a and 3b), serve as a comprehensive overview comparing the severity pattern of nine dermatitis markers for 15 different skin regions between two *FLG* genotypes. At figure 3b the localizations are grouped according to Table S1 except for the two groups *Hand area front* and *-back* which are kept as (six) individual regions. For the plot based on the original 32 skin regions, see Figure S2.

Severity

The skin was examined at 905 separate visits of which 276 (30.5%) were unscheduled visits for acute skin symptoms. Children with the *FLG* null mutations had more unscheduled visits than wild type children (mean 3.6 vs. 2.7 visits, p = 0.036) and *FLG* null children presented a higher SCORAD score than wild type children, albeit not statistically significant (44% vs. 31% with moderate-severe SCORAD, p = 0.14). Similar, non-significant trends were found in SCORAD values at unscheduled and scheduled visits separately (results not shown).

FLG null carriers had earlier onset of dermatitis (median age 128 vs. age 299 days, p<0.0001) and a more widespread dermatitis at each visit compared to wild type children (median 10% vs. 6% of the body, p<0.001). A similar difference was seen at both scheduled and unscheduled visits (results not shown).

Discussion

Main Finding

Primarily, this study showed that in our cohort of at-risk children, the *FLG* null driven AD endotype is characterized by dermatitis at anatomical localizations that tend to be exposed to drying conditions (e.g. wind, cold, sun and radiations from indoor heating), especially the back of the hands and the cheeks (figure 2) and with dermatitis lesions characterized by an up-regulation in

both acute and chronic markers when compared to wild type children. Moreover, this endotype had a higher frequency of acute dermatitis episodes, as illustrated by more unscheduled visits to our clinic, and also a more generalized, and severe dermatitis (higher SCORAD) when compared to *FLG* wild type children with AD, although the differences in severity were marginal.

Strengths and Limitations

The COPSAC cohort consists of prospective collection of data during the first 7 years of life. The diagnosis, detailed phenotype and management of skin lesions have been controlled solely by the clinical research unit physicians from standard operating procedures and treatment algorithms, and not by the general practitioner or others. Hence, the specificity of the AD diagnosis is high and the risk of misclassification is expected to be low. This is of particular importance in the clinical evaluation of AD where inter-observer variation may be a problem [24]. The children were followed every 6 months and were also seen in case of acute flare-up of dermatitis. Such prospective data collection reduces the risk of recall bias.

Our study is limited by all children being of Caucasian descent and it is possible that *FLG* mutations may not exert the same effect in other races. Furthermore, they are at-risk children with mothers suffering from asthma, thereby risking interaction with asthma genetics. Therefore, our results need replication in an unselected population.

Because of the project protocol, with the children being followed closely by trained physicians when having acute flare-ups, these children are more likely to receive better treatment than the general population. This optimized care is a potential confounder, which may dilute the differences between *FLG* null and wild type children with AD. However, this would support the genuine difference between the two groups regarding the anatomical localization and morphological presentation of their dermatitis. Despite our modest sample size we are the first to report a prospective registration of the dermatitis morphology and localization in AD patients stratified by *FLG* mutations. Since we find differences between the two strata, study size did not cause a type 2 error.

We used classic bar charts to illustrate our main findings and confirmed them by multivariate pattern analysis, i.e. PLSDA and PCA. This approach facilitates the handling of many variables in the same analysis, which is especially important for complex phenotypic data. Multivariate pattern analysis makes it possible to study the systematic variation, while filtering out uncorrelated random variation and hence observe patterns not otherwise recognized by traditional univariate statistical analysis. We were able to extract plausible acute and chronic components from the morphological data and characterize different skin regions. In this way, we use a data analytical approach more in line with the clinicians approach to clinical problems which is more often characterized by pattern recognition rather than any single markers.

Interpretation

AD has traditionally been classified as acute vs. chronic, intrinsic vs. extrinsic, associated with ichthyosis vulgaris, based on morphology (nummular, atopic prurigo, lichen planus-like, pityriasis alba) or based on localization (hand, juvenile plantar and palmar, eyelid, cheilitis, nipple, periorificial). However, none of these classifications seem to be satisfying, because patients often experience dynamic changes between the suggested categories and with affection of different sites [25]. Our data suggest that *FLG* null mutations, the cause of ichthyosis vulgaris, are associated with

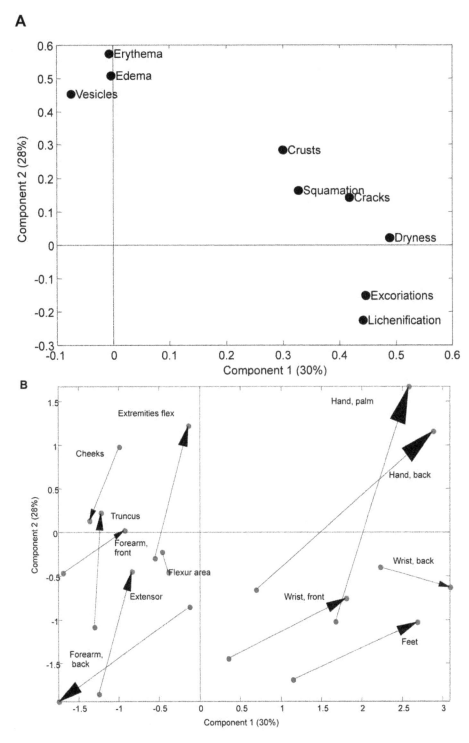

Figure 3. Morphology of the individual skin localizations. A: PCA loading plot for the first two components. Morphological characteristics such as fissures, lichenification and crust were found correlated as seen by the grouping at the x-axis (component 1, chronic markers), whereas edema, erythema and vesicles were grouped at the y-axis (component 2, acute markers). **B:** PCA score plot showing the morphology of the individual localizations. Each region is shown as two points ("blue circles": *FLG* wild type, "red circles": *FLG* null) connected with an arrow from *FLG* wild type to *FLG* null. E.g. hand (back) obtained higher values with respect to chronically inflammatory markers than e.g. forearm (front). A general up-regulation of both acute and chronic markers was observed for *FLG* null children across almost all regions.

dermatitis at "exposed areas", especially the cheeks and the back of the hands, but also the feet and extensor areas. These sites are typically exposed to drying and irritant factors such as water, sun, wind, child's play, changes in temperatures and radiation from indoor heating. It is likely that these factors may act as local triggers, resulting in further dry skin than dictated by the inherited skin constitution, and then dermatitis. In contrast, dermatitis in wild type children was not located on these rather exposed sites.

Supporting this interpretation, *FLG* deficient flaky tail mice bred in cages with contact to the environment, had a higher level of dermatitis and skin inflammation when compared to mice bred in cages with no environmental contact [26]. Other mechanisms, rather than primary barrier abnormality, might be responsible for the *FLG* wild type children's dermatitis. This could be changes in immunomodulatory factors, heat or bacterial growth.

Our study's suggested association between *FLG* null carrier status and hand dermatitis, is in line with a recent general population study, showing that the *FLG* null genotype significantly increased the risk of hand dermatitis in individuals with AD and that it was associated with early onset (before age 6) and persistence into adulthood [27]. Furthermore, the clinical observation was recently made, that adult patients with the *FLG* null genotype had a distinct phenotype of hand dermatitis characterized by fissured eruptions on the back of the hands and wrists with only sparse involvement of the palmar aspects, similar to the clinical description of hand dermatitis among atopic individuals previously described by other groups [28,29]. It is interesting that we could partly confirm this finding in our cohort of children, as *FLG* null carriers mainly had chronic markers of dermatitis on the back of their hands, whereas acute markers were upregulated in the palms as well as the back of the hands. Hence, the "dorsal hand eczema" as seen in patients with AD might indeed be associated with the *FLG* null genotype.

As a secondary finding we showed that *FLG* null children had more severe dermatitis, characterized by a higher number of visits in the clinical research unit, a more generalized dermatitis and a non-significant trend of higher SCORAD value. Also, *FLG* null mutations were associated with an earlier onset of disease. These observations are in agreement with previous cross-sectional reports [12,13,25,30] and suggest that *FLG* genotyping should be considered in the initial diagnostic work of patients suspected with AD and that it may be useful for classification.

Conclusion

In this study of at-risk children with AD, we find that the *FLG* null defines an endotype characterized by dermatitis with a predilection site at exposed areas of the body, in particular hands and cheeks, and an up-regulation in both acute and chronic morphological markers. Furthermore this endotype is characterized by an early onset of dermatitis and a more severe course with more generalized dermatitis resulting in more frequent medical consultations. These findings will hopefully help us segmenting AD patients and promise individualized treatment in the future, as well as improved disease prediction and research into novel preventive approaches. This is the first study reporting a prospectively characterizing of the morphology and localization of childhood dermatitis and stratifying it by *FLG* mutation status. However, future studies including replication in an unselected population are needed to confirm our findings.

Supporting Information

Figure S1   Figure S1A (PLSDA score plot) and Figure S1B (PLSDA loading plot): Skin localizations. PLSDA score- (**A**) and loading (**B**) plot for having dermatitis on a given localization in relation to number of visits in the clinic. Ellipsoids are centered at population mean with half axis corresponding to the standard deviation and under normality assumption hence cover ~50% of data. Red and blue represents *FLG* wild type and null mutation carriers, respectively.

Figure S2   Morphology of the individual skin localizations. Original PCA score plot showing the morphology of the individual localizations. Each region is shown as two points ("blue circles": *FLG* wild type, "red circles": *FLG* null) connected with an arrow from *FLG* wild type to *FLG* null. E.g. hand (back) obtained higher values with respect to chronically inflammatory markers than e.g. forearm (front). A general up-regulation of both acute and chronic markers was observed for *FLG* null children.

Table S1   Grouping the 35 predefined localizations into 11 groups.

Supporting Information S1 "Materials and methods" Elaborated statistical explanation for the multivariate analysis PLSDA.

Acknowledgments

The authors wish to thank the children and parents participating in the COPSAC cohorts as well as the COPSAC study teams.

Author Contributions

Conceived and designed the experiments: HB. Performed the experiments: HB CGC. Analyzed the data: CGC MAR. Wrote the paper: HB CGC MAR JPT TM. None.

References

1. Irvine AD (2007) Fleshing out filaggrin phenotypes. J Invest Dermatol 127: 504–507.

2. Candi E, Schmidt R, Melino G (2005) The cornified envelope: a model of cell death in the skin. Nat Rev Mol Cell Biol 6: 328–340.

3. Gruber R, Elias PM, Crumrine D, Lin TK, Brandner JM, et al. (2011) Filaggrin genotype in ichthyosis vulgaris predicts abnormalities in epidermal structure and function. Am J Pathol 178: 2252–2263.

4. Sergeant A, Campbell LE, Hull PR, Porter M, Palmer CN, et al. (2009) Heterozygous null alleles in filaggrin contribute to clinical dry skin in young adults and the elderly. J Invest Dermatol 129: 1042–1045.

5. Thyssen JP, Ross-Hansen K, Johansen JD, Zachariae C, Carlsen BC, et al. (2012) Filaggrin loss-of-function mutation R501X and 2282del4 carrier status is associated with fissured skin on the hands: results from a cross-sectional population study. Br J Dermatol 166: 46–53.

6. O'Regan GM, Kemperman PM, Sandilands A, Chen H, Campbell LE, et al. (2010) Raman profiles of the stratum corneum define 3 filaggrin genotype-determined atopic dermatitis endophenotypes. J Allergy Clin Immunol 126: 574–580.

7. Kezic S, O'Regan GM, Yau N, Sandilands A, Chen H, et al. (2011) Levels of filaggrin degradation products are influenced by both filaggrin genotype and atopic dermatitis severity. Allergy.

8. Palmer CN, Irvine AD, Terron-Kwiatkowski A, Zhao Y, Liao H, et al. (2006) Common loss-of-function variants of the epidermal barrier protein filaggrin are a major predisposing factor for atopic dermatitis. Nat Genet 38: 441–446.

9. Marenholz I, Nickel R, Ruschendorf F, Schulz F, Esparza-Gordillo J, et al. (2006) Filaggrin loss-of-function mutations predispose to phenotypes involved in the atopic march. J Allergy Clin Immunol 118: 866–871.

10. Weidinger S, Illig T, Baurecht H, Irvine AD, Rodriguez E, et al. (2006) Loss-of-function variations within the filaggrin gene predispose for atopic dermatitis with allergic sensitizations. J Allergy Clin Immunol 118: 214–219.

11. (1998) Worldwide variation in prevalence of symptoms of asthma, allergic rhinoconjunctivitis, and atopic eczema: ISAAC. The International Study of Asthma and Allergies in Childhood (ISAAC) Steering Committee. Lancet 351: 1225–1232.

12. Barker JN, Palmer CN, Zhao Y, Liao H, Hull PR, et al. (2007) Null mutations in the filaggrin gene (FLG) determine major susceptibility to early-onset atopic dermatitis that persists into adulthood. J Invest Dermatol 127: 564–567.

13. Brown SJ, Sandilands A, Zhao Y, Liao H, Relton CL, et al. (2007) Prevalent and Low-Frequency Null Mutations in the Filaggrin Gene Are Associated with Early-Onset and Persistent Atopic Eczema. J Invest Dermatol.

14. Bonnelykke K, Pipper CB, Tavendale R, Palmer CN, Bisgaard H (2010) Filaggrin gene variants and atopic diseases in early childhood assessed longitudinally from birth. Pediatr Allergy Immunol 21: 954–961.

15. Smith FJ, Irvine AD, Terron-Kwiatkowski A, Sandilands A, Campbell LE, et al. (2006) Loss-of-function mutations in the gene encoding filaggrin cause ichthyosis vulgaris. Nat Genet 38: 337–342.

16. Thyssen JP, Carlsen BC, Bisgaard H, Giwercman C, Johansen JD, et al. (2012) Individuals who are homozygous for the 2282del4 and R501X filaggrin null mutations do not always develop dermatitis and complete long-term remission is possible. J Eur Acad Dermatol Venereol 26: 386–389. 10.1111/j.1468–3083.2011.04073.x [doi].

17. Bisgaard H, Hermansen MN, Buchvald F, Loland L, Halkjaer LB, et al. (2007) Childhood asthma after bacterial colonization of the airway in neonates. N Engl J Med 357: 1487–1495.

18. Bisgaard H (2004) The Copenhagen Prospective Study on Asthma in Childhood (COPSAC): design, rationale, and baseline data from a longitudinal birth cohort study. Ann Allergy Asthma Immunol 93: 381–389.

19. Bisgaard H, Hermansen MN, Loland L, Halkjaer LB, Buchvald F (2006) Intermittent inhaled corticosteroids in infants with episodic wheezing. N Engl J Med 354: 1998–2005.

20. Hanifin JM, Rajka G (1980) Diagnostic features of atopic dermatitis. Acta Derm Venereol 92: 44–47.

21. (1993) Severity scoring of atopic dermatitis: the SCORAD index. Consensus Report of the European Task Force on Atopic Dermatitis. Dermatology 186: 23–31.

22. Barker M, Rayens W (2003) Partial least squares for discrimination. J Chemometrics 17: 166–173. 10.1002/cem.785.

23. Kaiser Henry F (1958) The varimax criterion for analytic rotation in factor analysis. Psychometrica 23: 187–200.

24. Williams HC, Burney PG, Strachan D, Hay RJ (1994) The U.K. Working Party's Diagnostic Criteria for Atopic Dermatitis. II. Observer variation of clinical diagnosis and signs of atopic dermatitis. Br J Dermatol 131: 397–405.

25. Pugliarello S, Cozzi A, Gisondi P, Girolomoni G (2011) Phenotypes of atopic dermatitis. J Dtsch Dermatol Ges 9: 12–20.

26. Fahy CMR, McLean WHI, Irvine AD (2011) Variation in the development of phenotype in filaggrin-deficiency: a murine model of atopic dermatitis. Poster at British Association of Dermatologists annual meeting.

27. Thyssen JP, Carlsen BC, Menne T, Linneberg A, Nielsen NH, et al. (2010) Filaggrin null mutations increase the risk and persistence of hand eczema in subjects with atopic dermatitis: results from a general population study. Br J Dermatol 163: 115–120.

28. Thyssen JP, Carlsen BC, Johansen JD, Meldgaard M, Szecsi PB, et al. (2010) Filaggrin null-mutations may be associated with a distinct subtype of atopic hand eczema. Acta Derm Venereol 90: 528.

29. Simpson EL, Thompson MM, Hanifin JM (2006) Prevalence and morphology of hand eczema in patients with atopic dermatitis. Dermatitis 17: 123–127.

30. Brown SJ, Relton CL, Liao H, Zhao Y, Sandilands A, et al. (2009) Filaggrin haploinsufficiency is highly penetrant and is associated with increased severity of eczema: further delineation of the skin phenotype in a prospective epidemiological study of 792 school children. Br J Dermatol 161: 884–889.

18

LD-Aminopterin in the Canine Homologue of Human Atopic Dermatitis: A Randomized, Controlled Trial Reveals Dosing Factors Affecting Optimal Therapy

John A. Zebala[1]*, **Alan Mundell**[2], **Linda Messinger**[3], **Craig E. Griffin**[4], **Aaron D. Schuler**[1], **Stuart J. Kahn**[1]

1 Syntrix Biosystems, Inc., Auburn, Washington, United States of America, 2 Animal Dermatology Service, Edmonds, Washington, United States of America, 3 Veterinary Referral Center of Colorado, Englewood, Colorado, United States of America, 4 Animal Dermatology Clinic, San Diego, California, United States of America

Abstract

Background: Options are limited for patients with atopic dermatitis (AD) who do not respond to topical treatments. Antifolate therapy with systemic methotrexate improves the disease, but is associated with adverse effects. The investigational antifolate LD-aminopterin may offer improved safety. It is not known how antifolate dose and dosing frequency affect efficacy in AD, but a primary mechanism is thought to involve the antifolate-mediated accumulation of 5-aminoimidazole-4-carboxamide ribonucleotide (AICAR). However, recent *in vitro* studies indicate that AICAR increases then decreases as a function of antifolate concentration. To address this issue and understand how dosing affects antifolate efficacy in AD, we examined the efficacy and safety of different oral doses and schedules of LD-aminopterin in the canine model of AD.

Methods and Findings: This was a multi-center, double-blind trial involving 75 subjects with canine AD randomized to receive up to 12 weeks of placebo, once-weekly (0.007, 0.014, 0.021 mg/kg) or twice-weekly (0.007 mg/kg) LD-aminopterin. The primary efficacy outcome was the Global Score (GS), a composite of validated measures of disease severity and itch. GS improved in all once-weekly cohorts, with 0.014 mg/kg being optimal and significant (43%, $P < 0.01$). The majority of improvement was seen by 8 weeks. In contrast, GS in the twice-weekly cohort was similar to placebo and worse than all once-weekly cohorts. Adverse events were similar across all treated cohorts and placebo.

Conclusions: Once-weekly LD-aminopterin was safe and efficacious in canine AD. Twice-weekly dosing negated efficacy despite having the same daily and weekly dose as effective once-weekly regimens. Optimal dosing in this homologue of human AD correlated with the concentration-selective accumulation of AICAR *in vitro*, consistent with AICAR mediating LD-aminopterin efficacy in AD.

Editor: Douglas Thamm, Colorado State University, United States of America

Funding: This study was supported by the National Institutes of Health (no. AR 056547 to SK and JZ). The funders had no role in study design, data collection and analysis, decision to publish, or preparation of the manuscript.

Competing Interests: SJK and JAZ are employees of Syntrix Biosystems and JAZ holds stock in Syntrix Biosystems. LD-aminopterin is a product in development at Syntrix Biosystems. LM is a paid consultant for Antech Diagnostics, and has received research or speaker support from AB Science, Dechra, Greer Laboratories, Novartis Animal Health, Virbac and Zoetis. CG has been a paid consultant, speaker or received research support from the following companies: Elanco, Merck, Novartis Animal Health, Pinnaclife, Sogeval, TEVA animal health, Veterinary Allergy Reference Laboratory and Zoetis.

* Email: jzebala@syntrixbio.com

Introduction

Atopic dermatitis (AD) affects approximately 3% to 5% of the adult population in the western world, and 30% of the worldwide pediatric population [1]. It is a complex, relapsing disease arising from interactions between genes and the environment and is characterized by pruritus, disruption of the epidermal barrier, and IgE-mediated sensitization to food and environmental allergens [2]. The pathogenesis of AD may involve an aberrant Th2 adaptive immune response to innocuous environmental antigens, skin barrier abnormalities, and an inadequate host response to cutaneous microbes [3].

Patients with AD who fail to respond to topical corticosteroids or topical calcineurin inhibitors may require second-line systemic immunosuppressive therapy [4]. Systemic treatment options include cyclosporine, corticosteroids, azathioprine and methotrexate [5,6]. Cyclosporine and prednisolone are appropriate as short-term treatments [5], the former being nephrotoxic and the latter predisposing to osteoporosis, hypertension and other side-effects [7]. Cyclosporine is also almost entirely metabolized by the liver cytochrome P450 IIIA system, and clinically significant sustained drug-drug interactions can occur during long-term therapy [8]. Caution in the use of azathioprine has been highlighted as well [5], given the heightened risk for hepatosplenic T-cell lymphoma, a rare but frequently lethal form of lymphoma [9]. Despite its well-established record of safety and efficacy, methotrexate is not well tolerated in many patients [10]. The limitations of current systemic treatments have prompted the search for improved treatments that might expand the armamentarium of therapeutic options for patients with AD.

LD-Aminopterin (Syntrix Biosystems, Auburn, WA) is the L- and D-enantiomer of N-[4-[[(2,4-diamino-6-pterdinyl)methyl]amino]benzoyl]-glutamic acid (Figure 1A) [11]. The L-enantiomer is an antifolate congener of methotrexate that is stereoselectively absorbed from LD-aminopterin by the intestinal proton coupled folate transporter [12]. Preclinical and clinical studies indicate it may provide improvements on methotrexate, including better bioavailability [13,14], greater cell uptake and conversion to active polyglutamylated metabolites [13,15], less central nervous system toxicity [16,17,18,19,20], and less liver toxicity [13]. Unlike cyclosporine, LD-aminopterin is not metabolized by human liver microsomes, and thus drug-drug interactions at the cytochrome P450 system are unlikely [12].

Methotrexate, L-aminopterin, and their polyglutamylated metabolites inhibit dihydrofolate reductase and enzymes involved in de novo purine and thymidylate synthesis (Figure 1B) [21,22]. Proposed anti-inflammatory mechanisms have centered on inhibition of de novo thymidylate synthesis [23,24,25], and inhibition of aminoimidazolecarboxamide ribonucleotide transformylase (AICART), an enzyme involved in de novo purine synthesis [26,27,28]. Inhibition of de novo thymidylate synthesis prevents cell-cycle progression of activated T-cells and induces their apoptosis by a Fas-independent pathway [23,24,25], an effect reproduced by several groups [29,30,31,32]. Inhibition of AICART causes increased levels of its substrate, 5-aminoimidazole-4-carboxamide-1-β-D-ribofuranosyl 5′-monophosphate (AICAR), which together with its dephosphorylated metabolite 5-aminoimidazole-4-carboxamide-1-β-D-ribofuranoside (AICA), inhibit AMP deaminase and adenosine deaminase [33,34], effects that cause an increase in extracellular adenosine [26]. Extracellular adenosine binds adenosine receptors to affect a reduction in

inflammation [35]. AICA is also cytotoxic to T lymphocytes, potentiates the cytotoxicity of methotrexate added to cultured T lymphocytes [34,36,37] and activates AMP-activated kinase [38,39].

Funk et al. recently demonstrated AICAR increased 115-fold following exposure of an erythroblastoid cell line to 10 nM methotrexate, but decreased with increasing methotrexate concentrations, declining to baseline with 1000 nM methotrexate [40]. In contrast, the substrate for thymidylate synthase, 2′-deoxyuridine 5′-monophosphate (dUMP), displayed concentration-dependent accumulation over the same range of methotrexate concentration. It was suggested that if clinical response is dependent on the accumulation of AICAR, that these in vitro findings might predict a clinical therapeutic response paradoxically related to dose.

Initial trials of methotrexate in AD simply adopted the dose and regimen commonly used to treat psoriasis and rheumatoid arthritis [41,42]. However, given the different underlying pathologic mechanisms between AD and these other autoimmune diseases, it is not clear that the same dosing strategy would be equally applicable. In fact, no study has examined how dose and regimen affect antifolate efficacy in AD, and thus how to best administer antifolate therapy in AD remains a significant unresolved question.

Although mouse models of AD have many practical benefits in the laboratory, they also have significant limitations in how clinically similar their disease is to human AD. In contrast, dogs naturally and commonly develop a pruritic dermatitis that is clinically and immunologically extremely similar to human AD [43]. Like human AD, canine AD is associated with severe pruritus, skin xerosis and increased transepidermal water loss, face and skin fold involvement, spongiotic dermatitis, skin-infiltrating eosinophils, skin infiltration by IgE(+) and CD1c(+) dendritic cells, Th2-dominated immune responses, positive atopy patch test, and IgE-specific responses. Owing to the remarkable similarity with the

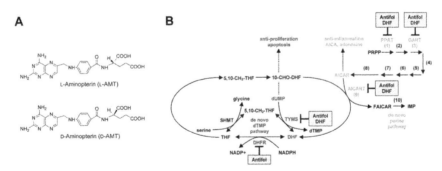

Figure 1. LD-Aminopterin composition and mechanistic model in anti-inflammation. (A) Chemical structure of L-aminopterin (*top*) and D-aminopterin (*bottom*). (B) The anti-inflammatory activity of L-aminopterin and methotrexate have been attributed to inhibition of thymidylate (*red*) and purine (*green*) de novo biosynthesis. In the de novo pathway of thymidylate (dTMP) synthesis, serine hydroxymethyltransferase (SHMT) catalyzes the conversion of serine and tetrahydrofolate polyglutamates (THF) to 5,10-CH$_2$-THF and glycine. Thymidylate synthase (TYMS) converts 5,10-CH$_2$-THF and deoxyuridine monophosphate (dUMP) to dihydrofolate polyglutamates (DHF) and dTMP. Dihydrofolate reductase (DHFR) completes the cycle by catalyzing the conversion of DHF to THF in an NADPH-dependent reaction. The purine, inosine monophosphate (IMP), is synthesized de novo in 10 chemical steps (shown numbered) catalyzed by six enzymes. The six enzymes are phosphoribosylpyrophosphate amidotransferase (PPAT; 1); a trifunctional enzyme composed of glycinamide ribonucleotide synthetase (GARS; 2), GAR formyltransferase (GART; 3) and aminoimidazole ribonucleotide synthetase (AIRS; 5); formylglycinamidine ribonucleotide synthase (FGAMS; 4); a bifunctional enzyme composed of carboxyaminoimidazole ribonucleotide synthase (CAIRS; 6) and succinoaminoimidazolecarboxamide ribonucleotide synthetase (SAICARS; 7); adenylosuccinate lyase (ASL; 8); and a bifunctional enzyme composed of aminoimidazolecarboxamide ribonucleotide transformylase (AICART; 9) and inosine monophosphate cyclohydrolase (IMPCH; 10). Evidence indicates that 10-formyl-7,8-dihydrofolate (10-CHO-DHF) is the predominant in vivo substrate for AICART, making AICART and TYMS the only enzymes to produce the DHFR substrate DHF [69]. Inside the cell, L-aminopterin and methotrexate and their polyglutamate metabolites (antifol) bind with high affinity to DHFR, resulting in accumulation of DHF and depletion of the reduced folate pool. Depletion of folates, as well as the direct inhibition by antifol and DHF, have all been implicated in the inhibition of PPAT, GART, AICART and TYMS [22,33,54,70]. In the case of AICART, the accumulation of DHF may cause this reaction to run backwards, since AICAR is normally driven towards the biosynthesis of FAICAR and IMP by the DHFR-catalyzed reduction of DHF to THF, as the equilibrium of this step actually lies in the direction of AICAR formation [60].

human disease, it has been suggested that canine AD can not only help answer mechanistic questions related to disease pathogenesis, but also serve as a model for testing of drugs with clinical potential in humans [43].

Here we report the efficacy and safety results from a 12-week dose-ranging randomized, double-blind, placebo-controlled, multi-center trial that tested the efficacy and safety of orally administered LD-aminopterin given once- or twice-weekly to subjects with canine AD. The objective was to examine how efficacy and safety of antifolate therapy varies as a function of dose and schedule. This study provides insights into how to administer antifolate therapy in canine AD that has implications for treating the human disease with LD-aminopterin based on a mechanism aimed at maximizing AICAR accumulation.

Materials and Methods

Ethics statement

The study was conducted in compliance with the Veterinary International Committee for Harmonization guidance for good clinical practice and was overseen and approved by a local Institutional Animal Care and Use Committee (North Carolina State University) and a centralized Institutional Animal Care and Use Committee (Infectious Disease Research Institute). Owners of subjects provided written consent for subjects to participate in the study and could withdraw from the study at any time.

Study design

Blinded trial. The study was performed as a double-blinded, randomized, placebo-controlled, parallel-group study conducted

at four referral-based specialty practices located in the United States (California, Colorado, North Carolina and Washington) (Figure 2).

Subjects were randomized in a 1:1:1:1:1 ratio to receive oral doses of placebo, or LD-aminopterin once-weekly (0.007, 0.014 or 0.021 mg/kg) or twice-weekly (0.007×2 mg/kg). Doses are for the free acid of the L-enantiomer. Study drug consisted of either a gelatin capsule containing microcrystalline cellulose (placebo), or a gelatin capsule containing 0.25 mg LD-aminopterin tablets in an appropriate number of whole and/or half tablets to provide the desired dose per subject weight, and backfilled with microcrystalline cellulose. Owners were not required to take any special handling precautions of study drug.

A pre-planned interim efficacy checkpoint at day 56 was instituted based on pilot trial data that indicated responsive subjects achieved the majority of benefit by 4–8 weeks, whereas unresponsive subjects failed to improve with further treatment [44]. Subjects achieving at least 25% GS improvement passed the checkpoint and continued to receive treatment up to day 84. Subjects unable to meet the minimum GS response exited to avoid further futile treatment; their day 56 evaluation became their efficacy endpoint. Efficacy endpoints were therefore from day 56 or 84 per protocol.

Each arm employed a twice-weekly dosing using dummy doses to keep the blind, where the second weekly dose was given 3 days after the first. See below for details on randomization, blinding and dosing compliance. Daily prednisolone (0.5 mg/kg) was offered for the first 14 days without taper to maintain enrollment due to the delayed onset of LD-aminopterin action [44]. No folic

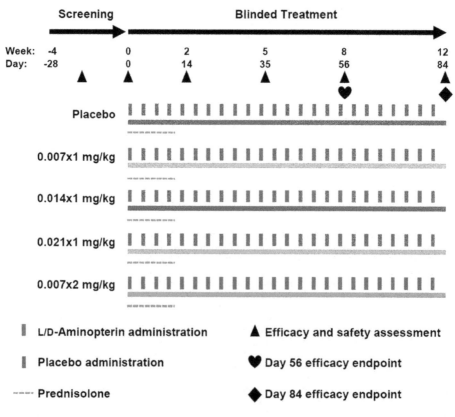

Figure 2. Study flow chart. Randomized subjects with AD were orally administered placebo, or LD-aminopterin once-weekly (0.007×1 mg/kg, 0.014×1 mg/kg, 0.021×1 mg/kg) or twice-weekly (0.007×2 mg/kg).

Table 1. Subject demographics and baseline AD characteristics.

| | | LD-Aminopterin | | | | |
| | Placebo | 0.007×1 mg/kg | 0.014×1 mg/kg | 0.021×1 mg/kg | 0.007×2 mg/kg | |
Variable	N = 15	N = 15	N = 15	N = 15	N = 15	P-value[a]
Age, y	6.7±3.5	4.9±2.5	6.8±3.7	6.0±2.6	5.9±3.0	0.48
Male, N (%)	9 (60.0)	10 (66.6)	10 (66.6)	10 (66.6)	8 (53.3)	0.91
Body weight, kg	28.7±10.1	23.3±12.2	22.7±12.0	26.1±14.3	17.1±10.9	0.11
GS	11.3±8.5	11.4±4.7	12.3±9.0	10.0±5.9	11.9±7.6	0.93
CADESI	160±105	170±64	159±94	130±56	173±99	0.66
PVAS	6.5±1.5	6.7±1.2	7.4±1.5	7.5±1.5	6.6±1.4	0.19
Nonseasonal, N (%)	15 (100.0)	15 (100.0)	14 (93.3)	15 (100.0)	14 (93.3)	0.54

Abbreviations: GS, Global Score; CADESI, Canine Atopic Dermatitis Extent and Severity Index 03; PVAS, Pruritus Visual Analogue Scale.
Data are mean ± SD for continuous variables.
[a]P-values were calculated by chi-square test for categorical data and one-way ANOVA for continuous data.

acid supplementation was specified. Disease activity was assessed at days 0, 14, 35, 56 and 84.

Open-label extension. Subjects from the blinded trial were optionally able to continue on LD-aminopterin in an open-label extension lasting up to 104 weeks. Subjects received other treatments within the standard of care at the discretion of the clinician. Dosing was 0.007–0.021 mg/kg once-weekly at the clinician's discretion.

Study population

Inclusion criteria were (i) a diagnosis of canine AD [45,46]; (ii) moderate-to-severe disease defined by a CADESI score ≥60 and <500 [47]; (iii) age >6 months; (iv) weight 7 to 50 kg; (v) testing to rule out food allergy, flea bite hypersensitivity and external parasites; (vi) absence of fleas and use of a long acting flea adulticide; and (vii) intradermal skin testing or allergen-specific IgE determination confirming the presence of immediate or late-phase hypersensitivity reactions, or reagin immunoglobulins to environmental allergens such as house dust or storage mites, pollens or molds.

Subjects were excluded for (i) pregnancy or lactation; (ii) malignant neoplasia; (iii) diet augmented with fatty acid supplements if the diet was not continued throughout trial; (iv) treatment with long-acting corticosteroids within 6 weeks, oral corticosteroids or cyclosporine within 3 weeks, or oral anti-histamines within 1 week of enrollment; (v) use of anti-allergenic or antipruritic shampoos or conditioners, topical corticosteroids, tacrolimus or cyclosporine within 1 week of enrollment; and (vi) allergen-specific

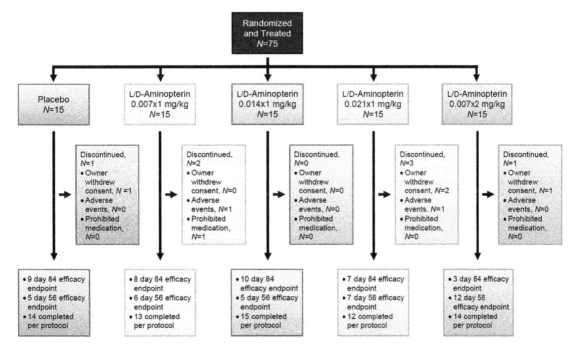

Figure 3. Disposition of subjects. A total of 68 subjects (91%) completed the study per protocol. Discontinuations (9%) were for withdrawal of owner consent (N = 2), owner perceived AE (N = 2), and prohibited medication (N = 1).

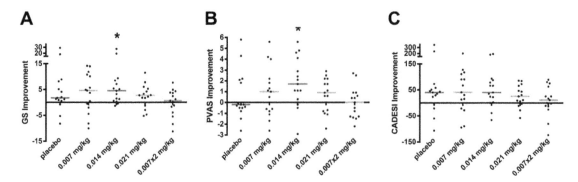

Figure 4. Effect of placebo and LD-aminopterin on canine AD disease measures. Subjects ($N = 75$) with AD were randomized equally to receive placebo, or LD-aminopterin once-weekly (0.007, 0.014 or 0.021 mg/kg) or twice-weekly (0.007×2 mg/kg). Improvement in baseline disease measures were determined for (A) GS, (B) PVAS and (C) CADESI (see Materials and Methods). GS and PVAS improved significantly in the 0.014 mg/kg cohort. *$P < 0.05$. Horizontal bars are medians. Abbreviations: GS, Global Score; PVAS, Pruritus Visual Analogue Scale; CADESI, Canine Atopic Dermatitis Extent and Severity Index 03.

immunotherapy started or changed within 6 months of enrollment, or if the allergen-specific immunotherapy was changed during the study. Antibiotics were permitted per protocol to treat skin infections at the discretion of investigators.

Assessments

Blinded trial. Disease activity was assessed using validated disease measures: PVAS to measure itch [48] and the CADESI to measure disease severity [47]. PVAS yields a possible score from 0 to 10, and CADESI yields a possible score from 0 to 1,240. CADESI and PVAS were assessed at study days 0 (baseline), 14, 35, 56 and 84 (i.e. end of weeks 2, 5, 8 and 12). GS is a composite score that is the product of CADESI and PVAS and thus captures the proportional change in CADESI and PVAS, where GS = (CADESI×PVAS)/100.

Safety assessments were performed at study days 0, 14, 35, 56 and 84 and consisted of recording all AEs and serious AEs and noting their severity and relationship to study drug. They included the regular monitoring of hematology, blood chemistry, and urine and physical examination. A central laboratory (Antech Diagnostic GLP, Morrisville, NC) was used for analysis of all specimens

collected and listed below. Hemoglobin, hematocrit, red blood cell (RBC) count, white blood cell (WBC) count with differential (neutrophils including bands, lymphocytes, monocytes, eosinophils, and basophils), and platelet count were measured at all scheduled study visits within the visit window. Serum chemistries including blood urea nitrogen (BUN), creatinine,, alanine transaminase/serum glutamic pyruvate transaminase (ALT/SGPT), alkaline phosphatase, lactate dehydrogenase (LDH), total protein, and albumin, were measured at all scheduled study visits within the visit window. Urinalysis for specific gravity, protein, glucose, blood, ketones, bilirubin and urobilinogen were performed at scheduled visits on day 0 and 84, or day 56 for subjects who exited the study at the interim efficacy checkpoint.

Open-label extension. Safety assessments were every 3 months in the first year and every 6 months in the second year using the same assessments as in the blinded trial.

Study endpoints

Per protocol, the primary efficacy endpoint was the change in baseline GS at study day 56 or 84. The primary study outcome was to assess the efficacy of four LD-aminopterin dosages in

Table 2. Concomitant medications.

		LD-Aminopterin				
	Placebo	0.007×1 mg/kg	0.014×1 mg/kg	0.021×1 mg/kg	0.007×2 mg/kg	
Medication	$N = 15$	$N = 15$	$N = 15$	$N = 15$	$N = 15$	P-value[a]
Prednisolone, N (%)[b]						
Yes	13 (86.6)	13 (86.6)	13 (86.6)	12 (80.0)	11 (73.3)	
No	2 (13.3)	2 (13.3)	2 (13.3)	3 (20.0)	4 (26.6)	0.83
Antibiotics, N (%)						
Weeks 0–4	11 (73.3)	12 (80.0)	3 (20.0)	12 (80.0)	12 (80.0)	0.001
Weeks 5–8	7 (46.7)	7 (46.7)	3 (20.0)	6 (40.0)	8 (53.3)	0.397
Weeks 9–12	6 (40.0)	6 (40.0)	3 (20.0)	5 (33.3)	5 (33.3)	0.772
Prohibited, N (%)						
Yes	0 (0.0)	1 (6.7)	0 (0.0)	0 (0.0)	0 (0.0)	
No	15 (100.0)	14 (93.3)	15 (100.0)	15 (100.0)	15 (100.0)	0.40

[a]P-values calculated by chi-square test.
[b]During first 14 days.

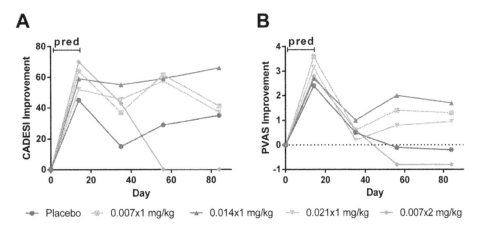

Figure 5. Change in CADESI and PVAS as a function of time in subjects treated with prednisolone and either placebo or LD-aminopterin. Subjects treated with prednisolone (pred) in the first 14 days ($N=62$) were treated with either placebo ($N=13$), or LD-aminopterin once-weekly (0.007×1 mg/kg, $N=13$; 0.014×1 mg/kg, $N=13$; 0.021×1 mg/kg, $N=12$) or twice-weekly (0.007×2 mg/kg, $N=11$). Median improvement in baseline (A) CADESI and (B) PVAS was determined at days 14, 35, 56 and 84. Abbreviations: CADESI, Canine Atopic Dermatitis Extent and Severity Index 03; PVAS, Pruritus Visual Analogue Scale; pred, prednisolone.

subjects with moderate-to-severe canine AD with respect to the primary efficacy endpoint, and determine the most (or least) effective dosage.

Secondary efficacy endpoints evaluated at study day 56 or 84 were the change in baseline CADESI and PVAS. Secondary outcomes included assessing the efficacy of four LD-aminopterin dosages in subjects with moderate-to-severe canine atopic dermatitis with respect to secondary efficacy endpoints, and determine the most (or least) effective dosage; the effect of LD-aminopterin on each secondary efficacy endpoint over time; the safety of LD-aminopterin by clinical and laboratory AEs as a function of dosage and time.

Randomization, blinding and dosing compliance

Randomization was performed centrally by Syntrix Biosystems Drug Supply Management. Subjects were randomized 1:1:1:1:1 into five treatment arms in blocks of five. Randomized blocks were generated using GraphPad QuickCalcs online software (www.graphpad.com/quickcalcs, GraphPad Software, Inc., La Jolla, CA). At randomization, each subject was assigned an identification number that was linked to a treatment arm and a sequentially numbered bottle of blinded study drug. Subject owners did not have contact with one another. All weekly study drug doses were provided in a single similar appearing capsule filled with microcrystalline cellulose. Dosing instructions specified only clear liquids for two hours before taking capsules, except for a small quantity of food to assist in administration. Weight-band-dosing tables were stratified by 1.0 kg increments. To preserve the blind, each arm maintained a schedule of twice-weekly dosing using a dummy dose in the once-weekly treatment schedules, and two dummy doses in the placebo cohort. Dosing compliance was determined by site monitoring and drug accountability (assigned capsules returned). Subject owners, investigator staff, and persons performing the assessments, were blinded to the identity of the treatment.

Statistical analyses

The sample size calculation was based on assessing four dosages of LD-aminopterin and placebo to determine the most or least effective dosage with respect to the primary efficacy endpoint using Hsu's multiple comparisons with the best (Hsu's MCB) test [49].

Assuming a minimum clinically meaningful change in GS of 1.5 (Dr. Thierry Olivry of North Carolina State University), and mean baseline GS of 5.5 and standard deviation of 0.8, both obtained from pilot trial data in subjects (n = 6) with moderate disease [44], a sample size of 15 subjects per cohort was required to achieve a power of 0.9.

The full analysis set consisted of all subjects who were randomized, using the initial randomized dosage, whether the subject ultimately dropped out of the trial or had their dose reduced per protocol. Subjects with missing day 56 or day 84 data were analyzed by the last observation carried forward. Balance in baseline characteristics between cohorts was analyzed by chi-square test for categorical data and one-way ANOVA for continuous data.

The primary outcome, change in baseline GS (absolute and percent change), was analyzed in each cohort by repeated-measures ANOVA. The two-sided type I error was adjusted for multiple cohort comparisons using the Bonferroni correction. The most effective dosage was analyzed using Hsu's MCB [49]. Hsu's MCB compares each cohort mean and the "best" of all the other cohort means to identify the best dosage, or reject a dosage as the best dosage. Hsu's MCB provides joint simultaneous confidence intervals for the differences between the mean baseline change of a dosage cohort minus the maximum of the mean baseline change in each of the other cohorts. If a cohort mean is significantly separated above all other cohort means, it is regarded as 'the best' (i.e., lower confidence limit >0). If a cohort mean has at least one cohort mean significantly separated above it, it is rejected as the best dosage (i.e., upper confidence limit <0). Secondary outcomes for CADESI and PVAS were analyzed as above.

Post hoc testing was by t-test and Mann-Whitney tests, and categorical data on concomitant medications were analyzed by chi-square test with significance claimed at $\alpha = 0.05$. Analyses and sample size calculations were performed with commercial software (PASS and NCSS, NCSS, LLC, Kaysville, UT; and GraphPad Prism version 6.00 for Windows, GraphPad Software, La Jolla, CA).

The safety set included all subjects who took at least one dose of study drug and had at least one post-baseline assessment. AEs were summarized by absolute and relative frequencies stratified by cohort and duration treated.

Table 3. Summary of clinical AEs by cohort[a].

| | | LD-Aminopterin | | | |
| | Placebo | 0.007×1 mg/kg | 0.014×1 mg/kg | 0.021×1 mg/kg | 0.007×2 mg/kg |
Preferred Term	N=15	N=15	N=15	N=15	N=15
Subjects with any AE(s)	**10 (66.6)**	**8 (53.3)**	**7 (46.7)**	**10 (66.6)**	**5 (33.3)**
Death	0	0	0	0	0
Serious AEs	0	0	0	0	0
AE led to discontinuation	0	1 (6.7)[b]	0	1 (6.7)[b]	0
All AEs in any cohort	**11 (73.3)**	**12 (80.0)**	**13 (86.7)**	**17 (113.3)**	**8 (53.3)**
Fatigue	1 (6.7)	1 (6.7)	1 (6.7)	2 (13.3)	0
Weight loss	0	0	0	1 (6.7)	0
Diarrhea	2 (13.3)	4 (26.7)	3 (20.0)	5 (33.3)	2 (13.3)
Anorexia	0	1 (6.7)	1 (6.7)	1 (6.7)	1 (6.7)
Vomiting	0	0	1 (6.7)	1 (6.7)	0
Constipation	0	0	1 (6.7)	0	0
Stool increased	1 (6.7)	0	0	0	0
Stool dark color	1 (6.7)	0	0	0	0
Thirst increased	0	2 (13.3)	0	0	0
Halitosis	0	0	1 (6.7)	0	0
Keratoconjunctivitis sicca	0	0	0	1 (6.7)	0
Eye discharge	0	0	0	0	1 (6.7)
Demodicosis[c]	0	1 (6.7)	0	0	1 (6.7)
Pyotraumatic dermatitis	0	0	0	0	1 (6.7)
Skin infection	1 (6.7)	2 (13.3)	2 (13.3)	2 (13.3)	1 (6.7)
Otitis externa	1 (6.7)	0	0	1 (6.7)	1 (6.7)
Urinary incontinence	1 (6.7)	0	1 (6.7)	1 (6.7)	0
Aural hematoma	0	1 (6.7)	0	0	0
Epistaxis	0	0	1 (6.7)	0	0
Anxiety	0	0	0	0	1 (6.7)
Irritability	1 (6.7)	0	0	0	0
Stomach pain	0	0	0	1 (6.7)	0
Dermatitis	1 (6.7)	0	0	0	0
Urticaria	1 (6.7)	0	0	0	0
Tail dysfunction	0	0	0	1 (6.7)	0

Abbreviations: AE, adverse event.
[a]Expressed as n and percent of total subjects in each cohort.
[b]AE led to discontinuation by subject owner, not by investigator.
[c]0.007×1 mg/kg cohort: *Demodex canis* at day 44 post 0.5 mg/kg prednisolone on days 0 to 14; and 0.007×2 mg/kg cohort: *Demodex injai* at day 56 post 1.0 mg/kg prednisolone on days 0 to 14. Demodicosis cleared after one dose of milbemycin oxime, and each subject treated with LD-aminopterin for 24 (0.007×1 mg/kg cohort) and 9 (0.007×2 mg/kg cohort) months in the open-label segment without recurrence.

Results

Subject baseline characteristics and disposition in the study

Treatment cohorts were balanced with respect to demographic features and baseline disease characteristics (Table 1). The average disease activity in each cohort was severe, defined by a CADESI≥ 120 [50]. The total population was balanced between moderate ($N = 36$) and severe ($N = 39$) disease. A total of 75 subjects were randomly assigned to receive oral LD-aminopterin or placebo (Figure 3). Four study sites enrolled 5 to 44 subjects each. A total of 68 subjects (90.7%) completed the study per protocol, with 37 subjects treated for 12 weeks and 31 subjects treated up to the interim 8 week efficacy checkpoint. Seven subjects (9.3%) discontinued the study. Drug accountability indicated that 95% ($N = 71$) of all subjects had taken 90% or more of the assigned doses, and this percentage was similar across cohorts.

Administration of weekly oral LD-aminopterin is efficacious in canine AD

The Global Score (GS) improved significantly in the 0.014×1 mg/kg cohort (Figure 4A). The GS improved by a mean ($\pm$SD) of 6.1$\pm$7.6 points (95% CI, 1.9–10.3), decreasing from 12.3$\pm$9.0 at baseline to 6.2$\pm$4.8 after treatment ($P<0.05$). The mean ($\pm$SD) percent reduction in baseline GS in the

Table 4. Summary of laboratory AEs by cohort[a].

		LD-Aminopterin			
	Placebo	0.007×1 mg/kg	0.014×1 mg/kg	0.021×1 mg/kg	0.007×2 mg/kg
Laboratory Abnormality	$N=15$	$N=15$	$N=15$	$N=15$	$N=15$
Hematocrit Decreased	0	1 (1.3)	1 (1.3)	2 (2.7)	1 (1.3)
RBC Count Decreased	0	0	2 (2.7)	1 (1.3)	0
Thrombocytopenia	1 (1.3)	0	0	0	1 (1.3)
Thrombocytosis	6 (8.0)	7 (9.3)	7 (9.3)	9 (12.0)	4 (5.3)
Leukopenia	1 (1.3)	0	0	0	0
Lymphopenia	2 (2.7)	0	0	1 (1.3)	0
Neutropenia	0	0	1 (1.3)	0	0
Eosinophilia	0	1 (1.3)	0	0	0
BUN Increased	4 (5.3)	4 (5.3)	3 (4.0)	2 (2.7)	2 (2.7)
Creatinine Increased	0	3 (4.0)	1 (1.3)	0	1 (1.3)
Alkaline Phosphatase Increased	6 (8.0)	5 (6.7)	7 (9.3)	6 (8.0)	7 (9.3)
ALT Increased	5 (6.7)	2 (2.7)	3 (4.0)	1 (1.3)	1 (1.3)
Serum Protein Decreased	0	1 (1.3)	0	1 (1.3)	0
Serum Albumin Decreased	2 (2.7)	3 (4.0)	2 (2.7)	1 (1.3)	1 (1.3)
Total	27 (36.0)	27 (36.0)	27 (36.0)	24 (32.0)	18 (24.0)

Abbreviations: RBC, red blood cell; BUN, blood urea nitrogen; ALT, alanine transaminase.
[a]Expressed as N and percent of 75 total subjects.

$0.014 \times 1 \times$ mg/kg cohort was $43.2 \pm 38.0\%$ (95% CI, 22–64%; $P < 0.01$).

Treatment with LD-aminopterin also resulted in a significant reduction ($P < 0.05$) in itch in the 0.014×1 mg/kg cohort (Figure 4B). The Pruritus Visual Analogue Scale (PVAS) improved by a mean ($\pm$SD) of 1.9 ± 2.3 points (95% CI, 0.6–3.2), decreasing from 7.4 ± 1.5 at baseline to 5.5 ± 2.5 after treatment. The mean percent reduction in PVAS in the 0.014×1 mg/kg cohort was 26% (95% CI, 7–43%). Pruritus in 4 of 15 subjects (27%) in the cohort responded with a robust reduction in baseline PVAS≥4 (mean [percent] reduction = 4.8 [65%]).

The change in baseline Canine Atopic Dermatitis Extent and Severity Index 03 (CADESI) was not significant in any cohort, although the 0.014×1 and 0.021×1 mg/kg cohorts had mean ($\pm$SD) changes (53 ± 71 and 26 ± 42, respectively) that were significant before adjusting the type I error for multiple comparisons (Figure 4C). There was improvement in mean ($\pm$SD) CADESI in the placebo cohort (52 ± 109), but it was not significant even prior to adjusting the type I error for multiple comparisons.

Antibiotics were permitted per protocol to treat skin infections at the discretion of investigators. The mean ($\pm$SE) duration of antibiotic treatment was 6.2+3.7 weeks. Antibiotic use was not a confounding factor in the significant efficacy responses to LD-aminopterin in the 0.014×1 mg/kg cohort because antibiotic use was similar across all treatment cohorts and placebo in each consecutive four week treatment period, except in the 0.014×1 mg/kg cohort, where it was lower (Table 2).

Dosing frequency determines optimal efficacy in canine AD

In addition to examining how varying LD-aminopterin dose impacted efficacy in canine AD, this study also examined how the schedule or frequency of administration affected efficacy. Inter-estingly, all endpoints for twice-weekly LD-aminopterin were no better than placebo, and worse than all once-weekly schedules (Figure 4). CADESI in the twice-weekly regimen was notable for being clearly worse than placebo, though not significantly. The 0.007×2 mg/kg cohort was statistically rejected as the best dosage based on GS and PVAS; each endpoint mean was smaller than, and significantly separated from the corresponding endpoint mean in the 0.014×1 mg/kg cohort ($P < 0.05$, Hsu's MCB).

A *post hoc* comparison with two weeks of daily prednisolone suggests LD-aminopterin may be highly effective in a subpopulation of canine AD

Per protocol, subjects were optionally treated with prednisolone in the first 14 days (see Materials and Methods). Subjects treated with prednisolone constituted 83% ($N = 62$), and were distributed similarly across cohorts (Table 2). Two independent time-response profiles were clearly evident for CADESI and PVAS in this sub-population, consistent with prednisolone and LD-aminopterin having distinctly different onsets of action (Figure 5). Whereas the action of LD-aminopterin on PVAS required 56 to 84 days to come to full prominence, prednisolone caused a rapid improvement in PVAS by day 14 that was lost by the time of the primary efficacy endpoint for LD-aminopterin.

The median (mean$\pm$SD) improvement in PVAS at day 14 in the prednisolone-treated population ($N = 62$) was 2.8 (2.9 ± 2.4) points, a treatment effect that was notably consistent among all cohorts (Figure 5). In contrast, the median (mean$\pm$SD) improvement in PVAS at day 14 in the population not treated with prednisolone ($N = 13$) was 0.0 (0.05 ± 0.6) points. The improvement in PVAS at day 14 in the populations treated and not treated with prednisolone were significantly different ($P < 0.0001$ for median and mean). Prednisolone treatment thus served not only to maintain enrollment during the onset of LD-aminopterin efficacy, it also provided an internal positive efficacy control that

Table 5. Summary of clinical AEs as a function of 4-week intervals[a].

Preferred Term	0 to 4 Weeks	5 to 8 Weeks	9 to 12 Weeks
All Categories	33 (54.1)	21 (34.4)	7 (11.5)
Constitutional	3 (4.9)	2 (3.3)	1 (1.6)
Fatigue	3 (4.9)	2 (3.3)	0
Weight loss	0	0	1 (1.6)
Gastrointestinal	17 (27.9)	7 (11.5)	4 (6.6)
Diarrhea	10 (16.4)	3 (4.9)	3 (4.9)
Anorexia	2 (3.3)	1 (1.6)	1 (1.6)
Vomiting	1 (1.6)	1 (1.6)	0
ConstipationN	1 (1.6)	0	0
Stool increased	1 (1.6)	0	0
Stool dark color	0	1 (1.6)	0
Thirst increased	2 (3.3)	0	0
Halitosis	0	1 (1.6)	0
Ocular	1 (1.6)	1 (1.6)	0
Keratoconjunctivitis sicca	0	1 (1.6)	0
Eye discharge	1 (1.6)	0	0
Infection	3 (4.9)	9 (14.8)	2 (3.3)
Demodicosis	0	2 (3.3)	0
Pyotraumatic dermatitis	1 (1.6)	0	0
Skin infection	2 (3.3)	5 (8.2)	1 (1.6)
Otitis externa	0	2 (3.3)	1 (1.6)
Renal/Genitourinary	3 (4.9)	0	0
Urinary incontinence	3 (4.9)	0	0
Hemorrhage	2 (3.3)	0	0
Aural hematoma	1 (1.6)	0	0
Epistaxis	1 (1.6)	0	0
Neurology	2 (3.3)	0	0
Anxiety	1 (1.6)	0	0
Irritability	1 (1.6)	0	0
Pain	1 (1.6)	0	0
Stomach pain	1 (1.6)	0	0
Allergy	0	1 (1.6)	0
Dermatitis	0	1 (1.6)	0
Dermatology	0	1 (1.6)	0
Urticaria	0	1 (1.6)	0
Musculoskeletal	1 (1.6)	0	0
Tail dysfunction	1 (1.6)	0	0

[a]Expressed as N and percent of 61 total AEs.

confirmed the reliability and reproducibility of blinded owner-assessed itch using PVAS.

The median PVAS improvement in the 0.014×1 mg/kg cohort ($N = 15$) due to LD-aminopterin was 61% of the median day 14 PVAS improvement due to prednisolone in the total prednisolone-treated population ($N = 62$). However, this difference was not significant ($P = 0.22$). Of the 62 prednisolone-treated subjects, 21 (33.9%) had robust improvement in PVAS$\geq$4 points at day 14. Among the 0.007×1 mg/kg and 0.014×1 mg/kg cohorts, 7 of 30 subjects (23.3%, all with nonseasonal disease) responded at day 84 with improvement in PVAS$\geq$4 points. The fraction of subjects with improvement in PVAS$\geq$4 after LD-aminopterin was not

significantly different than after prednisolone ($P = 0.34$). Of the 7 subjects with improvement in PVAS$\geq$4 after LD-aminopterin, 6 were treated with prednisolone, and had a mean improvement due to prednisolone substantially the same as that seen for the larger ($N = 62$) prednisolone-treated population (2.7 ± 2.1 versus 2.9 ± 2.4, respectively). In these 6 subjects, the mean ($\pm$SD) improvement in PVAS due to LD-aminopterin was significantly (77%) greater than from prednisolone (4.8 ± 0.7 versus 2.7 ± 2.1, $P<0.05$).

LD-Aminopterin is safe and well-tolerated in canine AD

Blinded trial. There was no relationship between clinical (Table 3) or laboratory (Table 4) adverse events (AEs), and either dose or schedule. The incidence of AEs in LD-aminopterin treated cohorts was similar to placebo. The most frequently reported AEs ($\geq$5% of 61 total) across all cohorts were gastrointestinal in nature (45.9% [$N = 28$]): diarrhea (26.2% [$N = 16$]) and anorexia (6.6% [$N = 4$]). All were mild in intensity and self-limiting. Abnormalities in liver function as measured by elevations in serum alanine transaminase were most common in placebo, and in all cases were mild and transient (Table 4). The incidence of AEs decreased as a function of time (Table 5). There were no serious AEs, or AEs that led investigators to discontinue study drug, reduce dose, or deviate from protocol.

Open-label extension.   Of the 75 subjects enrolled in the blinded trial, 62 (83%) enrolled in the open-label extension. The doses used in the open-label extension were 0.007 mg/kg (19%), 0.014 mg/kg (57%) and 0.021 mg/kg (24%). Including the 12 weeks of treatment in the blinded trial, 40 (65%) and 23 (37%) subjects were treated for more than 57 and 84 weeks, respectively. The drug was well-tolerated during chronic therapy. There were no clinical serious adverse events or deaths. No clinically significant laboratory adverse events occurred, and there was no dose-dependent trend in the incidence of adverse events for any laboratory test (Table S1). There was no laboratory adverse events that required discontinuation of study drug.

Discussion

This placebo-controlled study examined how dose and schedule of the investigational antifolate LD-aminopterin affected efficacy and safety in canine AD. Oral LD-aminopterin 0.014 mg/kg given once weekly resulted in efficacy in moderate-to-severe canine AD after 8–12 weeks of treatment, causing a significant reduction in GS and PVAS. An exploratory analysis identified ~25% of subjects who were highly responsive to the anti-pruritic effect of LD-aminopterin, and enjoyed a significantly larger mean reduction in itch (65%) than from two weeks of daily prednisolone (4.8 versus 2.7 point reduction, or 77% greater). CADESI was also significantly reduced, but only before correcting for multiple comparisons. CADESI was reduced in placebo but not significantly, an effect likely due to permitted antimicrobials [51], and/or carry-over effects of prednisolone used in the first 14 days per protocol [52].

Surprisingly, all efficacy endpoints for twice-weekly 0.007 mg/kg LD-aminopterin were no better than placebo, and worse than all once-weekly schedules. This held whether the once-weekly schedule provided the same daily (0.007 mg/kg) or total weekly (0.014 mg/kg) dose. Based on CADESI, twice-weekly dosing was even worse than placebo, though not significantly. These findings were unexpected and suggest that the schedule of antifolate administration is critical, with a minimum interval between dosings required for efficacy in canine AD.

Like methotrexate, the L-enantiomer of LD-aminopterin potently inhibits dihydrofolate reductase (Figure 1B) [17,53], which results in the rapid accumulation of dihydrofolate poly-glutamates that may reach 20% (~2 μM) of total intracellular folates from an initial undetectable level [21]. Dihydrofolate polyglutamates at these concentrations are capable of inhibiting the first committed step of purine biosynthesis catalyzed by PPAT and the two transformylase reactions catalyzed by GART and AICART [22]. In addition to dihydrofolate polyglutamates, methotrexate polyglutamates have also been implicated as effectors of inhibition of these three steps of *de novo* purine synthesis [22,33,34,54]. Although AICART inhibition and the accumulation of AICAR and its metabolite AICA have been proposed to mediate anti-inflammatory effects

[26,27,28,34,36,37,39], *in vitro* studies with leukemia cells and primary human T lymphocytes indicate that PPAT is the primary site of inhibition of purine biosynthesis by methotrexate [22,55]. In particular, levels of 5-phosphoribosyl-1-pyrophosphate, the natural PPAT substrate, increase 5-10-fold from 3 to 12 hours in cells exposed in culture to methotrexate at a concentration (0.1 μM) obtained in the plasma of patients undergoing therapy for inflammation, before decreasing to control levels after 24 hours [56,57]. Thus, methotrexate inhibits PPAT, GART and AICART, but empirically induces AICAR accumulation in patients [58,59]. Accumulated AICAR may therefore be derived from either selective inhibition of AICART at low antifolate concentrations [40], or from the pools of intermediates that exist between GART and AICART if both enzymes are inhibited non-selectively [22]. In the latter case, the abundance of intermediates may vary from patient to patient, potentially accounting in part for the variability in antifolate clinical efficacy. Another possibility is that AICAR is derived from FAICAR if the accumulation of dihydrofolate polyglutamates causes the AICART reaction to run backward, as suggested by the fact that the equilibrium of this reaction actually lies in the direction of AICAR formation [60].

Persistent inhibition of PPAT, GART and AICART in subjects would be expected to abrogate the downstream accumulation of AICAR and its AICA metabolite, since each would be eliminated from the body without precursors available for the synthesis of additional AICAR [61]. In patients given a single standard anti-inflammatory dose of methotrexate, Smolenska *et al.* demonstrated rapid inhibition of *de novo* purine biosynthesis that was sustained for at least 24–48 hours but that fully reversed by one week after dosing, kinetics that suggest twice-weekly dosing may lead to persistent inhibition of *de novo* purine synthesis [62]. If the anti-inflammatory effect of LD-aminopterin in AD is due to AICAR, an optimal schedule of therapy would require sufficient time between drug pulses to allow enzymes to cycle between states of complete and incomplete inhibition in order to regenerate intermediates in *de novo* purine synthesis and maintain optimally elevated and efficacious levels of AICAR. This mechanism could explain why twice-weekly dosing in this study negated efficacy in AD, despite having the same daily and weekly dose as effective once-weekly regimens.

Support for this model comes from recent *in vitro* studies carried out by Funk *et al.*, who demonstrated a 115-fold increase in AICAR following exposure of an erythroblastoid cell line to 10 nM MTX, but subsequently decreased with increasing MTX concentrations, declining to baseline levels with 1000 nM MTX [40]. In contrast, dUMP displayed concentration-dependent accumulation. These observations led these investigators to predict clinical anti-inflammatory responses due to AICAR might be paradoxically related to antifolate dose, whereas a dose-proportional response would be seen if due to inhibition of thymidylate synthase. Toxicity is observed in all subjects administered a sufficiently high dose of LD-aminopterin or methotrexate [12,14], consistent with the proposal that antifolate toxicity is mediated by thymidylate synthase inhibition [40]. In contrast, the dose-response data for efficacy in this study mirrors the *in vitro* concentration-response findings for AICAR described by Funk *et al.* [40], suggesting that LD-aminopterin efficacy in AD is mediated by AICAR accumulation.

Clinical evidence supportive of this model in humans comes from Radmanesh and colleagues, who observed greater efficacy in psoriatics treated with weekly methotrexate given on a single day in three doses (3×5 mg) than when the same weekly dose was administered equally over six days (6×2.5 mg) [63]. Likewise, stepwise increases in methotrexate dose in patients with juvenile idiopathic arthritis who were nonresponders to standard low-dose methotrexate did not result in improved clinical outcomes [64].

The safety of LD-aminopterin in canine AD was also examined. In contrast to efficacy, there was no relationship between safety and either dose or schedule of administration. As discussed above, the discordance between efficacy and toxicity in relation to dose supports distinct mechanisms for each, as previously suggested by *in vitro* studies [40]. The incidence of AEs in cohorts treated with LD-aminopterin were similar to one another and to the placebo-treated group. In a previous dose-ranging toxicology study in the canine [12], we determined that 0.2 mg/kg L-aminopterin given once-weekly was the lowest dose that caused the first signs of mild toxicity. Thus, the optimal therapeutic dose identified in this trial establishes a therapeutic index with a 14-fold margin of safety.

Subjects from the blinded trial were also optionally able to continue on LD-aminopterin in an open-label extension lasting up to 104 weeks. Of the 75 subjects enrolled in the blinded trial, 62 (83%) enrolled in the extension. The doses used in the extension were 0.007 mg/kg (19%), 0.014 mg/kg (57%) and 0.021 mg/kg (24%). Including the 12 weeks of treatment in the blinded trial, 40 (65%) and 23 (37%) subjects were treated for more than 57 and 84 weeks, respectively. The drug was well-tolerated during chronic therapy and no adverse event required discontinuation of study drug.

The safety profile of weekly methotrexate in the canine at anti-inflammatory doses is not well defined. Weekly treatment of five dogs with CAD with an oral anti-inflammatory dose of methotrexate (0.2 mg/kg) for four weeks resulted in severe vomiting in one subject and fatal hepatic necrosis in two subjects (personal communication by Dr. Thierry Olivry, North Carolina State University). Pond and Morrow reported a similar case of fatal hepatic necrosis in a dog with osteosarcoma treated with methotrexate at an oral dose of 5 mg/m^2 (0.25 mg/kg) on the first four days of each week [65]. A four-week toxicology study of LD-aminopterin, L-aminopterin and D-aminopterin in beagle dogs ($N = 6$ per cohort, once-weekly oral gavage of 0.5 mg/kg of each enantiomer or 35-fold the anti-inflammatory dose) found no liver histopathology in any cohort (unpublished data). Although data from controlled studies are needed, these observations suggest methotrexate and LD-aminopterin may have different therapeutic indices in the canine.

Options for systemic treatment of human AD include azathioprine, cyclosporine, and methotrexate [5]. A systematic review and meta-analysis of 15 studies and 602 patients determined that cyclosporine consistently decreased the severity of AD [66]. The pooled mean decrease in disease severity was 22% (95% CI, 8–36%) under low-dose cyclosporine (3 mg/kg), and 40% (95%-CI 29–51%) at dosages ≥4 mg/kg. Although effective, a proportion of patients discontinue cyclosporine because of ineffectiveness or side effects, and long-term use raises concerns of nephrotoxicity [67].

Methotrexate has fewer safety concerns than cyclosporine in humans, and was shown in open-label and randomized controlled trials to be an effective treatment of AD [42,68]. An open-label study evaluated the efficacy and safety of low-dose methotrexate (7.5 mg/week) and cyclosporine (2.5 mg/kg/day) in the treatment of severe AD, and determined there was no statistically significant difference in disease reduction between treatments [41].

Cyclosporine is FDA approved in the United States and elsewhere in the world for the control of CAD. In the pivotal efficacy field trial, four weeks of daily cyclosporine (5 mg/kg) gave a mean (baseline:endpoint) reduction in CADESI (0–360 scale) and PVAS (0–5 scale) in the intent-to-treat population ($N = 262$) of 31.5 (79.0:47.5) and 1.36 (3.75:2.39), respectively [51]. The data from this study show that once-weekly LD-aminopterin (0.014 mg/kg, $N = 15$) resulted in a mean (baseline:endpoint) reduction in CADESI of 53 (159:107), and a reduction in PVAS of 1.9 (7.4:5.5). Qualitatively, cyclosporine and LD-aminopterin appear to have a similar effect on CAD disease activity. Any formal comparison would require a well-controlled and properly powered head-to-head study.

LD-aminopterin may thus provide an additional therapeutic option to treat AD, but with a better safety profile than either methotrexate [16,17,18,19,20], or cyclosporine. The efficacy and safety data for LD-aminopterin from this study go toward supporting the rationale for a human trial and provide insights for optimal antifolate dosing in human AD.

Supporting Information

Table S1 Clinical laboratory adverse events in the open-label trial segment.

Dataset S1 GS scores.

Dataset S2 Percent change in baseline GS scores.

Dataset S3 PVAS scores.

Dataset S4 CADESI scores.

Acknowledgments

We thank Dr. Thierry Olivry and staff at North Carolina State University for enrolling subjects and Dr. Hong Yee and David Coblentz at DF/Net Research, Inc. for biostatistical advice.

Author Contributions

Conceived and designed the experiments: JAZ SJK. Performed the experiments: AM LM CEG. Analyzed the data: JAZ SJK ADS. Contributed reagents/materials/analysis tools: ADS SJK. Wrote the paper: JAZ SJK. Contributed to critical revisions: AM LM CEG ADS.

References

1. Williams H, Robertson C, Stewart A, Ait-Khaled N, Anabwani G, et al. (1999) Worldwide variations in the prevalence of symptoms of atopic eczema in the International Study of Asthma and Allergies in Childhood. J Allergy Clin Immunol 103: 125–138.
2. Sohn A, Frankel A, Patel RV, Goldenberg G (2011) Eczema. Mt Sinai J Med 78: 730–739.
3. Leung DY, Boguniewicz M, Howell MD, Nomura I, Hamid QA (2004) New insights into atopic dermatitis. J Clin Invest 113: 651–657.
4. Brown S, Reynolds NJ (2006) Atopic and non-atopic eczema. BMJ 332: 584–588.
5. Denby KS, Beck LA (2012) Update on systemic therapies for atopic dermatitis. Curr Opin Allergy Clin Immunol 12: 421–426.
6. Proudfoot LE, Powell AM, Ayis S, Barbarot S, Baselgatorres E, et al. (2013) The European treatment of severe atopic eczema in children taskforce (TREAT) survey. Br J Dermatol advance online publication, 16 Jul 2013 doi:10.1111/bjd.12505.
7. Chakravarty K, McDonald H, Pullar T, Taggart A, Chalmers R, et al. (2008) BSR/BHPR guideline for disease-modifying anti-rheumatic drug (DMARD) therapy in consultation with the British Association of Dermatologists. Rheumatology (Oxford) 47: 924–925.

8. Ryan C, Amor KT, Menter A (2010) The use of cyclosporine in dermatology: part II. J Am Acad Dermatol 63: 949–972; quiz 973–944.

9. Parakkal D, Sifuentes H, Semer R, Ehrenpreis ED (2011) Hepatosplenic T-cell lymphoma in patients receiving TNF-alpha inhibitor therapy: expanding the groups at risk. Eur J Gastroenterol Hepatol 23: 1150–1156.

10. Barker J, Horn EJ, Lebwohl M, Warren RB, Nast A, et al. (2011) Assessment and management of methotrexate hepatotoxicity in psoriasis patients: report from a consensus conference to evaluate current practice and identify key questions toward optimizing methotrexate use in the clinic. J Eur Acad Dermatol Venereol 25: 758–764.

11. Zebala J, Maeda DY, Morgan JR, Kahn SJ (2013) Pharmaceutical composition comprising racemic aminopterin. U.S. Patent No. 8,349,837.

12. Menter A, Thrash B, Cherian C, Matherly LH, Wang L, et al. (2012) Intestinal transport of aminopterin enantiomers in dogs and humans with psoriasis is stereoselective: evidence for a mechanism involving the proton-coupled folate transporter. J Pharmacol Exp Ther 342: 696–708.

13. Cole PD, Drachtman RA, Smith AK, Cate S, Larson RA, et al. (2005) Phase II trial of oral aminopterin for adults and children with refractory acute leukemia. Clin Cancer Res 11: 8089–8096.

14. Ratliff AF, Wilson J, Hum M, Marling-Cason M, Rose K, et al. (1998) Phase I and pharmacokinetic trial of aminopterin in patients with refractory malignancies. J Clin Oncol 16: 1458–1464.

15. Smith A, Hum M, Winick NJ, Kamen BA (1996) A case for the use of aminopterin in treatment of patients with leukemia based on metabolic studies of blasts in vitro. Clin Cancer Res 2: 69–73.

16. Cole PD, Beckwith KA, Vijayanathan V, Roychowdhury S, Smith AK, et al. (2009) Folate homeostasis in cerebrospinal fluid during therapy for acute lymphoblastic leukemia. Pediatr Neurol 40: 34–41.

17. Cole PD, Zebala JA, Alcaraz MJ, Smith AK, Tan J, et al. (2006) Pharmacodynamic properties of methotrexate and Aminotrexate during weekly therapy. Cancer Chemother Pharmacol 57: 826–834.

18. Li Y, Vijayanathan V, Gulinello M, Cole PD (2010) Intrathecal methotrexate induces focal cognitive deficits and increases cerebrospinal fluid homocysteine. Pharmacol Biochem Behav 95: 428–433.

19. Li Y, Vijayanathan V, Gulinello ME, Cole PD (2010) Systemic methotrexate induces spatial memory deficits and depletes cerebrospinal fluid folate in rats. Pharmacol Biochem Behav 94: 454–463.

20. Vijayanathan V, Gulinello M, Ali N, Cole PD (2011) Persistent cognitive deficits, induced by intrathecal methotrexate, are associated with elevated CSF concentrations of excitotoxic glutamate analogs and can be reversed by an NMDA antagonist. Behav Brain Res 225: 491–497.

21. Allegra CJ, Fine RL, Drake JC, Chabner BA (1986) The effect of methotrexate on intracellular folate pools in human MCF-7 breast cancer cells. J Biol Chem 261: 6478–6485.

22. Sant ME, Lyons SD, Phillips L, Christopherson RI (1992) Antifolates induce inhibition of amido phosphoribosyltransferase in leukemia cells. J Biol Chem 267: 11038–11045.

23. Genestier L, Paillot R, Fournel S, Ferraro C, Miossec P, et al. (1998) Immunosuppressive properties of methotrexate: apoptosis and clonal deletion of activated peripheral T cells. J Clin Invest 102: 322–328.

24. Paillot R, Genestier L, Fournel S, Ferraro C, Miossec P, et al. (1998) Activation-dependent lymphocyte apoptosis induced by methotrexate. Transplant Proc 30: 2348–2350.

25. Quemeneur L, Gerland LM, Flacher M, Ffrench M, Revillard JP, et al. (2003) Differential control of cell cycle, proliferation, and survival of primary T lymphocytes by purine and pyrimidine nucleotides. J Immunol 170: 4986–4995.

26. Cronstein BN, Eberle MA, Gruber HE, Levin RI (1991) Methotrexate inhibits neutrophil function by stimulating adenosine release from connective tissue cells. Proc Natl Acad Sci USA 88: 2441–2445.

27. Cronstein BN, Naime D, Ostad E (1993) The antiinflammatory mechanism of methotrexate. Increased adenosine release at inflamed sites diminishes leukocyte accumulation in an in vivo model of inflammation. J Clin Invest 92: 2675–2682.

28. Cutolo M, Sulli A, Pizzorni C, Seriolo B, Straub RH (2001) Anti-inflammatory mechanisms of methotrexate in rheumatoid arthritis. Ann Rheum Dis 60: 729–735.

29. Heijden JV, Assaraf Y, Gerards A, Oerlemans R, Lems W, et al. (2013) Methotrexate analogues display enhanced inhibition of TNF-alpha production in whole blood from RA patients. Scand J Rheumatol.

30. Herman S, Zurgil N, Langevitz P, Ehrenfeld M, Deutsch M (2003) The induction of apoptosis by methotrexate in activated lymphocytes as indicated by fluorescence hyperpolarization: a possible model for predicting methotrexate therapy for rheumatoid arthritis patients. Cell Struct Funct 28: 113–122.

31. Spurlock CF 3rd, Aune ZT, Tossberg JT, Collins PL, Aune JP, et al. (2011) Increased sensitivity to apoptosis induced by methotrexate is mediated by JNK. Arthritis Rheum 63: 2606–2616.

32. Swierkot J, Miedzybrodzki R, Szymaniec S, Szechinski J (2004) Activation dependent apoptosis of peripheral blood mononuclear cells from patients with rheumatoid arthritis treated with methotrexate. Ann Rheum Dis 63: 599–600.

33. Allegra CJ, Drake JC, Jolivet J, Chabner BA (1985) Inhibition of phosphoribosylaminoimidazolecarboxamide transformylase by methotrexate and dihydrofolic acid polyglutamates. Proc Natl Acad Sci USA 82: 4881–4885.

34. Baggott JE, Vaughn WH, Hudson BB (1986) Inhibition of 5-aminoimidazole-4-carboxamide ribotide transformylase, adenosine deaminase and 5-adenylate

deaminase by polyglutamates of methotrexate and oxidized folates and by 5-aminoimidazole-4-carboxamide riboside and ribotide. Biochem J 236: 193–200.

35. Chan ES, Cronstein BN (2010) Methotrexate–how does it really work? Nat Rev Rheumatol 6: 175–178.

36. Baggott JE, Morgan SL, Ha TS, Alarcon GS, Koopman WJ, et al. (1993) Antifolates in rheumatoid arthritis: a hypothetical mechanism of action. Clin Exp Rheumatol 11 Suppl 8: S101–105.

37. Ha T, Baggott JE (1994) 5-aminoimidazole-4-carboxamide ribotide (AICAR) and its metabolites: metabolic and cytotoxic effects and accumulation during methotrexate treatment. J Nutr Biochem 5: 522.

38. Guigas B, Taleux N, Foretz M, Detaille D, Andreelli F, et al. (2007) AMP-activated protein kinase-independent inhibition of hepatic mitochondrial oxidative phosphorylation by AICA riboside. Biochem J 404: 499–507.

39. Katerelos M, Mudge SJ, Stapleton D, Auwardt RB, Fraser SA, et al. (2010) 5-aminoimidazole-4-carboxamide ribonucleoside and AMP-activated protein kinase inhibit signalling through NF-kappaB. Immunol Cell Biol 88: 754–760.

40. Funk RS, van Haandel L, Becker ML, Leeder JS (2013) Low-dose methotrexate results in the selective accumulation of aminoimidazole carboxamide ribotide in an erythroblastoid cell line. J Pharmacol Exp Ther 347: 154–163.

41. El-Khalawany MA, Hassan H, Shaaban D, Ghonaim N, Eassa B (2013) Methotrexate versus cyclosporine in the treatment of severe atopic dermatitis in children: a multicenter experience from Egypt. Eur J Pediatr 172: 351–356.

42. Schram ME, Roekevisch E, Leeflang MM, Bos JD, Schmitt J, et al. (2011) A randomized trial of methotrexate versus azathioprine for severe atopic eczema. J Allergy Clin Immunol 128: 353–359.

43. Marsella R, Girolomoni G (2009) Canine models of atopic dermatitis: a useful tool with untapped potential. J Invest Dermatol 129: 2351–2357.

44. Olivry T, Paps JS, Bizikova P, Murphy KM, Jackson HA, et al. (2007) A pilot open trial evaluating the efficacy of low-dose aminopterin in the canine homologue of human atopic dermatitis. Br J Dermatol 157: 1040–1042.

45. DeBoer DJ, Hillier A (2001) The ACVD task force on canine atopic dermatitis (XV): fundamental concepts in clinical diagnosis. Vet Immunol Immunopathol 81: 271–276.

46. Willemse T (1986) Atopic skin disease: a review and a reconsideration of diagnostic criteria. J Small Anim Pract 27: 771–778.

47. Olivry T, Marsella R, Iwasaki T, Mueller R, International Task Force On Canine Atopic Dermatitis (2007) Validation of CADESI-03, a severity scale for clinical trials enrolling dogs with atopic dermatitis. Vet Dermatol 18: 78–86.

48. Rybnicek J, Lau-Gillard PJ, Harvey R, Hill PB (2009) Further validation of a pruritus severity scale for use in dogs. Vet Dermatol 20: 115–122.

49. Hsu JC (1996) Multiple Comparisons: Theory and Methods. London: Chapman & Hall. 277 p.

50. Olivry T, Mueller R, Nuttall T, Favrot C, Prelaud P, et al. (2008) Determination of CADESI-03 thresholds for increasing severity levels of canine atopic dermatitis. Vet Dermatol 19: 115–119.

51. Steffan J, Parks C, Seewald W, North American Veterinary Dermatology Cyclosporine Study Group (2005) Clinical trial evaluating the efficacy and safety of cyclosporine in dogs with atopic dermatitis. J Am Vet Med Assoc 226: 1855–1863.

52. Steffan J, Horn J, Gruet P, Strehlau G, Fondati A, et al. (2004) Remission of the clinical signs of atopic dermatitis in dogs after cessation of treatment with cyclosporin A or methylprednisolone. Vet Rec 154: 681–684.

53. Skipper HE, Mitchell JH, Bennett LL (1950) Inhibition of nucleic acid synthesis by folic acid antagonists. Cancer Res 10: 510–512.

54. Lyons SD, Christopherson RI (1991) Antifolates induce primary inhibition of the de novo purine pathway prior to 5-aminoimidazole-4-carboxamide ribotide transformylase in leukemia cells. Biochem Int 24: 187–197.

55. Fairbanks LD, Ruckemann K, Qiu Y, Hawrylowicz CM, Richards DF, et al. (1999) Methotrexate inhibits the first committed step of purine biosynthesis in mitogen-stimulated human T-lymphocytes: a metabolic basis for efficacy in rheumatoid arthritis? Biochem J 342 (Pt 1): 143–152.

56. Buesa-Perez JM, Leyva A, Pinedo HM (1980) Effect of methotrexate on 5-phosphoribosyl 1-pyrophosphate levels in L1210 leukemia cells in vitro. Cancer Res 40: 139–144.

57. Kamal MA, Christopherson RI (2004) Accumulation of 5-phosphoribosyl-1-pyrophosphate in human CCRF-CEM leukaemia cells treated with antifolates. Int J Biochem Cell Biol 36: 545–551.

58. Baggott JE, Morgan SL, Sams WM, Linden J (1999) Urinary adenosine and aminoimidazolecarboxamide excretion in methotrexate-treated patients with psoriasis. Arch Dermatol 135: 813–817.

59. Morgan SL, Oster RA, Lee JY, Alarcon GS, Baggott JE (2004) The effect of folic acid and folinic acid supplements on purine metabolism in methotrexate-treated rheumatoid arthritis. Arthritis Rheum 50: 3104–3111.

60. Wall M, Shim JH, Benkovic SJ (2000) Human AICAR transformylase: role of the 4-carboxamide of AICAR in binding and catalysis. Biochemistry 39: 11303–11311.

61. Dixon R, Fujitaki J, Sandoval T, Kisicki J (1993) Acadesine (AICA-riboside): disposition of an adenosine-regulating agent. J Clin Pharmacol 33: 955–958.

62. Smolenska Z, Kaznowska Z, Zarowny D, Simmonds HA, Smolenski RT (1999) Effect of methotrexate on blood purine and pyrimidine levels in patients with rheumatoid arthritis. Rheumatology (Oxford) 38: 997–1002.

63. Radmanesh M, Rafiei B, Moosavi ZB, Sina N (2011) Weekly vs. daily administration of oral methotrexate (MTX) for generalized plaque psoriasis: a randomized controlled clinical trial. Int J Dermatol 50: 1291–1293.

64. Ruperto N, Murray KJ, Gerloni V, Wulffraat N, de Oliveira SK, et al. (2004) A randomized trial of parenteral methotrexate comparing an intermediate dose with a higher dose in children with juvenile idiopathic arthritis who failed to respond to standard doses of methotrexate. Arthritis Rheum 50: 2191–2201.

65. Pond EC, Morrow D (1982) Hepatotoxicity associated with methotrexate therapy in a dog. J small Anim Pract 23: 659–666.

66. Schmitt J, Schmitt N, Meurer M (2007) Cyclosporin in the treatment of patients with atopic eczema - a systematic review and meta-analysis. J Eur Acad Dermatol Venereol 21: 606–619.

67. Behnam SM, Behnam SE, Koo JY (2005) Review of cyclosporine immunosuppressive safety data in dermatology patients after two decades of use. J Drugs Dermatol 4: 189–194.

68. Weatherhead SC, Wahie S, Reynolds NJ, Meggitt SJ (2007) An open-label, dose-ranging study of methotrexate for moderate-to-severe adult atopic eczema. Br J Dermatol 156: 346–351.

69. Baggott JE, Tamura T (2010) Evidence for the hypothesis that 10-formyldihydrofolate is the in vivo substrate for aminoimidazolecarboxamide ribotide transformylase. Exp Biol Med (Maywood) 235: 271–277.

70. Seither RL, Trent DF, Mikulecky DC, Rape TJ, Goldman ID (1989) Folate-pool interconversions and inhibition of biosynthetic processes after exposure of L1210 leukemia cells to antifolates. Experimental and network thermodynamic analyses of the role of dihydrofolate polyglutamylates in antifolate action in cells. J Biol Chem 264: 17016–17023.

19

Comparative Effectiveness of Homoeopathic vs. Conventional Therapy in Usual Care of Atopic Eczema in Children: Long-Term Medical and Economic Outcomes

Stephanie Roll[1]*, Thomas Reinhold[1], Daniel Pach[1], Benno Brinkhaus[1], Katja Icke[1], Doris Staab[2], Tanja Jäckel[1], Karl Wegscheider[3], Stefan N. Willich[1], Claudia M. Witt[1,4]

1 Institute for Social Medicine, Epidemiology, and Health Economics, Charité University Medical Centre, Berlin, Germany, 2 Department of Paediatric Pulmonology and Immunology, Charité University Medical Centre, Berlin, Germany, 3 Department of Medical Biometry and Epidemiology, University Medical Centre, Hamburg-Eppendorf, Germany, 4 Centre for Integrative Medicine, University of Maryland School of Medicine, Baltimore, Maryland, United States of America

Abstract

Background: One in five children visiting a homeopathic physician suffers from atopic eczema.

Objectives: We aimed to examine the long-term effectiveness, safety and costs of homoeopathic vs. conventional treatment in usual medical care of children with atopic eczema.

Methods: In this prospective multi-centre comparative observational non-randomized rater-blinded study, 135 children (48 homoeopathy, 87 conventional) with mild to moderate atopic eczema were included by their respective physicians. Depending on the specialisation of the physician, the primary treatment was either standard conventional treatment or individualized homeopathy as delivered in routine medical care. The main outcome was the SCORAD (SCORing Atopic Dermatitis) at 36 months by a blinded rater. Further outcomes included quality of life, conventional medicine consumption, safety and disease related costs at six, 12 and 36 months after baseline. A multilevel ANCOVA was used, with physician as random effect and the following fixed effects: age, gender, baseline value, severity score, social class and parents' expectation.

Results: The adjusted mean SCORAD showed no significant differences between the groups at 36 months (13.7 95% CI [7.9–19.5] vs. 14.9 [10.4–19.4], p = 0.741). The SCORAD response rates at 36 months were similar in both groups (33% response: homoeopathic 63.9% vs. conventional 64.5%, p = 0.94; 50% response: 52.0% vs. 52.3%, p = 0.974). Total costs were higher in the homoeopathic versus the conventional group (months 31–36 200.54 Euro [132.33–268.76] vs. 68.86 Euro [9.13–128.58], p = 0.005).

Conclusions: Taking patient preferences into account, while being unable to rule out residual confounding, in this long-term observational study, the effects of homoeopathic treatment were not superior to conventional treatment for children with mild to moderate atopic eczema, but involved higher costs.

Editor: Monica da Silva Nunes, Universidade Federal do Acre (Federal University of Acre), Brazil

Funding: Funding source: Robert Bosch Foundation (grant number 12.5.1060.0083.1). The funders had no role in study design, data collection and analysis, decision to publish, or preparation of the manuscript.

Competing Interests: The authors have declared that no competing interests exist.

* E-mail: stephanie.roll@charite.de

Introduction

Comparative Effectiveness Research (CER) is a growing field in health care research; it has considerable potential to inform stakeholders on decision-making. Different definitions for CER have been published. In this paper we use the working definition as established by the Institute of Medicine (IOM) Committee, which defines CER as "the generation and synthesis of evidence that compares the benefits and harms of alternative methods to prevent, diagnose, treat, and monitor a clinical condition or to improve the delivery of care". The purpose of CER is to assist consumers, clinicians, purchasers, and policy makers to make informed decisions that will improve health care at both the individual and population levels [1]. CER is especially valuable for disorders that are most common and most costly to society, have the highest morbidity rates and have a great degree of variation in the treatment of the disorder [2].

Atopic eczema is a chronic inflammatory skin disease associated with pruritus, which occurs predominantly in children [3,4]. Atopic eczema, as well as other atopic diseases, has become even more prevalent in Western industrialized countries in recent years, affecting around 7 to 8% children aged 6 to 7 and 13 to 14 with current eczema symptoms, and up to 22 to 25% worldwide [4]. The nationwide population-based German Health Interview and Examination Survey for Children and Adolescents (KIGGS) found a life-time prevalence of 13% and a point prevalence of 7% for atopic eczema in children and adolescents [5].

Atopic eczema can impose great burden on both the child's and their parents' overall wellbeing and has relevant economic impact on both the individual and to society [6,7] with estimated annual costs of 1.1 to 3.6 Billion Euro [8,9] in Germany alone.

Complementary medicine is increasingly asked for in the treatment of atopic eczema, as well as other allergic conditions [10–12]. Homoeopathy, for example, is widely used in Germany for treating atopic eczema, although official guidelines do not recommend it. Data from a cohort study showed that one in five children who sought a homoeopathic medical doctor suffer from atopic eczema [13]. However, very little data on the efficacy or effectiveness of homoeopathy for eczema is available. A meta-analysis on homeopathy included nine dermatological studies, none of which looked specifically at atopic eczema [14]. A small randomized, placebo-controlled trial could not show a superior effect of individualized homeopathic treatment over placebo [15]. In addition, most trials focus on the short-term effects, however this yields little insight into the longer treatment options for this chronic condition.

A comparative effectiveness research study (ADEV study) was performed to examine the effectiveness, safety and cost of homoeopathic vs. conventional treatment in usual care of children with atopic eczema taking patient preferences into account [16].

Children were included and followed between January 2005 and October 2009. The primary endpoint of the study was a symptom score after six months (SCORAD; SCORing-Atopic-Dermatitis). Those results (including a follow-up after 12-months) have already been published [16]. After six and 12 months homoeopathic treatment was not superior to conventional treatment and higher costs were observed in the homoeopathic compared to the conventional group.

Information on the long-term effects is of great interest, especially for chronic conditions. Thus, the aim of the present analysis was to describe the effectiveness and the costs involved in the long-term follow-up after 36 months.

Materials and Methods

Study Design and Participants

Children were recruited from January 2005 to June 2006 in Berlin, Germany for this non-randomized prospective multicentre open comparative observational study. Data was collected up until October 2009 for the long-term follow-up, allowing a total observation period of 36 months per patient. Children and their parents were recruited at either homoeopathic or conventional doctors' practices and had already made their own choice of therapy. Thus, the parents' preference towards treatment of atopic eczema generated the groups to be compared. The recruitment of homoeopathic doctors was through the association of homoeopathic doctors in Berlin, while doctors for conventional treatment (paediatricians or dermatologists) were chosen from address lists or by recommendation. Further methods of this study have been described in detail previously [16]. Inclusion and exclusion criteria, intervention details and outcome measures are summarized in Fig. 1. The study was compliant with Good Epidemiological Practice (GEP) and applicable data-protection laws. Oral and written informed consent was obtained from the parent accompanying the child after verbal information about the study was provided by the physician. The signed consent form was sent to the central study center, and a copy was kept at the physician's office. The study and the consent procedure were approved by the Ethics Committee of the Charité-Universitätsmedizin Berlin, Germany.

Study Procedures

At baseline, a conventional case history, screening and recruitment took place at the physicians' practice before the patients were enrolled in the study. Patients were then asked to complete a questionnaire on socio-demographic characteristics, outcome measures, and adverse events. The main outcome was the SCORAD (SCORing-Atopic-Dermatitis) score, which includes the rating of the extent and intensity of AD, as well as subjective items on pruritus and sleeplessness. To reduce bias, the SCORAD was centrally assessed by two specially trained staff members who were blinded of the treatment group. Patients were asked to respect the blinding of the rater. Each patient was assigned to one rater only for the whole study period to ensure intra-rater stability. After the central rating had taken place, patients could visit their respective physician and start with either the homoeopathic case history taking and the subsequent individualised treatment or the conventional treatment. The children's physicians documented the treatment over a 12 months period. To reflect usual care, patients visited their physician whenever needed. At each visit, data was obtained by filling out questionnaires and ratings. For the final three-year follow-up, all patients that had attended at least one of the prior follow-up visits (at six or 12 months) were invited. After 36 months no follow-up data was retrieved from the physicians.

Economic Analysis

The cost-comparison analysis was made from a societal perspective and was performed from a diagnosis specific view (only costs with direct relation to atopic eczema were considered). We summarized costs for 12 months before study onset (months −12 to months 0), and for the following 6 month periods after study onset: 1–6 months, 7–12 months and 31–36 months, where available. Data on resource consumption such as hospital stays, use of medication and days on sick leave were obtained from the patient questionnaires and diaries. Costs of days spent in hospitals were based on the appropriate dermatological German DRGs. The cost of medication was based on consumed units and package prices. If this data was not available, daily defined dosage [17] was multiplied by the number of days of intake. Outpatient visits were valued by multiplying the number of visits and the mean contact-costs depending on the physician's profession (data provided by the Association of German Statutory Health Insurance Physicians). For the follow-up between months 31 and 36, the costs were discounted by 3% per year. For the first 12 months of the study, the costs incurred due to visits to the ADEV-study physician were directly extracted from the doctors' documentation. For the long-term follow-up for the months 31 to 36, no physicians' documentation was available. The mean cost values from the respective treatment group at months 7–12 were used for those patients who documented that they still visited their study physician. As a post-hoc sensitivity analysis we calculated the costs for these visits in months 31 to 36 for the treatment group to be 40% of the costs at months 7–12, as there is evidence for a reduction in costs in homoeopathic treatments over time [18].The cost for patients who had no further contact with their ADEV-study physician was valued at 0€.

Indirect costs were calculated by adopting the human capital approach. In cases of disease-related absence from work, the indirect costs were measured according to the parents' income level.

Inclusion criteria
- children (aged 1-14 years) with atopic eczema
- disease duration at least 6 months
- fulfilling 3 out of 4 Williams' criteria [30, 31]
- Three Item Severity (TIS) Score: 2-7 (mild/moderate symptoms [32])

Exclusion criteria
- other dermal disease, or severe medical or psychological disease
- oral or intravenous corticosteroids during the last 3 months
- psychotherapy, allergy desensitization, or additional complementary therapy during the last 3 months

Treatments

Homoeopathic group
- classical homoeopathy defined as a homoeopathic case history taking and a prescription of a single remedy according to the simile law
- emollient creams were recommended
- corticosteroids were reserved for rescue medication only

Conventional group
- routine treatment according to German guidelines

Outcomes

Main outcome
- SCORAD (SCORing Atopic Dermatitis; evaluated outcome measure for atopic eczema [33-35])

Other outcomes
- self-rated skin condition, pruritus, sleep disturbance, general well being (by visual analogue scale (VAS) from 0 to 100)
- parents' quality of life [36, 37]
- childrens' quality of life (CDLQI: Children Dermatology Life Quality Index; validated for age 3 to 16) [38]
- use of conventional medicine
- response rates
- safety measures
- disease related costs

Figure 1. Description of inclusion and exclusion criteria, treatments and outcome measures.

Statistics

Statistical analyses were based on the intention-to-treat (ITT) principle, including all patients with baseline values who received treatment and with assessed outcome using multilevel models (analysis of covariance (ANCOVA) or generalized estimating equations (GEE)). In these models, physicians were considered random effect and fixed effects were: baseline value (continuous), Three item severity (TIS) Score (continuous), social class (high, average, low), parents' expectation of a good outcome (high, low), children's age (continuous) and gender (male/female). Results are presented as adjusted mean or proportion with a standard error (SE) and/or 95% confidence interval (CI). All tests were exploratory and two-sided with a level of significance of 5%. Adverse events and intake of corticosteroids of different potency groups [19] were analyzed descriptively by frequencies, percentages and by Chi-squared or Fisher's exact test (if feasible). As a sensitivity analysis, analysis was additionally performed with replacing missing outcome data by the last observation carried forward (LOCF) method.

As a post-hoc analysis on a subset of patients with SCORAD data available for all time points, a repeated measures ANCOVA for differences to baseline of SCORAD values was used to test if changes over time were different for the two groups (time by group effect).

The nonparametric bootstrapping method was used to generate a picture of variability around the arithmetic mean for the cost-effectiveness analyses. The original sample was bootstrapped 1000 times in order to obtain 1000 means for costs and effect differences. Each bootstrap sample was adjusted for confounding variables as previously described.

For detailed description and sample size calculation, see the previously published article [16]. Statistical analyses were performed according to a predefined statistical analysis plan using PASW Statistics 18.0 (SPSS Chicago, IL) and SAS for Windows, version 9.2 (SAS Institute, Cary, NC, USA).

Results

Population

135 children were included into the study and analyzed in the primary analysis after 6 months (mean age 4.01 ± 2.97 (SD), 48% girls, conventional group n = 87, homoeopathic group n = 48, Table 1). Children were recruited by 26 physicians experienced in the treatment of atopic eczema in children (10 homoeopaths and 16 conventional doctors). For details on the doctors'

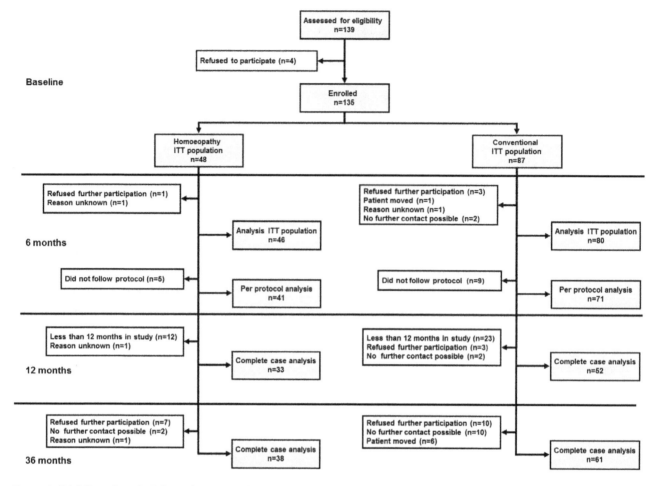

Figure 2. Trial flow chart (ITT: intention to treat).

specialisations please see the previously published article [16]. After 36 months, data from 99 participants (38 in the homeopathic and 61 in the conventional group) were available (Fig. 2). Reasons for missing follow-up data included refusal of further participation, relocation, or not contactable.

Patient preferences resulted in the following baseline differences: patients in the homeopathic group showed more severe SCORAD scores and a trend to a longer symptom duration, while the TIS score was higher in the conventional group. On average, the parents of the homoeopathic group were older, had a higher income level and were better educated, i.e. had a higher social status than the parents of the conventional group (Table 1). In addition, higher baseline costs in the homeopathic group were seen. These differences in baseline characteristics were similar for the patients who were still available to be assessed at 36 months.

Outcome Parameters

After 36 months the primary outcome parameter SCORAD showed no significant differences between groups: homeopathy group 13.68±2.91 (adjusted mean±SE) 95% CI [7.88–19.48] vs. conventional group 14.90±2.25 [10.41–19.40], p = 0.741) (Table 2, Fig. 3). When replacing missing SCORAD values at 36 months by LOCF as a sensitivity analysis, results remained similar (homeopathy group 13.29±2.51 [8.30–18.28] vs. conventional group 15.24±1.92 [11.43–19.05], p = 0.541). Neither the

SCORAD at six or 12 months [29] nor the SCORAD subscales showed significant differences (Table 2; and Witt et.al [16]).

No significant overall group effect was found between homoeopathy and conventional treatment in the repeated measures analysis when analyzing SCORAD differences to baseline for the subset of patients with SCORAD data available for all time points (p = 0.908). However, SCORAD values in general decreased significantly over time (p<0.001). This change in time seemed different for the two groups with a faster improvement in the conventional treatment group at 6 months, and a catching up of the homoeopathy group after 12 months (p = 0.055, Fig. 4).

No significant differences could be observed at any time point for adjusted response rates based on SCORAD values. At 36 months a 33% response (defined as an improvement of at least 33% in the SCORAD) of 63.9% was seen in the homoeopathic and 64.5% in the conventional group (p = 0.949). A 50% response was seen at 36 months in 52.0% of patients in the homoeopathic and 52.3% of patients in the conventional group (p = 0.974).

At 36 months the quality of life of the children and parents was similar in both groups in the short and long-term (Table 2).

Conventional Treatment

At 36 months the frequency of daily basic skin care was reduced compared to baseline, and comparable in both groups, as was the number of different medications (including corticosteroids and antihistamines) according to the patients' documentation (Table 2).

Table 1. Baseline characteristics of study participants.

	Homoeopathy			Conventional			
	n	mean±SD or n (%)	Median	n	mean±SD or n (%)	Median	P-value
PATIENTS							
Age (years)	48	4.3±2.9	4.0	87	3.9±3.0	3.0	0.300
Gender female	48	26 (54.2%)		87	39 (44.8%)		0.369
Siblings	47	1.1±1.0	1.0	84	1.0±1.2	1.0	0.530
Symptom duration (years)	48	3.5±2.6	3.0	86	2.9±2.7	2.0	0.057
Treatment duration (years)	46	3.0±2.7	2.0	83	2.7±2.9	1.0	0.364
Additional atopic disease							
Allergic rhinitis	47	4 (8.5%)		84	8 (9.5%)		1.000
Allergic asthma	47	2 (4.3%)		84	8 (9.5%)		0.330
Food allergy	47	10 (21.3%)		84	10 (11.9%)		0.205
Other	47	6 (12.8%)		84	8 (9.5%)		0.568
Allergy test	48	21 (43.8%)		87	36 (41.4%)		0.856
Allergen positive	19	11 (57.9%)		30	14 (46.7%)		0.561
Three item severity score (TIS) (0–9)[a]	48	3.8±1.6	3.0	87	4.5±1.5	4.0	0.010
Therapy for AE during previous 12 months							
Basic skin care	47	40 (85.1%)		84	73 (86.9%)		0.795
Avoidance of certain food	47	25 (53.2%)		84	33 (39.3%)		0.144
Alternative therapies	47	19 (40.4%)		84	3 (3.6%)		<0.001
Drug therapy	47	42 (89.4%)		84	71 (84.5%)		0.598
Number of different medications	47	2.2±1.7	2.0	84	2.3±1.9	2.0	0.852
Corticosteroids	47	12 (25.5%)		84	40 (47.6%)		0.016
Topical calcineurin inhibitors	47	18 (38.3%)		84	26 (31.0%)		0.443
Antihistamines	47	9 (19.1%)		84	18 (21.4%)		0.825
SCORAD Total score[b]	48	31.3±14.1	30.9	87	22.8±13.4	19.9	0.001
SCORAD Extent	48	18.7±19.4	13.3	87	12.9±16.0	7.0	0.066
SCORAD Intensity	48	6.1±2.7	6.5	87	4.1±2.6	3.0	<0.001
SCORAD Subjective symptoms	48	6.1±4.6	5.0	87	5.9±5.0	5.0	0.856
Children's QoL CDLQI[c]	28	3.8±2.6	3.5	49	4.8±3.6	4.0	0.189
ACCOMPANYING PARENT							
Age (years)	47	36.7±6.1	36.0	84	32.7±6.3	32.5	<0.001
Gender female	47	41 (87.2%)		84	76 (90.5%)		0.568
Single parent	47	7 (14.9%)		84	21 (25.0%)		0.192
Education	47			84			<0.001
A-level		31 (66.0%)			22 (26.2%)		
University, College		20 (42.6%)			13 (15.5%)		
Net income per month	38			61			<0.001
<2000 Euro		16 (42.1%)			41 (67.2%)		
2000–4000 Euro		18 (47.4%)			20 (32.8%)		
>4000 Euro		4 (10.5%)			0 (0.0%)		
Social class	47			84			<0.001
Low		2 (4.3%)			29 (34.5%)		
Middle		17 (36.2%)			34 (40.5%)		
High		28 (59.6%)			21 (25.0%)		
Parents' QoL[d]							
Psychosomatic wellbeing	47	65.0±20.9	69.4	84	64.4±21.3	69.4	0.890
Effects on social life	47	87.2±16.7	91.7	84	84.6±15.4	87.5	0.384
Confidence in medical treatment	45	62.8±21.6	60.0	84	67.4±18.1	65.0	0.195

Table 1. Cont.

Emotional coping	47	72.9±19.3	75.0	84	71.7±21.5	75.0	0.762
Acceptance of the disease	46	70.4±22.1	75.0	84	68.6±24.4	75.0	0.682
Expected symptom improvement (0–6)[e]	46	4.4±1.2	4.0	83	3.8±1.2	4.0	0.013
Costs during 12 months before study [in EURO]		mean±SD	95% CI		mean±SD	95% CI	
Medication	48	119.5±146.5	77.0;162.1	87	109.6±150.7	77.5;141.7	0.493
Hospital	48	22.6±156.2	−22.8;67.9	87	12.4±81.6	−5.0;29.8	0.950
Physician contact	48	86.6±68.0	66.9;106.4	87	102.3±95.0	82.1;122.6	0.190
Medical aids and adjuvant therapies	48	254.6±563.2	91.0;418.1	87	113.5±264.2	57.1;169.8	0.032
Indirect costs	48	134.0±460.9	0.2;267.9	87	32.2±105.1	9.8;54.5	0.527
Total	48	617.3±841.2	373.0;861.6	87	370.0±380.8	288.8;451.1	0.164

[a]high score = high intensity;
[b]<25 mild, 25–50 moderate, >50 severe disease;
[c]high score = low QoL (only children of age 3 to 16 could be questioned, because CDLQI was only validated for that age group);
[d]high score = high QoL;
[e]0 = not sure, 6 = very sure;
AE: atopic eczema, QoL: quality of life, SD: standard deviation, CI: confidence interval.

One patient (2.6%) in the homoeopathic group and one patient (1.6%) in the conventional group took corticosteroids of the weak group (group I according [19]), while one patient (1.6%) in the in the conventional group took moderately potent corticosteroids (group II). Three patients (7.9%) in the homoeopathic and 11 patients (18.0%) in the conventional group took potent cortico-steroids (group III). Details of the homeopathic treatment within the first 12 months of the study have previously been described [16].

Subgroups

Considering only patients still treated by the study doctor they have chosen at study start at 36 months (n = 62), SCORAD values showed no differences between the groups (homeopathic 14.28±3.46, 95% CI [7.36–21.21] vs. conventional group 15.89±2.72 [10.46–21.33], p = 0.722). Similar results were found for patients no longer receiving study therapy at 36 months (n = 33) (homeopathic 12.26±4.17 [3.92–20.60] vs. conventional group 14.33±3.09 [8.16–20.50], p = 0.686). A test of interaction (effect modification) from still receiving study therapy was not significant (p = 0.937).

Adverse Events

The number of patients reporting adverse events at 36 months was similar in both groups. Two patients (5.3%) in the homoeopathy group and five (8.2%) in the conventional group reported adverse events (p = 0.704). The following eight adverse events were reported in the homoeopathy group: pruritus (n = 2),

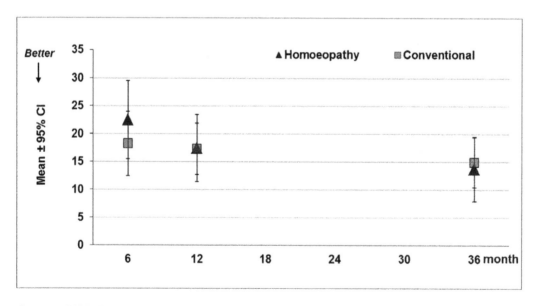

Figure 3. SCORAD at 6, 12 and 36 months, adjusted mean ±95% confidence interval (CI) per group from multilevel models (ANCOVA) with fixed effects age, gender, baseline value, TIS-score, social status, expectation of the parents, and random effect physician (lower values indicate lower disease severity).

Table 2. Intention to treat analyses of SCORAD and secondary outcomes at 36 months (adjusted means or proportions and confidence intervals (CI) from multilevel models (ANCOVA or GEE) with fixed effects age, gender, baseline value, TIS-score, social status, expectation of the parents, and random effect physician).

	Homoeopathy n = 37		Conventional n = 61		
	Mean	95% CI	Mean	95% CI	P-value
PATIENTS					
SCORAD Total score[a]	13.7	7.9–19.5	14.9	10.4–19.4	0.741
SCORAD Extent	5.0	2.1–7.8	3.4	1.1–5.8	0.406
SCORAD Intensity	3.1	1.9–4.4	3.4	2.4–4.3	0.777
SCORAD Subjective symptoms	2.0	0.8–3.2	2.3	1.4–3.3	0.682
Children's QoL CDLQI (0–30)[b]	2.2	1.4–3.4	1.8	1.2–2.8	0.627
Different medications per patient	0.7	0.4–1.4	0.7	0.5–0.9	0.904
Other physician visits	1.7	0.4–3.0	1.5	0.5–2.4	0.754
MEDICATION (31–36 months)	Proportion of patients (%)	95% CI	Proportion of patients (%)	95% CI	P-value
Corticosteroids	9.5	2.9–27.1	10.2	3.8–24.8	0.889
Topical calcineurin inhibitors	n.c.	n.c.	n.c.	n.c.	n.c.
Antihistamines	1.3	0.2–10.9	4.0	1.7–9.1	0.304
Basic skin care	66.9	53.0–78.4	61.0	50.0–70.9	0.557
Still treated by study doctor	71.7	47.6–87.6	62.9	50.1–74.0	0.5068
ACCOMPANYING PARENT	Mean	95% CI	Mean	95% CI	P-value
Parents' QoL[c]					
Psychosomatic wellbeing	82.4	76.8–88.0	77.1	73.0–81.1	0.136
Effects on social life	94.8	91.8–97.9	94.1	91.8–96.5	0.726
Confidence in medical treatment	77.7	71.1–84.3	77.5	72.7–82.4	0.959
Emotional coping	87.0	81.1–92.8	85.0	80.8–89.2	0.597
Acceptance of the disease	83.3	76.0–90.6	84.0	78.4–89.6	0.869
COSTS (31–36 months)					
Medication	36.0	7.3–64.7	36.7	14.4–59.1	0.969
Hospital	n.c.	n.c.	n.c.	n.c.	n.c.
Physician contact	119.8	95.1–144.5	45.4	27.5–63.4	<0.001
Study doctor	83.8	63.8–103.9	17.1	0.8–33.5	<0.001
Other physicians	35.1	12.8–57.5	26.6	10.3–43.0	0.546
Medical aids and adjuvant therapies	53.0	18.6–87.3	16.1	0.0–41.0	0.093
Indirect costs	9.3	0.0–22.1	1.9	0–11.7	0.369
Total costs	217.0	154.1–279.9	99.9	53.7–146.1	0.005

[a] <25: mild, 25–50: moderate, >50: severe disease.
[b] higher scores refer to lower QoL.
[c] higher scores refer to higher QoL.
SCORAD: Scoring atopic dermatitis; CDLQI: Children Dermatology Life Quality Index; QoL: quality of life; CI: confidence interval, n.c.: not computable.

burning sensation (1), reddening (1), dry skin/flaky skin (2), burns (1), herpes zoster (1); and 12 adverse events in the conventional group: pruritus (3), burning sensation (3), reddening (2), dry skin/flaky skin (3), and allergic reaction (1). The number of adverse events reported was also similar in the two groups at six and 12 months, with one child in the conventional group needing hospitalisation due of a worsening of the atopic eczema with additional streptococcal infection [16].

Economic Analyses

Economic data from the patients' questionnaires were available for 135 patients at baseline and for 98 patients for the study period from 31 to 36 months. During the 12 months before baseline costs

were 617.28 Euro 95%CI [373.02–861.55] in the homoeopathic group and 369.96 Euro [288.80–451.13] in the conventional group (p = 0.164, Table 1).

Cost-comparison analyses

Significant total cost differences were found at the long-term follow-up from 31 to 36 months after baseline (homoeopathic group: 216.99 Euro [154.12–279.87]; conventional group: 99.93 Euro [53.75–146.12], p = 0.004; Table 2). The respective physician's contacts were one of the main cost drivers (homoeopathic group: Euro 119.77 [95.06–144.49]; conventional group: Euro 45.44 [27.48–63.41], p<0.001), particularly contacts with the study doctor (homoeopathic group: 83.84 Euro [63.84–103.85];

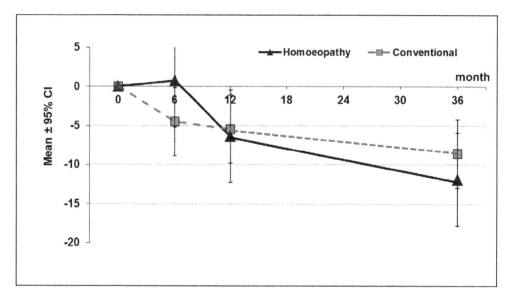

Figure 4. SCORAD differences to baseline at 6, 12, and 36 months, adjusted mean ±95% confidence interval (CI) per group from repeated measures multilevel model with time and time-by-group interaction and fixed effects age, gender, baseline value, TIS-score, social status, expectation of the parents, and random effect physician; post-hoc analysis on complete cases (patients with SCORAD data available for all time points); lower mean values indicate greater improvement.

conventional group: 17.12 Euro [0.75–33.49], p<0.001). In the sensitivity analysis the total costs were 183.17 Euro [119.65–246.69] in the homoeopathic, and 100.18 Euro [53.19–147.17] in the conventional group (p = 0.043).

Discussion

In this observational comparative effectiveness study, no significant long-term outcome differences were seen after 36 months in children with atopic eczema when treated conventionally compared to homoeopathic treatment; neither were short-term differences seen (at six or 12 months [16]). Both groups substantially improved during the observation period and in both groups every tenth patient used corticoids. Patients in the conventional groups showed a trend towards earlier improvements. Costs, however, were higher in the homoeopathic group.

The design of the study (observational, usual-care and multi-centre setting) allows evaluation of a therapy's comparative effectiveness considering the patients' own preferences and therapy choices. In our study the treatment was individualised and to reflect a more realistic care additional medication was not forbidden. Data collection was performed using a variety of sources including the affected child, their parents, study doctors and external blinded raters, to improve the objectivity and validity of the study outcomes.

The aim of this study was to reflect the real world situation and to compare conventional and homeopathic care provided by physicians in a usual care setting. Thus, we chose to take patients' and/or parents' therapy preferences into account, making randomisation not possible. The observational design resulted in relevant baseline differences between the two groups. In the homoeopathic group severity of disease appeared higher compared to the conventional group. Eczema conditions according to the SCORAD were less favourable (especially the intensity and extent of atopic eczema) and the disease duration was longer. In addition, parents in the homoeopathic group were older, had a higher social class background and a higher treatment expectation. To take baseline differences into account, we adjusted our analyses

for these factors. However, it is possible that other unknown and unmeasured factors might have influenced the results. If other confounding factors were present but not accounted for, or if the performed adjustments were not sufficient (e.g. due to broad value categories or measurement error), residual confounding might be present. If adjustments did not sufficiently balance disease severity, then results might be biased in favour of either the conventional or the homoeopathic group. Therefore, the non-randomised design is a clear limitation of our study regarding the internal validity of our results [16].

At six, 12 and 36 months SCORAD severity was comparable in both groups, although patients in the conventional group took more conventional medication in the first year, e.g. corticosteroids, antihistamines or pimecrolimus and tacrolimus [16]. Baseline use of pimecrolimus and tacrolimus was comparable in both groups, in contrast to less use of corticosteroids in the homoeopathic group than in the conventional group. While at six months, the use of these anti-inflammatory drugs was lower in the homoeopathic group, after 36 months around ten percent of patients in both groups used corticoids. Overall medication use decreased during the trial in both groups compared to baseline values. In both groups the frequency of basic skin care was comparable. However when interpreting these results, one should also take into account that atopic eczema can improve spontaneously in young children.

Although disease specific costs in both groups appear lower in the third year compared to the first year, the long-term costs were more than twice as high in the homeopathy group compared to the conventional group. Costs were mainly driven by doctors' fees and paying for medical aids. As described in the methods section, the mean costs during months 7–12 of the study were used to estimate the costs for the outpatient contact at the long-term follow-up for the main analysis. We chose this method as it also seems to be a conservative approach, in assuming that the intensity of medical contact (especially for homeopathic treatment) is much higher during the first year of treatment, and that the use of these costs for estimating follow-up expenditures might lead to an overestimation of costs. Data from another prospective observational study that included 3981 patients with different diagnoses showed that children with atopic eczema [18] visited their homeopathic doctor between month 7–12 40% more often (1.5±1,7 times) than a year later (0.9±1.2 times in months 19–24). These findings were used as the basis for a sensitivity analysis, resulting still in higher costs in the homoeopathic group.

The substantial and statistically significant cost-differences between the groups found during the first year of treatment were stable over time. The follow-up between 31 and 36 months lead to a comparable result compared to the analysis in the first year. While interpreting these differences, potential limitations should be kept in mind, particularly in regard to how the outpatient costs were estimated. Within the 31–36 months follow-up detailed therapeutic documentation was not available. However, the method of calculating the outpatient costs during the first year of the study was based on this kind of documentation.

Conclusion

In this long-term observational study after three years, while unable to rule out residual confounding but taking patient preferences into account, treatment at homoeopathic doctors was similar, yet not superior to treatment at conventional doctors for children with mild to moderate atopic eczema, but still had higher costs.

Acknowledgments

We would like to thank Beatrice Eden for her excellent performance at the study office, data collection, and rating. We also thank Angelina Bockelbrink for drafting the background section of the manuscript.

Author Contributions

Conceived and designed the experiments: CMW BB SNW. Performed the experiments: CMW BB DP DS TJ. Analyzed the data: SR TR KI KW. Wrote the paper: SR TR DP BB KW DS TJ KI SNW CMW.

References

1. Committee on Comparative Effectiveness Research Prioritization (2009) What is Comparative Effectiveness Research? In: Institute of Medicine, ed. Initial National Priorities for Comparative Effectiveness Research. Washington D.C.: The National Academies Press. 29.

2. Fineberg H (2009) Foreword. In: Institute of Medicine, ed. Initial National Priorities for Comparative Effectiveness Research. Washington D.C.: The National Academies Press.

3. Hoare DY, Wan Po AL, Williams H (2000) Systematic Review of treatment of atopic eczema. Health Technol Assess 4: 1–191.

4. Odhiambo JA, Williams HC, Clayton TO, Robertson CF, Asher MI (2009) Global variations in prevalence of eczema symptoms in children from ISAAC Phase Three. J Allergy Clin Immunol 124: 1251–1258.

5. Schlaud M, Atzpodien K, Thierfelder W (2007) Allergische Erkrankungen. Bundesgesundheitsblatt - Gesundheitsforschung - Gesundheitsschutz 50: 701–710.

6. Emerson RM, Williams HC, Allen BR (2001) What is the cost of atopic dermatitis in preschool children? Br J Dermatol 144: 514–522.

7. Herd RM (2002) The financial impact on families of children with atopic dermatitis. Arch Dermatol 138: 819–820.

8. Augustin M, Zschocke I (2001) Lebensqualität und Ökonomie bei allergischen Hauterkrankungen. Allergologie 24: 433–442.

9. Szucs T (1995) Sozioökonomische Aspekte der Neurodermitis in Deutschland. In: Riedl-Seifert R, ed. Expert Report zu Bufexamac. München: 49–66.

10. Anderson P, Dinulos JG (2009) Atopic dermatitis and alternative management strategies. Current Opinion in Pediatrics 21: 131–138.

11. Keil T, Witt CM, Roll S, Vance W, Weber K, et al. (2008) Homoeopathic versus conventional treatment of children with eczema: a comparative cohort study. Complement Ther Med 16: 15–21.

12. Schäfer T, Riehle A, Wichmann HE, Ring J (2002) Alternative medicine in allergies - prevalence, patterns of use, and costs. Allergy 57: 694–700.

13. Becker-Witt C, Lüdtke R, Weisshuhn TE, Willich SN (2004) Diagnoses and treatment in homeopathic medical practice. Forsch Komplementärmed Klass Naturheilkd 11: 98–103.

14. Linde K, Clausius N, Ramirez G, Melchart D, Eitel F, et al. (1997) Are the clinical effects of homeopathy placebo effects? A meta-analysis of placebo-controlled trials. Lancet 350: 834–843.

15. Siebenwirth J, Lüdtke R, Remy W, Rakoski J, Borelli S, et al. (2009) Wirksamkeit einer klassisch-homöopathischen Therapie bei atopischem Ekzem. Forsch Komplementärmed Klass Naturheilkd 16: 315–323.

16. Witt CM, Brinkhaus B, Pach D, Reinhold T, Wruck K, et al. (2009) Homoeopathic versus Conventional Therapy for Atopic Eczema in Children: Medical and Economic Results. Dermatology 219: 329–340.

17. Schwabe U, Paffrath D (2007) Arzneiverordnungsreport 2007 - Aktuelle Daten, Kosten, Trends und Kommentare. Heidelberg: Springer.

18. Witt CM, Lüdtke R, Willich SN (2009) Homeopathic treatment of children with atopic eczema: a prospcective observational study with 2 years follow-up. Acta Derm Venereol 89: 182–183.

19. WHO Collaborating Centre for Drug Statistics Methodology. Available from: www.whocc.no/atc_ddd_index/?code=D07A. Accessed at 16-7-22012.

20

Genetic Variation in the Epidermal Transglutaminase Genes Is Not Associated with Atopic Dermatitis

Agne Lidén[1,9], **Mårten C. G. Winge**[1,2*,9], **Annika Sääf**[1], **Ingrid Kockum**[3], **Elisabeth Ekelund**[1], **Elke Rodriguez**[4], **Regina Fölster-Holst**[4], **Andre Franke**[5], **Thomas Illig**[6,7], **Maria Tengvall-Linder**[8], **Hansjörg Baurecht**[4], **Stephan Weidinger**[4], **Carl-Fredrik Wahlgren**[2], **Magnus Nordenskjöld**[1], **Maria Bradley**[1,2]

1 Department of Molecular Medicine and Surgery, Karolinska Institutet, Stockholm, Sweden, **2** Dermatology Unit, Department of Medicine Solna, Karolinska University Hospital, Stockholm, Sweden, **3** Department of Clinical Neurosciences, Karolinska Institutet, Stockholm, Sweden, **4** Department of Dermatology, University of Kiel, Kiel, Germany, **5** Institute of Clinical Molecular Biology, Christian- Albrechts-Universität zu Kiel, Kiel, Germany, **6** Research Unit of Molecular Epidemiology, Helmholtz Zentrum München, German Research Center for Environmental Health, Neuherberg, Germany, **7** Hannover Unified Biobank, Hannover Medical School, Hannover, Germany, **8** Clinical Immunology and Allergy, Department of Medicine Solna, Karolinska Institutet, Stockholm, Sweden

Abstract

Background: Atopic dermatitis (AD) is a common chronic inflammatory skin disorder where epidermal barrier dysfunction is a major factor in the pathogenesis. The identification of AD susceptibility genes related to barrier dysfunction is therefore of importance. The epidermal transglutaminases (*TGM1, TGM3* and *TGM5*) encodes essential cross-linking enzymes in the epidermis.

Objective: To determine whether genetic variability in the epidermal transglutaminases contributes to AD susceptibility.

Methods: Forty-seven single nucleotide polymorphisms (SNPs) in the *TGM1, TGM3* and *TGM5* gene region were tested for genetic association with AD, independently and in relation to *FLG* genotype, using a pedigree disequilibrium test (PDT) in a Swedish material consisting of 1753 individuals from 539 families. In addition, a German case-control material, consisting of 533 AD cases and 1996 controls, was used for *in silico* analysis of the epidermal *TGM* regions. Gene expression of the *TGM1, TGM3* and *TGM5* gene was investigated by relative quantification with Real Time PCR (qRT-PCR). Immunohistochemical (IHC) analysis was performed to detect TG1, TG3 and TG5 protein expression in the skin of patients and healthy controls.

Results: PDT analysis identified a significant association between the *TGM1* SNP rs941505 and AD with allergen-specific IgE in the Swedish AD family material. However, the association was not replicated in the German case-control material. No significant association was detected for analyzed SNPs in relation to *FLG* genotype. TG1, TG3 and TG5 protein expression was detected in AD skin and a significantly increased *TGM3* mRNA expression was observed in lesional skin by qRT-PCR.

Conclusion: Although *TGM1* and *TGM3* may be differentially expressed in AD skin, the results from the genetic analysis suggest that genetic variation in the epidermal transglutaminases is not an important factor in AD susceptibility.

Editor: Johanna M. Brandner, University Hospital Hamburg-Eppendorf, Germany

Funding: Financial assistance is acknowledged from the Welander-Finsen Foundation, the Swedish Asthma and Allergy Association, the Centre for Allergy Research (CfA) at Karolinska Institutet, the Swedish Research Council and the regional agreement on medical training and clinical research (ALF) between Stockholm County Council and Karolinska Institutet. The funders had no role in study design, data collection and analysis, decision to publish, or preparation of the manuscript.

Competing Interests: The authors have declared that no competing interests exist.

* E-mail: marten.winge@ki.se

⊙ These authors contributed equally to this work.

Introduction

Atopic dermatitis (AD, OMIM#603165) also referred to as eczema [1], is a common chronic inflammatory skin disorder which results from a complex interaction of genetic and environmental factors [2,3,4]. Epidermal barrier dysfunction is a major component in the development of AD [2], most recently highlighted by the identification of the filaggrin (*FLG*) gene as a susceptibility gene in AD [5]. Filaggrin aggregates keratin intermediate filaments in the cornified envelope and is also believed to play additional roles in the formation of a functional epidermal barrier. However, a number of genes are likely to be responsible for the barrier dysfunction seen in AD patients and the identification of these genes would improve the understanding of AD pathogenesis and provide an important basis for improved therapeutics in AD.

Transglutaminases (TGs) are Ca^{2+}-dependent enzymes that catalyze the formation of Nε-(γ-glutamyl) lysine bonds between proteins and the covalent incorporation of biogenic polyamines into proteins through N,N-bis(γ-glutamyl) bonds. The TGs are important in many biological processes including the formation of the epidermal skin barrier [6]. Among the nine mammalian TGs, TG1, TG3 and TG5 are expressed in the epidermis and are known to be involved in the formation of the cornified cell envelope [7]. TGs are responsible for the cross linking of several structural proteins including envoplakin, periplakin, loricrin, small proline-rich proteins and the previously mentioned filaggrin protein. TG1 are also capable of attaching and cross link lipids on the already cross linked proteins [7].

Rare mutations in TGs have been identified in severe recessive epidermal disorders, with mutations in the *TGM1* gene causing lamellar ichthyosis [8,9] and mutations in the *TGM5* gene causing the acral form of "the peeling skin syndrome" [10]. Furthermore, in a previously published cDNA microarray study we showed increased expression of the *TGM1* and *TGM3* transcripts in the skin of AD patients sensitized to skin-colonizing yeast *Malassezia sympodialis (Mal s)* [11].

Although TGs are key players in forming the cornified envelope, and are linked to epidermal disorders, and map in genomic regions (14q12, 20p13 and 15q15) previously linked to AD and associated phenotypes [12,13,14], a more detailed study investigating a potential role in AD pathogenesis has to our knowledge not been performed. We therefore decided to test whether genetic variation at the *TGM1*, *TGM3* and *TGM5* gene loci might be associated with AD susceptibility and to study the expression of these genes in the skin of AD patients and healthy controls.

Materials and Methods

Genetic association analysis in the Swedish family material

The material consisted of 1753 individuals from 539 nuclear families with at least two AD affected sibs in each family and has been described previously [15,16]. Families including a sibling with allergen-specific IgE was used to form a subgroup (AD[IgE+]) in the analysis (n = 404). All patients in this subgroup had raised specific IgE against single or a panel of common aero-allergens (reported as positive or negative), using Phadiatop analysis (Phadia, Uppsala, Sweden).

Genotype data for SNPs in the *TGM1*, *TGM3* and *TGM5* gene region was downloaded from the HapMap project (release #23a, NCBI build 36, dbSNP b126). Selection of SNPs was mainly done by using the Tagger feature in Haploview program [17] with a minor allele frequency of 5% as cut-off. The pair wise and 2- and 3-marker tagging option was used with an r^2 threshold of 0.8. Genotyping was performed in two sets. The first set of SNPs was selected to cover the *TGM1* locus and typed with TaqMan® SNP Genotyping Assays (Applied Biosystems, Foster City, CA, USA). The second set included additional SNPs for the *TGM1* locus, included due to the LD pattern in this region, and SNPs covering the *TGM3* and *TGM5* loci. The second set was typed on a MALDI-TOF (Matrix Assisted Laser Desorption-Ionisation-Time Of Flight) platform (Sequenom). Information regarding the Sequenom methodology is provided elsewhere [18]. Population Hardy-Weinberg equilibrium was evaluated using the Haploview program and families with Mendelian errors were excluded. A complete list of SNPs, including quality assessment, is available in Table S1. In addition, association of all analyzed SNPs was compared to *FLG* genotype. Siblings in the family material were sub-grouped into either *FLG* wildtype (n = 998) or *FLG* heterozygote/compound heterozygote/homozygote (n = 277), determined by previously published genotype data for the study population for

mutations R501X and 2282del4 [19] combined with genotype data for R2447X and S3247X determined with previously described primers and PCR conditions [20].

In silico genetic association analysis in the German case-control material

SNP data from the *TGM1* region were extracted from a recently published genome-wide association study (GWAS) [21]. Variants within 100 kb up- or downstream of the candidate region were extracted and LD was investigated in the CEU population HapMap release 28 [22]. *In silico* analysis was performed for 533 AD cases (of which 335 had AD[IgE+]), recruited in Munich and Kiel, Germany, and 1996 healthy controls from the population-based KORA S4/F4 survey [23]. SNPs were filtered according to call rate>0.97, HWE deviation p>0.001 and minor allele frequency (MAF) in controls >0.05.

Gene expression and immunohistochemical analysis

For relative quantification with Real Time PCR (qRT-PCR), skin biopsies from 10 adult patients with AD and 10 healthy controls were collected and for the immunohistochemical analysis (IHC), skin biopsies from 10 adult patients with AD and 9 healthy controls were collected at the Department of Dermatology, Karolinska University Hospital Solna, Stockholm, Sweden. Punch biopsies from non-lesional AD skin and from healthy control skin were taken from the lower back region, whereas biopsies from lesional skin were taken from available areas with comparable skin thickness. Inclusion criteria for the AD patients were diagnosis according to the UK working party criteria [24]. The patients had not received treatment for the previous two months. All patients had raised specific IgE against a panel of common aero-allergens, Phadiatop analysis (Phadia, Uppsala, Sweden). The healthy controls had no clinical symptoms or history of allergy or skin diseases, had total serum IgE levels <122 kU/l, and were Phadiatop negative (<0.35 kU/l).

Biopsies were snap frozen and stored at −80°C. For IHC, six μm cryo sections were fixed in acetone, and blocked with 0.3% H_2O_2, normal goat serum (dilution 1/10) and avidin and biotin (Vector Laboratories Inc. Burlingame, CA, USA). A mouse monoclonal antibody against human TG1, dilution 1/250 (Biogenesis, Einköpngland, UK), was used for staining and a biotinylated horse-anti-mouse secondary antibody (dilution 1/400, Vector Laboratories Inc.) was used as a secondary antibody. TG3 and TG5, were detected by a goat polyclonal antibody against human TG3, dilution 1/200 (Santa Cruz, CA, USA), and a rabbit polyclonal antibody against human TG5, dilution 1/4000 (Novus, Cambridge, UK), respectively, and biotinylated horse-anti-goat and biotinylated goat-anti-rabbit (dilution 1/200, Vector Laboratories Inc.) were used as secondary antibodies. The sections were then incubated with preformed avidin-biotin-enzyme complex (ABC-ELITE reagent, Vector laboratories Inc.) and developed with 3-amino-9-ethylcarbazole (AEC) substrate. Counterstaining was made with Mayer's haematoxylin. Irrelevant mouse IgG2a was used as a control antibody. The results from the IHC analysis, including differences in staining between samples, were evaluated independently by two dermatologists (MB and CFW).

Total RNA was extracted from skin biopsies with the Trizol Reagent (Invitrogen, Carlsbad, CA, USA) and used for gene expression analysis. Total RNA quality was assessed by NanoDrop spectrophotometer and gel electrophoresis. One microgram of total RNA was used for cDNA synthesis with the SuperScript III System (Invitrogen) using random hexamers and oligo (dT) primers. qRT-PCR was performed using 18S as endogenous control, Power SYBR Green and the 7900HT Fast Real-Time

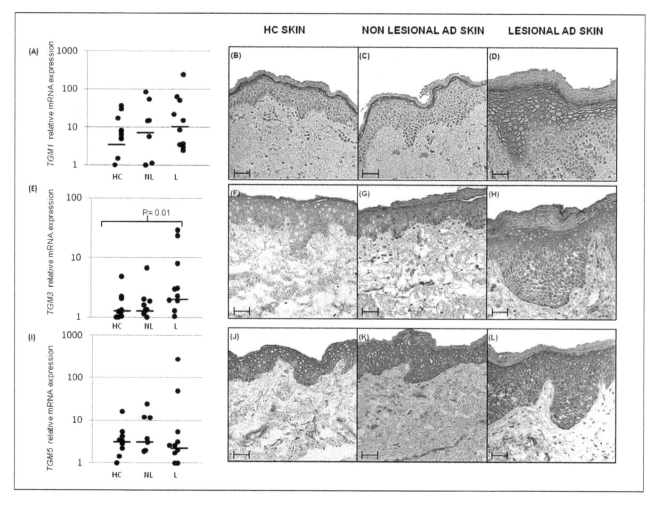

Figure 1. *TGM1*, *TGM3* and *TGM5* **gene expression in the skin of AD patients and healthy controls.** TGM transcript levels (A, E and I) of healthy controls (HC, n = 10) non lesional skin of AD patients (NL, n = 7) and lesional skin from AD patients (L, n = 10). Horizontal bars represent median values in each group and data is presented on a logaritmic scale. For IHC analysis of the TG protein expression, skin sections from nine AD patients and ten healthy controls were stained. Representative staining from one healthy control and one patient is shown in the figure for TG1 (B–D), TG3 (F–H) and TG5 (J–L) expression. Scale bar represents 50 μm.

PCR System (Applied Biosystems). Primer sequences are listed in table S2.

Statistical analysis

PDT and odds ratio (OR) estimates for the genetic association study conducted in the family material was performed using the Unphased (3.1.3) program [25]. Statistical power analysis was performed using the Genetic Power Calculator [26]. The statistical power was estimated to be above 80% for detecting a factor with an allele frequency of 0.10 and an OR of 1.5 in the family material. The case-control analysis was carried out with PLINK [27] using a chi-square test for the two by two table for each SNP [21]. For qRT-PCR analysis the Mann-Whitney U test was performed to evaluate difference in expression between the sample groups. P-values <0.05 were considered significant.

Ethics

All studies were approved by the local ethics committee, conducted according to the Declaration of Helsinki principles, and the subjects gave their written informed consent.

Results

Genetic association of the TGM1 gene in the Swedish family material

Genotyping was performed for 47 SNPs in total covering the *TGM1*, *TGM3* and *TGM5* locus (a complete list of SNPs is supplied in table S1) in a Swedish family material consisting 1753 individuals from 539 nuclear families. The success rate was above 85.5% for all genotype assays. The first set of eight SNPs selected for genotyping, with TaqMan® SNP Genotyping Assays, targeted the *TGM1* region. Analysis of the first set of *TGM1* SNPs identified one SNP in the 5′ region, rs941505, that was significantly associated with AD [IgE+], p = 0.002, showing an estimated OR of 0.60 (confidence interval (CI), 0.43–0.84) for the minor allele. Data from the HapMap CEU population indicates some level of LD between rs941505 and upstream SNPs. Additional SNPs in this region were therefore genotyped, with Sequenom methodology, in the second set of SNPs that also targeted the *TGM3* and *TGM5* region. Genotyping for the associated SNP rs941505 was also repeated with the Sequenom methodology, validating the results of TaqMan run. Analysis in RAVEN (http://www.cisreg.ca/cgi-bin/RAVEN/a) and the MAPPER database suggest that the rs941505 SNP could alter putative binding site of transcription factors overlapping this position. None of the SNPs analyzed in the *TGM3* and *TGM5* region provided p-values that would remain significant after correction for multiple testing (a complete list of p-values is presented in table S1). Similarly, no significant association remained after multiple testing of analyzed SNPs in relation to *FLG* genotype (data not shown).

In silico genetic association analysis in the German case-control material

According to data from the HapMap CEU population the *TGM1* SNP rs941505 SNP is in complete LD ($r^2 = 1$) with one SNP, rs2075530, previously analyzed in a recently published GWAS [21]. Also, the minor allele frequency for the rs2075530 SNP in the German material was the same as for the rs941505 SNP in the Swedish material ($\sim$0.095), i.e. in support of complete LD between these SNPs. However, *in silico* association analysis did not show any significant association with this SNP with AD ($p = 0.96$) or a subgroup of AD $^{IgE+}$ patients ($p = 0.80$).

Increased TGM3 mRNA levels in lesional AD skin

Expression of the *TGM1*, *TGM3 and TGM5* gene was measured by qRT-PCR and the results showed a significantly higher level of *TGM3* mRNA in lesional skin from AD patients ($n = 10$) compared to skin from healthy controls, $p = 0.01$. Further, a median increase of *TGM1* expression was noted in both non-lesional and lesional skin (Fig. 1). Four out of the seven samples, where a paired biopsy was available, showed a $\sim$2-fold increase (or more) for *TGM1* when comparing lesional to non-lesional samples. However, this trend did not reach statistical significance. Due to alternate splicing, expression of the *TGM5* gene was evaluated with two primer pairs specific for the different transcript isoforms. The results were very similar for both isoforms (data not shown) with no significant difference between the sample groups. The result for isoform 1 is presented in Figure 1.

TG1, TG3 and TG5 protein expression in AD skin

Finally, IHC analysis was used to study the expression of the TG1, TG3 and TG5 protein in lesional and non-lesional skin of AD patients and in healthy individuals. The results indicated a distinct TG1 and TG3 expression in a majority of lesional skin samples, while non-lesional skin samples appeared to have a less marked expression of these proteins compared to healthy controls (Fig. 1). Furthermore, in lesional skin, characterized by hyperplasia, TG1 and TG3 expression was found in several of the suprabasal layers, while in skin from healthy individuals the proteins was localized in the outermost granular layer of the epidermis. No apparent differences regarding TG5 expression was found.

Discussion

Epidermal barrier dysfunction is an important factor in AD pathogenesis and the identification of susceptibility genes in barrier dysfunction is therefore of major importance. The epidermal transglutaminases, *TGM1*, *TGM3* and *TGM5* encodes essential cross-linking enzymes in the epidermis and map in genomic regions that have previously been linked to AD and are therefore strong candidate genes for AD.

In this study we tested whether genetic variability at the epidermal transglutaminase loci may contribute to AD susceptibility and investigated gene expression in AD patients and healthy controls. We detected a significant genetic association for one SNP, rs941505, located upstream of the *TGM1* gene in the 14q12

region in a putative transcription binding site. The minor allele was under-transmitted to offspring with AD and allergen-specific IgE ($OR = 0.60$). To replicate our finding in an independent material, we used a German case-control material, previously used in a GWAS exploring AD in the European population [21]. Looking at the SNPs present on the arrays used in the GWAS, we conclude that the SNP rs2075530 in high LD with rs941505 were not significantly associated with AD or the subgroup with allergen-specific IgE.

Our observations from expression data indicate a marked protein expression of both TG1 and TG3 in the skin of AD patients compared to the skin of healthy controls. Also, although the increase of *TGM1* transcript levels unlike *TGM3* were non-significant, median expression was higher in both non-lesional and lesional skin compared to healthy skin. The limited sample size might explain why the levels did not reach statistical significance. Both TG1 and TG3 are thought to cooperatively cross-link proteins involved in CE formation residues at different cellular sites combining intramolecular crosslinks (*TGM3*) and formation of larger oligomers (*TGM1*) during cornification [28,29]. *TGM1* and *TGM3* are both expressed in the granular and spinous layers of the epidermis, but with more limited *TGM3* expression [30]. Interestingly, a recent study show reduced expression of *TGM3* in AD skin compared to control skin [31]. However, this study investigates protein extracted from stratum corneum, whereas our data represent semi-quantification based on all epidermal immunolocalization. It is possible that differences in expression and function vary based on epidermal localization, which cannot be excluded in our data.

An elevated *TGM1* expression would be in line with results from a previous study where we showed a significant increase in the expression of the *TGM1* mRNA and protein in the skin of AD patients sensitized to *Mal s* compared to healthy controls [11]. Furthermore, a recently published study has shown that *TGM1* and *TGM3* were up regulated in AD skin upon barrier disruption using a tape-stripping technique [32]. A disrupted barrier is evident in AD skin and may be concordant with our findings. The distinct expression observed in lesional AD skin may, at least in part, indicate that *TGM1* and *TGM3* activity may be susceptible to inflammatory mediators. This hypothesis is supported by previous data, showing that *TGM1* is susceptible to up regulation following pro-inflammatory cytokine stimulation [33]. However, it may be more likely that the observed expression patterns reflect epidermal hyper proliferation and/or a impaired differentiation process, and would be in line with the increase in TG1 that has been noted in other hyper-proliferatory disorders such as psoriasis [34].

In conclusion, although *TGM1* and *TGM3* may be differentially expressed in AD skin, the results from the genetic analysis suggest that genetic variation in the epidermal transglutaminases is not an important factor in AD susceptibility.

Supporting Information

Table S1 Genotyped SNPs. Positions are from dbSNP build 126, UCSC NCBI36/hg18. SNPs that failed quality assessment and were replaced have been omitted from the table. Please note that two SNPs, rs7151201 and rs941505, were re-typed on the Sequenom platform. Two replacement SNPs were from dbSNP with no HapMap data available (marked with N/A in the column for HapMap concordance). HWpval = Hardy-Weinberg equilibrium p-value calculated using Haploview. HapMap concordance rates were calculated by typing 40 individuals with known genotypes from the HapMap project. Furthermore, concordance rates were also evaluated by re-typing a set of 90 in house control samples (Mutation analysis facility, Karolinska Institutet). Presented are uncorrected p-values for all typed SNPs, AD = Atopic dermatitis, AD^{IgE+} = Atopic Dermatitis with allergen-specific IgE (positive in Phadiatope testing).

Acknowledgments

The authors would like to thank Sigrid Sahlén for help with sample preparation and Anna-Lena Kastman for performing immunohistochemical staining. The authors would also like to thank the participating patients and families.

Author Contributions

Conceived and designed the experiments: AL AS CFW MN MB. Performed the experiments: AL MCGW AS EE. Analyzed the data: MCGW AL AS CFW MB MN IK HB. Contributed reagents/materials/analysis tools: HB ER TI RFH AF SW MTL MCGW AS AL EE IK MB CFW. Wrote the paper: AL AS MCGW MN CFW MB.

References

1. Johansson SG, Bieber T, Dahl R, Friedmann PS, Lanier BQ, et al. (2004) Revised nomenclature for allergy for global use: Report of the Nomenclature Review Committee of the World Allergy Organization, October 2003. J Allergy Clin Immunol 113: 832–836.
2. Cork MJ, Robinson DA, Vasilopoulos Y, Ferguson A, Moustafa M, et al. (2006) New perspectives on epidermal barrier dysfunction in atopic dermatitis: Gene-environment interactions. Journal of Allergy and Clinical Immunology 118: 3–21.
3. Flohr C, Pascoe D, Williams HC (2005) Atopic dermatitis and the 'hygiene hypothesis': too clean to be true? Br J Dermatol 152: 202–216.
4. Morar N, Willis-Owen SAG, Moffatt MF, Cookson WOCM (2006) The genetics of atopic dermatitis. Journal of Allergy and Clinical Immunology 118: 24–34.
5. Palmer CN, Irvine AD, Terron-Kwiatkowski A, Zhao Y, Liao H, et al. (2006) Common loss-of-function variants of the epidermal barrier protein filaggrin are a major predisposing factor for atopic dermatitis. Nat Genet 38: 441–446.
6. Lorand L, Graham RM (2003) Transglutaminases: crosslinking enzymes with pleiotropic functions. Nat Rev Mol Cell Biol 4: 140–156.
7. Candi E, Schmidt R, Melino G (2005) The cornified envelope: a model of cell death in the skin. Nat Rev Mol Cell Biol 6: 328–340.
8. Huber M, Rettler I, Bernasconi K, Frenk E, Lavrijsen SP, et al. (1995) Mutations of keratinocyte transglutaminase in lamellar ichthyosis. Science 267: 525–528.
9. Russell LJ, DiGiovanna JJ, Rogers GR, Steinert PM, Hashem N, et al. (1995) Mutations in the gene for transglutaminase 1 in autosomal recessive lamellar ichthyosis. Nat Genet 9: 279–283.
10. Cassidy AJ, van Steensel MA, Steijlen PM, van Geel M, van der Velden J, et al. (2005) A homozygous missense mutation in TGM5 abolishes epidermal transglutaminase 5 activity and causes acral peeling skin syndrome. Am J Hum Genet 77: 909–917.
11. Saaf AM, Tengvall-Linder M, Chang HY, Adler AS, Wahlgren CF, et al. (2008) Global expression profiling in atopic eczema reveals reciprocal expression of inflammatory and lipid genes. PLoS One 3: e4017.
12. Bradley M, Soderhall C, Luthman H, Wahlgren CF, Kockum I, et al. (2002) Susceptibility loci for atopic dermatitis on chromosomes 3, 13, 15, 17 and 18 in a Swedish population. Hum Mol Genet 11: 1539–1548.
13. Cookson WO, Ubhi B, Lawrence R, Abecasis GR, Walley AJ, et al. (2001) Genetic linkage of childhood atopic dermatitis to psoriasis susceptibility loci. Nat Genet 27: 372–373.
14. Soderhall C, Bradley M, Kockum I, Wahlgren CF, Luthman H, et al. (2001) Linkage and association to candidate regions in Swedish atopic dermatitis families. Hum Genet 109: 129–135.
15. Bradley M, Kockum I, Soderhall C, Van Hage-Hamsten M, Luthman H, et al. (2000) Characterization by phenotype of families with atopic dermatitis. Acta Derm Venereol 80: 106–110.
16. Ekelund E, Saaf A, Tengvall-Linder M, Melen E, Link J, et al. (2006) Elevated expression and genetic association links the SOCS3 gene to atopic dermatitis. Am J Hum Genet 78: 1060–1065.
17. Barrett JC, Fry B, Maller J, Daly MJ (2005) Haploview: analysis and visualization of LD and haplotype maps. Bioinformatics 21: 263–265.
18. Melen E, Bruce S, Doekes G, Kabesch M, Laitinen T, et al. (2005) Haplotypes of G protein-coupled receptor 154 are associated with childhood allergy and asthma. Am J Respir Crit Care Med 171: 1089–1095.
19. Ekelund E, Lieden A, Link J, Lee SP, D'Amato M, et al. (2008) Loss-of-function variants of the filaggrin gene are associated with atopic eczema and associated phenotypes in Swedish families. Acta Derm Venereol 88: 15–19.
20. Sandilands A, Terron-Kwiatkowski A, Hull PR, O'Regan GM, Clayton TH, et al. (2007 May) Comprehensive analysis of the gene encoding filaggrin uncovers prevalent and rare mutations in ichthyosis vulgaris and atopic eczema. Nat Genet 39: 650–654.
21. Esparza-Gordillo J, Weidinger S, Folster-Holst R, Bauerfeind A, Ruschendorf F, et al. (2009) A common variant on chromosome 11q13 is associated with atopic dermatitis. Nat Genet 41: 596–601.
22. Frazer KA, Ballinger DG, Cox DR, Hinds DA, Stuve LL, et al. (2007) A second generation human haplotype map of over 3.1 million SNPs. Nature 449: 851–861.
23. Kollerits B, Coassin S, Beckmann ND, Teumer A, Kiechl S, et al. (2009) Genetic evidence for a role of adiponutrin in the metabolism of apolipoprotein B-containing lipoproteins. Hum Mol Genet 18: 4669–4676.
24. Williams HC, Burney PG, Hay RJ, Archer CB, Shipley MJ, et al. (1994) The U.K. Working Party's Diagnostic Criteria for Atopic Dermatitis. I. Derivation of a minimum set of discriminators for atopic dermatitis. Br J Dermatol 131: 383–396.
25. Dudbridge F (2003) Pedigree disequilibrium tests for multilocus haplotypes. Genet Epidemiol 25: 115–121.
26. Purcell S, Cherny SS, Sham PC (2003) Genetic Power Calculator: design of linkage and association genetic mapping studies of complex traits. Bioinformatics 19: 149–150.
27. Purcell S, Neale B, Todd-Brown K, Thomas L, Ferreira MA, et al. (2007) PLINK: a tool set for whole-genome association and population-based linkage analyses. Am J Hum Genet 81: 559–575.
28. Eckert RL, Sturniolo MT, Broome AM, Ruse M, Rorke EA (2005) Transglutaminase function in epidermis. J Invest Dermatol 124: 481–492.
29. Hitomi K (2005) Transglutaminases in skin epidermis. Eur J Dermatol 15: 313–319.
30. Yamane A, Fukui M, Sugimura Y, Itoh M, Alea MP, et al. (2010) Identification of a preferred substrate peptide for transglutaminase 3 and detection of in situ activity in skin and hair follicles. FEBS J 277: 3564–3574.
31. Broccardo CJ, Mahaffey S, Schwarz J, Wruck L, David G, et al. (2011) Comparative proteomic profiling of patients with atopic dermatitis based on history of eczema herpeticum infection and Staphylococcus aureus colonization. J Allergy Clin Immunol 127: 186–193, 193 e181–111.
32. de Koning HD, van den Bogaard EH, Bergboer JG, Kamsteeg M, van Vlijmen-Willems IM, et al. (2012) Expression profile of cornified envelope structural proteins and keratinocyte differentiation-regulating proteins during skin barrier repair. Br J Dermatol.
33. Yano S, Banno T, Walsh R, Blumenberg M (2008) Transcriptional responses of human epidermal keratinocytes to cytokine interleukin-1. J Cell Physiol 214: 1–13.
34. de Koning HD, van den Bogaard EH, Bergboer JGM, Kamsteeg M, van Vlijmen-Willems IMJJ, et al. (2012) Expression profile of cornified envelope structural proteins and keratinocyte differentiation-regulating proteins during skin barrier repair. British Journal of Dermatology 166: 1245–1254.

21

Mapping Systematic Reviews on Atopic Eczema—An Essential Resource for Dermatology Professionals and Researchers

Masaki Futamura[1,2]*, Kim S. Thomas[1], Douglas J. C. Grindlay[3], Elizabeth J. Doney[1], Donna Torley[4], Hywel C. Williams[1]

1 Centre of Evidence Based Dermatology, University of Nottingham, King's Meadow Campus, Nottingham, United Kingdom, 2 Division of Allergy, National Center for Child Health and Development, Tokyo Japan, 3 Centre for Evidence-based Veterinary Medicine, University of Nottingham, Sutton Bonington Campus, Leicestershire, United Kingdom, 4 Alan Lyell Centre for Dermatology, Southern General Hospital Glasgow, Glasgow, United Kingdom

Abstract

Background: Many research studies have been published on atopic eczema and these are often summarised in systematic reviews (SRs). Identifying SRs can be time-consuming for health professionals, and researchers. In order to facilitate the identification of important research, we have compiled an on-line resource that includes all relevant eczema reviews published since 2000.

Methods: SRs were searched for in MEDLINE (Ovid), EMBASE (Ovid), PubMed, the Cochrane Database of Systematic Reviews, DARE and NHS Evidence. Selected SRs were assessed against the pre-defined eligibility criteria and relevant articles were grouped by treatment category for the included interventions. All identified systematic reviews are included in the Global Resource of EczemA Trials (GREAT) database (www.greatdatabase.org.uk) and key clinical messages are summarised here.

Results: A total of 128 SRs reviews were identified, including three clinical guidelines. Of these, 46 (36%) were found in the Cochrane Library. No single database contained all of the SRs found. The number of SRs published per year has increased substantially over the last thirteen years, and reviews were published in a variety of clinical journals. Of the 128 SRs, 1 (1%) was on mechanism, 37 (29%) were on epidemiology, 40 (31%) were on eczema prevention, 29 (23%) were on topical treatments, 31 (24%) were on systemic treatments, and 24 (19%) were on other treatments. All SRs included searches of MEDLINE in their search methods. One hundred six SRs (83%) searched more than one electronic database. There were no language restrictions reported in the search methods of 52 of the SRs (41%).

Conclusions: This mapping of atopic eczema reviews is a valuable resource. It will help healthcare practitioners, guideline writers, information specialists, and researchers to quickly identify relevant up-to-date evidence in the field for improving patient care.

Editor: Michel Simon, CNRS-University of Toulouse, France

Funding: MF conducted this work as part of a research sabbatical funded by the National Center for Child Health and Development. Some of the searches for systematic reviews included in this study were carried out by DG in his previous role producing Annual Evidence Updates for the National Library for Health and NHS Evidence. The GREAT Database has been developed as part of independent research commissioned by the National Institute for Health Research (NIHR) under its Programme Grants for Applied Research funding scheme (RP-PG-0407-10177). The views expressed in this publication are those of the author(s) and not necessarily those of the NHS, the NIHR or the Department of Health. This work was partially supported by NHS evidence. No other external funding was received for this study. The funders had no role in study design, data collection and analysis, decision to publish, or preparation of the manuscript.

Competing Interests: The authors have declared that no competing interests exist.

* E-mail: masaki.futamura@nottingham.ac.uk

Background

Atopic eczema (AE), also known as atopic dermatitis, is a common disease that attracts considerable research interest [1,2]. Data from published epidemiological research and clinical trials, including randomized controlled trials (RCTs), are exponentially increasing [3]. RCTs are the recognised gold standard for assessing the effectiveness of interventions [4], and these have recently been collated into an openly accessible on-line database of eczema trials, the Global Resource of EczemA Trials (GREAT) database (www.greatdatabase.org.uk) [5].

However, relying on single RCTs is hazardous [6], and systematic reviews (SRs) that collate information from individual studies to provide a more reliable form of evidence are an essential tool for healthcare practitioners.

The aim of this project was to identify and provide easy access to all atopic eczema systematic reviews in a convenient "one-stop shop" in order to facilitate the practice of evidence-based dermatology amongst healthcare practitioners, guideline writers, information specialists, and researchers. In ensuring the easy identification of all published SRs, we hope to reduce unnecessary duplication of effort, and to assist with the identification of potential areas that require an up-to-date review.

As part of the process to build a SR resource, we have been regularly reviewing all SRs on AE published since 2000 and these have been summarised as Annual Evidence Updates published each year [7–11]. A similar resource summarising SRs on acne vulgaris has been produced and maintained since 2007, and is available from the website for the Centre of Evidence Based Dermatology, University of Nottingham (www.nottingham.ac.uk/dermatology). This mapping of SRs has been used to produce clinical evidence updates in acne [12–14], and similar updates have been published for psoriasis [15,16] and skin cancer [17,18].

This paper provides an opportunity to direct healthcare practitioners and researchers to the relevant SRs on AE for different topic areas, and to highlight some of the key messages to have emerged from the last 13 years of AE research.

Methods

Search Dates

Searches were conducted for studies published from 1st January 2000 to 31st December 2012. The last search was conducted on 16th January 2013 in order to allow for the inclusion of studies published in 2012, although it is possible that some reviews published towards the end of 2012 may have been omitted if they have not been indexed yet.

Sources Searched

The following electronic databases were searched: MEDLINE (Ovid), EMBASE (Ovid), PubMed, Cochrane Database of Systematic Reviews, Database of Abstracts of Reviews of Effects (DARE) and NHS Evidence. Searches were conducted by a trained information specialist or librarian (DJCG or EJD).

Search Terms

The following search terms were used in all the databases: "eczema", "atopic dermatitis" and "neurodermatitis". The SIGN (Scottish Intercollegiate Guidelines Network) SR filters were used to identify SRs in MEDLINE and EMBASE (see Appendix S1 & S2 in Appendixes S1). The PubMed Clinical Queries SR filter was used for the PubMed search. There were no language restrictions in our searches.

Identification of SRs

An SR was defined from the Glossary of Terms in the Cochrane Collaboration as "A review of a clearly formulated question that uses systematic and explicit methods to identify, select, and critically appraise relevant research, and to collect and analyse data from the studies that are included in the review. Statistical methods (meta-analysis) may or may not be used to analyse and summarise the results of the included studies" [19].

All citations from the searches were handsearched by a single investigator (MF or DJCG) by reading titles and abstracts to identify SRs, and potential SRs, relevant to AE. The following exclusion criteria were used: 1) not relevant for the clinical topic, 2) non-review article, 3) conference abstract only, or 4) methodology unclear preventing potential replication or validation of results. Reviews that did not name the databases that had been searched or the dates of the search were also excluded. In order to be inclusive, we did not exclude SRs because they had 1) searched a single database, 2) used a single data extractor, 3) applied language restrictions, or 4) were not pre-registered. Clinical guidelines were included if a SR had been carried out and published as part of the

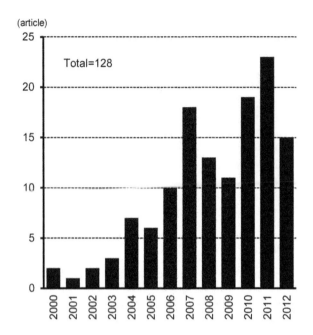

Figure 1. Numbers of published systematic reviews by year.

production process. The final decision on whether publications were to be included as a SR was made by HCW.

Mapping of Reviews

The identified SRs were sorted into six categories: mechanism, epidemiology, prevention, topical treatments, systemic treatments, and other treatments. Updated reviews were counted as a single SR if they were published in the same journal as the earlier version, and for these the latest publication date was used [20]. In the tables, citations (with links to on-line records) are given by

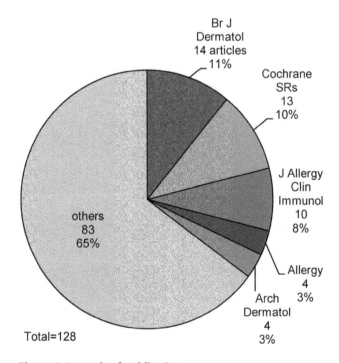

Figure 2. Journals of publication.

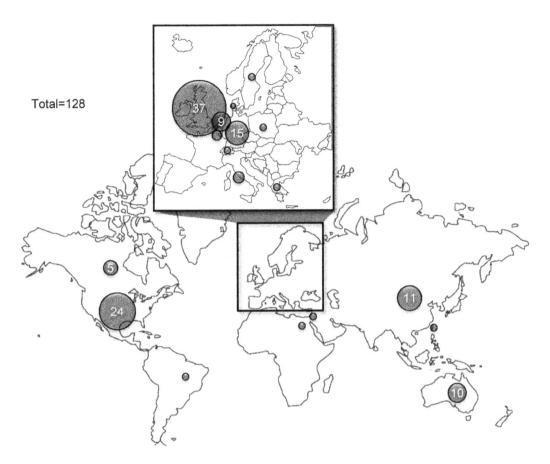

Figure 3. Geographic distribution of author's institutions.

category and topic area, and ordered according to the date of the last search. Where a SR covered more than one topic area, it was listed under all relevant topics. Details of databases used for the SR and any language restrictions applied are also listed. The country of origin for all SRs was defined as the location of the institution for the first author.

Current AE Guidelines

Current guidelines on AE were checked to confirm how many of the identified SRs had been used to inform relevant clinical guidelines. We searched for AE guidelines published since 2007 from the National Guidelines Clearing House website (http://guideline.gov/) in addition to PubMed. We selected guidelines which 1) were written in English or had references mainly written in English, 2) were published in medical journals or on a freely accessible website, and 3) were written on behalf of governmental or national organizations. For each identified guideline, the reference list was scrutinised in order to identify the number of relevant SRs that had been cited.

Value of the SR Mapping

In order to assess the potential value of this mapping of SRs in the dermatology community, we conducted an on-line survey between 19th November and 4th December 2012. This anonymous survey was open for two weeks and was performed on-line. Approach letters were sent to 480 members of the UK

Table 1. Number of systematic reviews by category.

Category	Topic (articles)
Mechanism	autoreactivity (1)
Epidemiology	aetiology/risk factor (15), disease impact/evaluation (14), prevalence/co-morbidity (12)
Prevention	dietary/supplement (28), breastfeeding (15), maternal diet (12), other prevention (4)
Topical treatments	calcineurin inhibitor (21), corticosteroid (12), emollient (7), antimicrobial (6), occlusive therapy (4), other topical (5)
Systemic treatments	dietary/supplement (20), immunotherapy/desensitisation (10), immune modulator (7), antimicrobial (6), anti-histamine/anti-allergic (5), corticosteroid (3), other systemic (4)
Other treatments	Chinese herb (10), psychological/education (9), complementary/alternative (9), phototherapy (6), clothing (6), environmental control (5)

Table 2. Evidence from recent systematic reviews.

	Epidemiology	Prevention	Treatment
2006–2007 [8]	✓ around a third of children with eczema developed asthma by 6 yrs old	? delayed introduction of solids	✓ educational support in a nurse-led clinic
	? textiles, irritants and detergents in causing eczema flares	X avoiding allergenic foods during pregnancy	✓ psychological and educational intervention
		X hydrolyzed formulae or soy formulae	✓ short term wet wraps for induction of remission in moderate/severe eczema
			✓ oral cyclosporine for induction of remission in severe eczema
			✓ UVA1 for acute eczema
			✓ narrowband UVB for chronic eczema
			? IVIG and infliximab
			X more than once daily application of TCS
			X evening primrose oil
2007–2008 [9,10]	✓ UK Working Party's diagnostic criteria are the most extensively validated	✓ probiotics in infants born to atopic parents	✓ tacrolimus more effective than weak TCS or pimecrolimus
	✓ sufficiently tested outcome measures are SCORAD, EASI and POEM	? prebiotics	✓ pimecrolimus better than plain grease
	✓ association with adverse psychological factors early in life	? breastfeeding	✓ pimecrolimus less effective than potent TCS or tacrolimus
	✓ association with FLG mutation	X keeping a furry pet early in life	? subcutaneous desensitization
	✓ decrease the risk of developing a glioma		? exclusion diets, few-food diets or elemental diets
	✓ leading family sleep loss, anxiety and depression		? anti-staphylococcus intervention for eczema
	✓ direct cost can be large		X probiotics
	X association with caesarean section		
2008–2009 [11]	✓ association with FLG mutation	X exclusive breastfeeding for more than 3 months	? dietary restrictions of certain foods
	? relationship with TGF level in breast milk	X omega-3 and omega-6 oils	? long term safety of tacrolimus
			X probiotics
2009–2010 [12]	✓ inverse relation with glioma/ALL	✓ partially hydrolysed formulas	✓ tacrolimus, pimecrolimus for children
	✓ association with ADHD	? organic foods	? bath emollients
	✓ increase risk when living in urban	? fish or fish-oil supplementation	? tacrolimus in treating pruritus
	? association with multiple sclerosis		? dry and wet occlusion
			? silk clothing
			? anti-staphylococcus intervention for eczema
2010–2011*	✓ inverse relation with meningioma	✓ probiotics with lactic acid bacteria	✓ proactive treatment for flare prevention
	✓ increase risk with antibiotics use	? prebiotics	✓ tacrolimus as effective as mild/moderate TCS
	✓ decrease risk when keeping dogs	X omega-3 oils during pregnancy	✓ tacrolimus more effective than pimecrolimus
	? association with antioxidant status		? patient education
	? increase risk with mould exposure		? coal tar
	X decrease risk with childhood vaccination		? azathioprine, Efalizumab
			? homeopathy, Chinese herb, botanical extracts
			? house dust immunotherapy
2012**	✓ increasing the prevalence in Africa, eastern Asia, western Europe and parts of northern Europe between1990 and 2010	✓ probiotics during pregnancy	✓ calicineurin inhibitor for pruritus
	✓ role of autoreactivity in driving disease exacerbation (Mechanism)	? probiotics only in infant	? immunotherapy
	? defining incident cases in prevention trials	? vitamin D during pregnancy	? omalizumab
		X avoiding allergenic foods during pregnancy	? homeopathy

Table 2. Cont.

Epidemiology	Prevention	Treatment
	X exclusive breastfeeding for more than 3 months	X dietary supplement (oils, zinc, vitamin)

ADHD, attention deficit hyperactivity disorder; ALL, acute lymphoblastic leukaemia; EASI, the Eczema Area and Severity Index; FLG, filaggrin; HDM, house dust mites; IVIG, intravenous immunoglobulin; POEM, the Patient Oriented Eczema Measure; SCORAD, SCORing Atopic Dermatitis; TCS, topical corticosteroid; TGF, transforming growth factor, * between August 2010 and December 2011, ** updated on 16th January 2013.
✓; probably effective based on systematic review evidence.
?; not clear, or limited evidence to recommendation.
X; unlikely to be effective based on systematic review evidence.

Dermatology Clinical Trial Network (UK DCTN) (http://www. ukdctn.org/) and to 140 members of the international Harmonizing Outcome Measures for Eczema (HOME) initiative (http://www.homeforeczema.org/). Participants were asked to comment on the potential uses of the map of SRs and to assess how useful the resource would be in their own work.

Results

Overall Characteristics

Our search identified 128 SRs on AE published between 2000 and 2012 (see Figure 1). None of the databases searched contained all of the 128 included SRs. Forty six (36%) were found in the Cochrane Library, 102 (80%) were found in MEDLINE, 113 (88%) were found in EMBASE, 107 (84%) from PubMed, and 53 (41%) from NHS Evidence.

Three non-English SRs (one German and four Chinese) were included. Three clinical guidelines were included as they fulfilled our inclusion criteria of being guidelines containing their own systematic reviews [21–23].

Eighty one SRs were published in the last five years alone – equating to an average of 16 SRs per year. The most common

places for SRs to be published were the *British Journal of Dermatology* (14) and the *Cochrane Database of Systematic Reviews* (13) (see Figure 2). However, SRs were published in many journals, and the five most commonly used journals accounted for less than 40% of the total number of reviews. Thirty seven (29%) of the SRs originated in the United Kingdom, while 24 (19%) came from the United States, and 15 (12%) were from Germany (see Figure 3).

Topic Areas of Systematic Reviews

The categories covered by the SRs were mechanism (1; 1%), epidemiology (37; 29%), prevention (40; 31%), topical treatments (29; 23%), systemic treatments (31; 24%), and other treatments (24; 19%). Each topic had between 1 and 24 relevant SRs (see Table 1). In recent years, there has been increasing interest in prevention (28% between 2000 and 2007, 33% between 2008 and 2012).

Quality of SRs

The number of databases search in a SR can be one indicator of quality of the review. Most of the included SRs searched more than one database (106 SRs; 83%). The most commonly searched

Table 3. Systematic reviews in guidelines on atopic dermatitis published since 2007.

Developer (Country/area)	Year	Target, Topics	Total references	Systematic Reviews (%)
NICE (UK) [22]	2007	Children	550	14 (2.5)
AAP (USA) [27]	2008	Prevention	63	5 (7.9)
AAP (USA) [28]	2008	Children	112	4 (3.6)
DSSA (South Africa) [29]	2008	Adults	168	10 (6.0)
DDG (German) [30]	2009	–	280	6 (2.1)
JDA (Japan) [31]	2009	–	66	0 (0.0)
EADV (Europe)* [32]	2010	–	135	5 (3.7)
AAAAI (USA)** [33]	2011	Immunotherapy	6[†]	1 (16.7)
JSA (Japan) [34]	2011	–	32	0 (0.0)
SIGN (UK) [23]	2011	Primary care	62	22 (35.5)
BAD (UK)*** [35]	2012	–	22	1 (4.5)
EDF (Europe)**** [36,37]	2012	–	363	7 (1.9)

AAAAI, American Academy of Allergy, Asthma and Immunology; AAP, American Academy of Pediatrics; BAD, British Association of Dermatologists; DDG, Deutschen Dermatologischen Gesellschaft [German Society of Dermatology]; DSSA, the Dermatological Society of South Africa; EADV, European Academy of Dermatology and Venereology; EDF, European Dermatology Forum; JAD, Japanese Dermatological Association; JSA, Japanese Society of Allergology; NICE, National Institute for Health and Clinical Excellence; SIGN, Scottish Intercollegiate Guidelines Network.
*also on behalf of the European Task Force on Atopic Dermatitis (ETFAD), **also on behalf of the American College of Allergy, Asthma & Immunology (ACAAI) and the Joint Council of Allergy, Asthma & Immunology (JCAAI), ***also on behalf of Royal College of General Practitioners (RCGP), ****also on behalf of EADV, ETFAD, European Federation of Allergy (EFA), European Society of Paediatric Dermatology (ESPD), and Global Allergy and Asthma European Network (GA2LEN), [†]relevant articles to atopic eczema.

database was MEDLINE (used in all SRs), followed by EMBASE (used in 78 SRs; 61%). No language restrictions were reported in 52 SRs (41%).

A meta-analysis was conducted in 71 of the SRs (56%). Five of the thirteen Cochrane SRs had been updated at least once [24–26]. None of the other SRs had been updated.

Summary of Clinical Implications from the Reviews

For the last five years, Annual Evidence Updates have been produced that summarise the recent evidence from published SRs [7–11]. The key clinical messages from these updates, and from other SRs published between August 2010 and December 2012 are briefly outlined in Table 2.

SRs in Guidelines

We reviewed 12 guideline references relevant to AE that had been published since 2007 (Table 3) [22,23,27–37]. The guidelines most likely to cite SRs were the SIGN guideline on the management of AE in primary care (22 SRs) and the NICE guideline for the management of children with AE (14 SRs). However, some guidelines cited very few or no SRs, the reasons for which are unclear.

Usefulness of the Resource

In response to an on-line survey of dermatology health care professionals, 123 participants responded (91 members of the UK DCTN and 32 non-UK DCTN members of the HOME initiative). Overall, 112 (91%) of responders felt that the ability to identify relevant SRs quickly would be useful for their work, and 110 (90%) rated the mapping of SRs as being either 'very useful' or 'somewhat useful'. General comments in response to the survey included: "This would be an invaluable source and a great asset for dermatologists" and "This is also useful for patients who can understand English".

Availability

Full links and citations to reviews relating to the treatment of eczema are included in the GREAT Database. This freely accessible database includes all RCTs of AE interventions published since 1966, and the SRs published since 2000 that are the topic of this paper. A full list of the SRs can be downloaded as a PDF file (available at http://www.nottingham.ac.uk/dermatology).

Discussion

Main Findings

For this review, we focused on one of the most prevalent and commonly researched skin diseases, and found 128 SRs published in the last thirteen years. The number of SRs published in recent years has increased significantly – more than 70% had been published since 2008. Although our eligibility criteria were broad, many articles were excluded because of unclear methodology, especially those published more than five years ago. To address the sub-optimal reporting of SRs, quality of reporting standards have been developed and published such as QUOROM (QUality Of Reporting Of Meta-analyses) in 1999 [38], and PRISMA (Preferred Reporting Items for Systematic reviews and Meta-Analyses) in 2009 [39]. Adherence to these reporting guidelines may explain the apparent increase in the number of eligible SRs included in this review in recent years.

In common with SRs of other diseases [40], the majority of SRs focused on treatments. However, prevention of AE was an increasingly frequent topic in recent years, possibly reflecting a growing research interest in public health.

SRs on AE were found in many different journals, making it difficult for health care practitioners and researchers to identify them easily. Although the Cochrane Library is a reliable source for identifying high-quality SRs [41,42], it did not contain all the relevant reviews. Similarly, MEDLINE, the most commonly searched bibliographic database [43], did not contain seven of our included reviews. It was time consuming to identify non-Cochrane SRs in the bibliographic databases, and distinguishing true systematic reviews from other clinical reviews was sometimes difficult. From this we conclude that, as when searching for clinical trials to include in a SR, multiple databases should be used to find all relevant SRs on a given topic.

It would seem that many clinical guidelines are produced without reference to relevant and up-to-date SRs. Although it is not possible to establish why this might be, it is clearly important to promote the availability of this mapping of reviews as a resource for future guideline writers in order to ensure that clinical practice is based on the best available evidence.

Strengths and Limitations

We searched six bibliographic databases. SRs were only included in this review if they fulfilled our eligibility criteria. Whilst we might have missed some SRs with non-English abstracts, we believe this review to be the most comprehensive summary of important SRs on AE in the world [44].

The importance of being able to identify relevant SRs quickly was supported by the dermatology professionals and researchers who responded to our survey, and so this resource will be maintained on an annual basis.

Conclusions

This paper describes a collection of SRs on AE which provide a unique resource that will substantially reduce the amount of time and effort spent in searching for high-quality information by healthcare practitioners, guideline writers, information specialists, and researchers. This paper also summarises the key clinical messages to have emerged from these reviews over the last decade. The resource will be continually updated in the future (available through the Centre of Evidence Based Dermatology's website and the GREAT Database), ensuring that the information remains up-to-date and relevant to the needs of the clinical community.

Supporting Information

Appendixes S1 Appendix S1. Search strategies of Ovid MEDLINE. Appendix S2. Search strategies of Ovid Embase.

Checklist S1 PRISMA checklist.

Acknowledgments

We thank Helen Nankervis, who supplied the data for the connection with the GREAT database. We also thank Dr Jonathan Batchelor, Dr Rosalind Simpson and Dr Viktoria Eleftheriadou for their helpful comments in assessing the usability of the review maps.

Author Contributions

Conceived and designed the experiments: KST HCW. Performed the experiments: MF DJCG EJD DT. Analyzed the data: MF DJCG DT. Wrote the paper: MF KST.

References

1. Hon KL, Yong V, Leung TF (2012) Research statistics in Atopic Eczema: what disease is this? Ital J Pediatr 38: 26.
2. Flohr C (2011) Atopic dermatitis diagnostic criteria and outcome measures for clinical trials: still a mess. J Invest Dermatol 131: 557–559.
3. Tsay MY, Yang YH (2005) Bibliometric analysis of the literature of randomized controlled trials. J Med Libr Assoc 93: 450–458.
4. Harbour R, Miller J (2001) A new system for grading recommendations in evidence based guidelines. BMJ 323: 334–336.
5. Nankervis H, Maplethorpe A, Williams HC (2011) Mapping randomized controlled trials of treatments for eczema–the GREAT database (the Global Resource of EczemA Trials: a collection of key data on randomized controlled trials of treatments for eczema from 2000 to 2010). BMC Dermatol 11: 10.
6. Schulz KF, Chalmers I, Hayes RJ, Altman DG (1995) Empirical evidence of bias. Dimensions of methodological quality associated with estimates of treatment effects in controlled trials. JAMA 273: 408–412.
7. Williams HC, Grindlay DJ (2008) What's new in atopic eczema? An analysis of the clinical significance of systematic reviews on atopic eczema published in 2006 and 2007. Clin Exp Dermatol 33: 685–688.
8. Williams HC, Grindlay DJ (2010) What's new in atopic eczema? An analysis of systematic reviews published in 2007 and 2008. Part 1. Definitions, causes and consequences of eczema. Clin Exp Dermatol 35: 12–15.
9. Williams HC, Grindlay DJ (2010) What's new in atopic eczema? An analysis of systematic reviews published in 2007 and 2008. Part 2. Disease prevention and treatment. Clin Exp Dermatol 35: 223–227.
10. Batchelor JM, Grindlay DJ, Williams HC (2010) What's new in atopic eczema? An analysis of systematic reviews published in 2008 and 2009. Clin Exp Dermatol 35: 823–827; quiz 827–828.
11. Shams K, Grindlay DJ, Williams HC (2011) What's new in atopic eczema? An analysis of systematic reviews published in 2009–2010. Clin Exp Dermatol 36: 573–577; quiz 577–578.
12. Ingram JR, Grindlay DJ, Williams HC (2010) Management of acne vulgaris: an evidence-based update. Clin Exp Dermatol 35: 351–354.
13. Smith EV, Grindlay DJ, Williams HC (2011) What's new in acne? An analysis of systematic reviews published in 2009–2010. Clin Exp Dermatol 36: 119–122; quiz 123.
14. Simpson RC, Grindlay DJ, Williams HC (2011) What's new in acne? An analysis of systematic reviews and clinically significant trials published in 2010–11. Clin Exp Dermatol 36: 840–843; quiz 843–844.
15. Foulkes AC, Grindlay DJ, Griffiths CE, Warren RB (2011) What's new in psoriasis? An analysis of guidelines and systematic reviews published in 2009–2010. Clin Exp Dermatol 36: 585–589; quiz 588–589.
16. Warren RB, Brown BC, Grindlay DJ, Griffiths CE (2010) What's new in psoriasis? Analysis of the clinical significance of new guidelines and systematic reviews on psoriasis published in 2008 and 2009. Clin Exp Dermatol 35: 688–691; quiz 692.
17. Macbeth AE, Grindlay DJ, Williams HC (2011) What's new in skin cancer? An analysis of guidelines and systematic reviews published in 2008–2009. Clin Exp Dermatol 36: 453–458.
18. National Institute for Health and Clinical Excellence (2011) Improving outcomes for people with skin tumours including melanoma: Evidence Update October 2011.
19. Higgins JPT, Green S, Cochrane Collaboration. (2008) Cochrane handbook for systematic reviews of interventions. Chichester, England; Hoboken, NJ: Wiley-Blackwell. xxi, 649 pp.
20. Moher D, Tsertsvadze A (2006) Systematic reviews: when is an update an update? Lancet 367: 881–883.
21. Hanifin JM, Cooper KD, Ho VC, Kang S, Krafchik BR, et al. (2004) Guidelines of care for atopic dermatitis, developed in accordance with the American Academy of Dermatology (AAD)/American Academy of Dermatology Association "Administrative Regulations for Evidence-Based Clinical Practice Guidelines". J Am Acad Dermatol 50: 391–404.
22. National Institute for Health and Clinical Excellence (2007) Atopic Eczema in Children: Management of atopic eczema in children from birth up to the age of 12 years.
23. Scottish Intercollegiate Guidelines Network (2011) Management of atopic eczema in primary care. Scottish Intercollegiate Guidelines Network.
24. Kramer MS, Kakuma R (2006) Maternal dietary antigen avoidance during pregnancy or lactation, or both, for preventing or treating atopic disease in the child. Cochrane Database Syst Rev: CD000133.
25. Osborn DA, Sinn J (2006) Soy formula for prevention of allergy and food intolerance in infants. Cochrane Database Syst Rev: CD003741.
26. Osborn DA, Sinn J (2006) Formulas containing hydrolysed protein for prevention of allergy and food intolerance in infants. Cochrane Database Syst Rev: CD003664.
27. Greer FR, Sicherer SH, Burks AW (2008) Effects of early nutritional interventions on the development of atopic disease in infants and children: the role of maternal dietary restriction, breastfeeding, timing of introduction of complementary foods, and hydrolyzed formulas. Pediatrics 121: 183–191.
28. Krakowski AC, Eichenfield LF, Dohil MA (2008) Management of atopic dermatitis in the pediatric population. Pediatrics 122: 812–824.
29. Sinclair W, Aboobaker J, Jordaan F, Modi D, Todd G (2008) Management of atopic dermatitis in adolescents and adults in South Africa. S Afr Med J 98: 303–319.
30. Werfel T, Erdmann S, Fuchs T, Henzgen M, Kleine-Tebbe J, et al. (2009) Approach to suspected food allergy in atopic dermatitis. Guideline of the Task Force on Food Allergy of the German Society of Allergology and Clinical Immunology (DGAKI) and the Medical Association of German Allergologists (ADA) and the German Society of Pediatric Allergology (GPA). J Dtsch Dermatol Ges 7: 265–271.
31. Saeki H, Furue M, Furukawa F, Hide M, Ohtsuki M, et al. (2009) Guidelines for management of atopic dermatitis. J Dermatol 36: 563–577.
32. Darsow U, Wollenberg A, Simon D, Taieb A, Werfel T, et al. (2010) ETFAD/EADV eczema task force 2009 position paper on diagnosis and treatment of atopic dermatitis. J Eur Acad Dermatol Venereol 24: 317–328.
33. Cox L, Nelson H, Lockey R, Calabria C, Chacko T, et al. (2011) Allergen immunotherapy: a practice parameter third update. J Allergy Clin Immunol 127: S1–55.
34. Katayama I, Kohno Y, Akiyama K, Ikezawa Z, Kondo N, et al. (2011) Japanese guideline for atopic dermatitis. Allergol Int 60: 205–220.
35. Baron SE, Cohen SN, Archer CB (2012) Guidance on the diagnosis and clinical management of atopic eczema. Clin Exp Dermatol 37 Suppl 1: 7–12.
36. Ring J, Alomar A, Bieber T, Deleuran M, Fink-Wagner A, et al. (2012) Guidelines for treatment of atopic eczema (atopic dermatitis) part I. J Eur Acad Dermatol Venereol 26: 1045–1060.
37. Ring J, Alomar A, Bieber T, Deleuran M, Fink-Wagner A, et al. (2012) Guidelines for treatment of atopic eczema (atopic dermatitis) Part II. J Eur Acad Dermatol Venereol 26: 1176–1193.
38. Moher D, Cook DJ, Eastwood S, Olkin I, Rennie D, et al. (1999) Improving the quality of reports of meta-analyses of randomised controlled trials: the QUOROM statement. Quality of Reporting of Meta-analyses. Lancet 354: 1896–1900.
39. Moher D, Liberati A, Tetzlaff J, Altman DG (2009) Preferred reporting items for systematic reviews and meta-analyses: the PRISMA statement. J Clin Epidemiol 62: 1006–1012.
40. Moher D, Tetzlaff J, Tricco AC, Sampson M, Altman DG (2007) Epidemiology and reporting characteristics of systematic reviews. PLoS Med 4: e78.
41. Collier A, Heilig L, Schilling L, Williams H, Dellavalle RP (2006) Cochrane Skin Group systematic reviews are more methodologically rigorous than other systematic reviews in dermatology. Br J Dermatol 155: 1230–1235.
42. Olsen O, Middleton P, Ezzo J, Gotzsche PC, Hadhazy V, et al. (2001) Quality of Cochrane reviews: assessment of sample from 1998. BMJ 323: 829–832.
43. Chiu YW, Weng YH, Lo HL, Ting HW, Hsu CC, et al. (2009) Physicians' characteristics in the usage of online database: a representative nationwide survey of regional hospitals in Taiwan. Inform Health Soc Care 34: 127–135.
44. Egger M, Zellweger-Zahner T, Schneider M, Junker C, Lengeler C, et al. (1997) Language bias in randomised controlled trials published in English and German. Lancet 350: 326–329.

22

Common *FLG* Mutation K4671X Not Associated with Atopic Dermatitis in Han Chinese in a Family Association Study

Ruhong Cheng[1]◐, Ming Li[1]◐, Hui Zhang[1], Yifeng Guo[1], Xilan Chen[1], Jianfeng Tao[1], Aifang Jiang[1], Jiecheng Gan[1], Huaishan Qi[1], Hong Yu[1], Wanqing Liao[2]*, Zhirong Yao[1]*

1 Department of Dermatology, Xinhua Hospital, Shanghai Jiaotong University School of Medicine, Shanghai, China, 2 Department of Dermatology, Changzheng Hospital, The Second Military Medical University, Shanghai, China

Abstract

Background: Filaggrin gene (*FLG*) mutations have been identified as the cause of ichthyosis vulgaris (IV) and major predisposing factors for atopic dermatitis (AD). The relationship among AD, IV and *FLG* mutations has not been clarified yet. Mutations 3321delA and K4671X, two of the most common mutations in Chinese patients, were both statistically associated with AD in case-control studies.

Materials and Methods: A group of 100 family trios (a total of 300 members with one affected AD proband and both parents) were recruited and screened for three filaggrin null mutations (3222del4, 3321delA and K4671X). The subjects' manifestations of AD and IV were assessed by two experienced dermatologists and recorded in detail. The relationship of common mutations to AD were assessed using both case-control and family-based tests of association. Filaggrin expression was measured in skin of 3 subjects with K4671X heterozygote and the normal control using quantitative real-time RT-PCR and immunohistochemistry.

Results: Of 100 probands for AD, 22 were carriers for common *FLG* mutations and only 2 of them were from 40 none-IV family trios (5.00%), consistent with that of the healthy control group (3.99%, $P>0.05$). Significant statistical associations were revealed between AD and 3321delA ($P<0.001$, odds ratio 12.28, 95% confidence interval 3.35–44.98) as well as K4671X ($P=0.002$, odds ratio 4.53, 95% confidence interval 1.77–11.60). The family-based approach revealed that 3321delA was over-transmitted to AD offspring from parents (T:U = 12:1, $P=0.003$) but failed to demonstrate transmission disequilibrium between K4671X and AD (T:U = 10:8, $P=0.815$). Moreover, compared to the normal control, filaggrin expression at both mRNA and protein levels in epidermis of subjects with K4671X^{heter} was not reduced.

Conclusions: AD patients from none-IV family trios have low probability of carrying *FLG* mutations. The present family samples confirmed the susceptibility of mutation 3321delA to AD in Han Chinese. K4671X was not a pathogenic mutation.

Editor: Michel Simon, CNRS-University of Toulouse, France

Funding: This study was funded by Science and Technology Commission of Shanghai Municipality (11jc1408400) and National Nature Science Foundation of China (81171544). The funders had no role in study design, data collection and analysis, decision to publish, or preparation of the manuscript.

Competing Interests: The authors have declared that no competing interests exist.

* E-mail: dermatology.yao@sohu.com (ZRY); Liaowanqing@sohu.com (WQL)

◐ These authors contributed equally to this work.

Introduction

Atopic dermatitis (AD) is characterized by skin dryness and chronic inflammation [1]. Ichthyosis vulgaris (IV, OMIM #146700) is the most common inherited disorder of keratinization, exhibiting palmar hyperlinearity, keratosis pilaris, and a fine scale that is prominent over the lower abdomen, arms, and legs [2,3]. Previous reports have shown that 2.5% to 37% of patients with AD have clinical evidence of IV [4]. Between 37% and 70% of patients with IV display clinical features of AD [5]. Mutations in the filaggrin gene (*FLG*), the gene encoding *profilaggrin/filaggrin*, have been identified as the underlying cause of IV and shown to predispose patients to AD [2,6]. However,

the relationship among AD, IV and *FLG* mutations has not been clarified yet.

Common *FLG* mutations in Europeans, R501X and 2282del4 in repeat 1 of exon 3, were demonstrated to be associated with AD both by case-control study and family-based analysis [7]. *FLG* null variants were also found to have strong association with AD among the Chinese. The associations of common mutations in Chinese, 3321delA and K4671X, with AD were both statistically significant in case-control studies [8,9], however, have not been evaluated in family-based association test.

Analysis of available detailed *FLG* genotype information gathered from a collection of carefully phenotyped family trios provides a useful tool to help investigate the relationship among

FLG mutations, AD, and IV as well as to reassess the association between *FLG* mutations and AD by family-based association test.

Results

Clinical Features

The clinical characteristics of the family trios were shown in Table 1. The average age of 100 AD probands was 2.87 ± 3.04 years compared with 13.90 ± 4.37 years of the 301 controls (104 girls and 197 boys without AD or IV) [9]. In 100 AD trios, there were 40 none-IV family trios(none of the AD probands and their parents were presented with the IV phenotype). The normal control was a 34-year-old man without AD or IV. Patient 1 and 2 were female parents at the age of 33 and 38. They were not presented with AD or IV. Patient 3 was a 26-year-old adult with mild AD but no IV.

Genotyping

The genotyping success rate was 100%. Analysis of Mendelian inheritance within the families revealed no significant errors. Of 100 AD probands, 22 (22%) were carriers for common *FLG* null alleles, including 20 heterozygous, 1 homozygote for 3321delA, and 1 compound heterozygote for 3321delA and K4671X. Among 200 AD parents, 31 (15.5%) were carriers for common *FLG* null alleles, 30 heterozygous along with 1 compound heterozygote for 3321delA and K4671X. Twenty-three out of 24 *FLG* null alleles carried by 22 probands were inherited from their parents. The patient with a spontaneous mutation K4671X was a 22-month-old boy with moderate AD but no IV phenotype. No homozygous for either K4671X or 3222del4 was observed in the present family cohort. (Table 2) Twelve out of 301 healthy controls were heterozygote carriers for common *FLG* mutations (1 for 3222del4, 3 for 3321delA, and 8 for K4671X).

No *FLG* mutation was found in the normal control. Patient 1, 2, and 3 were heterozygote for *FLG* mutation K4671X.(Figure1A)In addition, mutation K4671X was identified in cDNA of the skin from Patient 2 and 3.

Relationship Among AD, IV and *FLG* Mutations

Of 22 probands carrying *FLG* null alleles, 14 heterozygote carriers (7 for 3321delA and 7 for K4671X) did not exhibit the IV phenotype. But it was noted that 20 (33.33%) probands with common *FLG* mutations were from 60 families with at least one parent affected by IV whereas only 2 (5.00%) were from 40 none-IV family trios (P = 0.001, OR = 9.50, 95%CI:2.08–43.43), consistent with that of the healthy control group (3.99%, P > 0.05). (Table 3).

Relationship of Common *FLG* Mutations with AD-associated Phenotype as Well as the SCORAD

The compound genotypes for common *FLG* variants were associated with three co-existing phenotype, IV, keratosis pilaris, and palmar hyperlinearity. (Table 4) However, the compound genotypes for common *FLG* variants were not associated with the total SCORAD (46.2 ± 18.8 vs. 39.6 ± 17.7, P = 0.127) in an independent-samples T test.

Family-based Association Test

Significant statistical associations were revealed between AD and 3321delA (P<0.001, odds ratio 12.28, 95% confidence interval 3.35–44.98) as well as K4671X (P = 0.002, odds ratio 4.53, 95% confidence interval 1.77–11.60). Family-based approach revealed that 3321delA was over-transmitted to AD offspring from parents (T:U = 12:1, P = 0.003) but failed to demonstrate transmission disequilibrium between K4671X and AD (T:U = 10:8, P = 0.815) (Table 5).

Quantitative Real-time RT-PCR Analysis and Immunohistochemistry

FLG mRNA expression was not reduced in both Patient 2 and 3 in real-time RT-PCR analysis. (Figure 1 B) Immunohistochemical staining revealed that profilaggrin /filaggrin peptides were also not reduced in the epidermis of Patient 1, 2 and 3. (Figure 1C).

Table 1. Phenotype characteristics of 100 trios included in the analyses.

Clinical information	Trios(n = 100)	
	Parents(200)	Offspring(100)
Han Chinese, n* (%)	200 (100%)	100 (100%)
Male sex, n* (%)	100 (50%)	66 (66%)
Mean±SD age, y	ND	2.87±3.04
Simple atopic dermatitis, n* (%)	39 (19.5%)	87 (87%)
Isolated ichthyosis vulgaris, n* (%)	53 (26.5%)	–
atopic dermatitis + ichthyosis vulgaris, n* (%)	29 (14.5%)	13 (13%)
Keratosis pilaris, n* (%)	44 (22%)	4 (4%)
Palmar hyperlinearity, n* (%)	72 (36%)	31 (31%)
Cheilitis, n* (%)	22 (11%)	21 (21%)
Dyshidrosis, n* (%)	53 (26.5%)	8 (8%)
Mild atopic dermatitis (SCORAD,0–24points)	ND	20 (20%)
Moderate atopic dermatitis (SCORAD,25–50points)	ND	46 (46%)
Severe atopic dermatitis (SCORAD,51–103points)	ND	34 (34%)

*Number affected/total number with data available.
SCORAD, SCORing atopic dermatitis.
ND, not done.

Table 2. Frequencies of filaggrin gene null alleles in parents, offspring as well as normal controls.

Genotype	3321delA			K4671X			3222del4			Combined genotype		
	parents	offspring	control	parents	offspring	control	Parents	offspring	control	parents	offspring	control
AA	187(93.5%)	89(89%)	298(99%)	182(91%)	89(89%)	293(97.3%)	199(99.5%)	99(99%)	300(99.7%)	169(85.0%)	78(78%)	289(96%)
Aa	13(6.5%)	10(10%)	3(1.0%)	18(9%)	11(11%)	8(2.7%)	1(0.5%)	1(1%)	1(0.3%)	30(14.5%)	20(20%)	12(3.9%)
aa	0	1(1%)	0	0	0	0	0	0	0	1(0.5%)	2(2%)	0

AA, Wild-type/wild-type/wild-type *FLG* genotype for 3321delA, 3222del4, and K4671X variants;
Aa, Heterozygous genotype for 3321delA, 3222del4 or K4671X;
aa, Homozygous 3321delA, K4671X or 3222del4 genotype or compound heterozygous genotype.

Discussion

In 2006, Smith et al. succeeded in demonstrating that loss-of-function mutations encoding *FLG* cause IV in an incomplete-dominant pattern. Palmer et al. conducted a further research using the 15 families studied for the IV research and presented a new and striking theory that AD was inherited as an incomplete-dominant trait in these families with high penetrance in *FLG*-null homozygous or compound heterozygous and reduced penetrance in heterozygous [2,6,10]. Because of the incomplete dominant pattern of *FLG* gene in the pathogenesis of IV, it is conceivable that in our previous and current studies of 361 AD cases in total, 82 cases without the IV phenotype were carriers for common *FLG* mutations [11]. However, in the current study of 100 AD family trios, 40 were none-IV families, from which only 2 AD probands

were common *FLG* mutation carriers (5%). It was noted that the mutation rate of combined *FLG* mutations among these 40 probands was consistent with that of healthy control group (P>0.05). The data meant a convenient method for initial exclusion of AD patients without *FLG* mutations in clinic. In addition, *FLG* mutations were associated with palmar hyperlinearity and keratosis pilaris significantly. However, the severity of AD was not correlated with the *FLG* genotype, which has been demonstrated in our previous studies [8,9].

In the current study, we found that common *FLG* mutation 3321delA, located in repeat 2 of exon 3, was associated with AD both in the case-control and family-based studies. Therefore, the association of 3321delA with AD is further confirmed. The

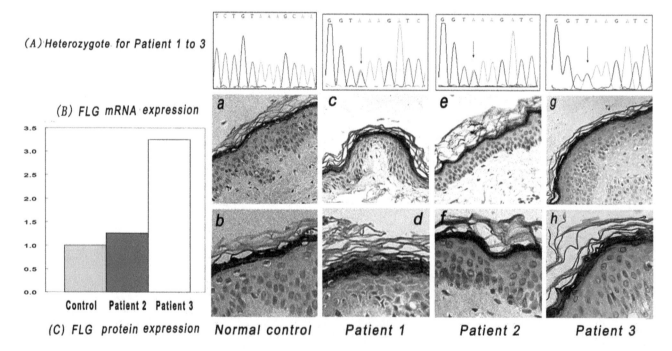

Figure 1. Filaggrin gene mutation analysis and comparison of filaggrin expression. The normal control was an *FLG*[wt] male adult. Patient 1 and 2 with K4671X[heter] variant were mothers of 2 atopic dermatitis (AD) patients. Patient 3 was an adult male AD patient with K4671X[heter] variant. Skin with normal appearance was got from the 4 subjects. (A) Identification of *FLG* mutations in 3 patients. Patient 1, 2, and 3 were all heterozygote for K4671X. (B) Quantitative Real-time reverse transcription–polymerase chain reaction analysis of *FLG* mRNA expression in the skin of normal control and 2 patients with K4671X[heter] variant. Direct sequence analysis of *FLG* cDNA from mRNA expressed in skin samples further confirmed that Patient 2 and 3 were heterozygote for K4671X. *FLG* mRNA expression was not reduced either in Patient 2 or 3: *FLG* mRNA expression in Patient 2/3: *FLG* mRNA expression in control was1.26 and 3.25, respectively. (C) Immunohistochemical staining using antifilaggrin monoclonal antibody in 4 subjects at the same time (a,c,e,g,i: Original magnification×100; b,d,f,h,j:Original magnification×200). Immunohistochemically, it was obvious that filaggrin was strongly positive in the epidermis of Patient 1, 2, and 3(c–h).

Table 3. Prevalance and comparison of compound genotype for common *FLG* mutations in various groups.

Probands and controls	Compound genotype for common *FLG* mutations			
	n(n%)	P-value	OR	95%CI
control (301)	12(3.99%)	–	–	–
All probands(100)	22(22.00%)	<0.001	6.79	3.22–14.33
Simple AD (87)	14(16.09%)	<0.001	4.62	2.05–10.41
AD with IV(13)	8(61.50%)	<0.001	38.53	10.96–135.54
AD from none-IV Family trios (40)	2(5.00%)	>0.05	–	–
AD from families with parental IV (60)	20(33.33%)	<0.001	12.04	5.47–26.49

FLG, filaggrin gene; AD, atopic dermatitis; IV, ichthyosis vulgaris.
OR: odds ratio; CI : confidence interval;

association test is not available for mutation 3222del4 as only one parent and a single proband are mutation carriers.

Unlike other mutations, such as 3321delA, R501X and 2282del4, mutation K4671X, primarily identified in the Japanese population as p.Lys4021X, is located in the C-terminal incomplete filaggrin repeat [12]. The current case-control study also demonstrated a significant association between K4671X and AD, consistent with our previous studies [8,9]. But an opposite result was produced from the family-based study. In order to further understand the effect of K4671X on skin barrier function, filaggrin expression in the skin with K4671X[heter] is required. Previous immunohistochemical staining performed by Nemoto-Hasebe I et al. on two AD patients bearing p.Lys4021X showed profilaggrin/filaggrin peptides were remarkably reduced in the patients' epidermis but real-time RT-PCR analysis revealed that mRNA expression of *FLG* was not reduced significantly [12], indicating that factors other than *FLG* mutations may lead to filaggrin deficiency in the epidermis of patients bearing mutation K4671X. Experimental evidence for such genetic and environmental modulation includes the demonstration that cytokines from Th2 cells can down-regulate filaggrin expression in AD skin [13]. To minimize factors other than *FLG* mutations on filaggrin

exression, we studied the filaggrin expression in skin with normal appearace in subjects with mutation K4671X. The results directly showed that filaggrin expression either at mRNA or protein level was not reduced in the epidemis of subjects with mutation K4671X.

Unlike mutation 3321delA, mutation K4671X could not be found in Taiwanese or Singaporean Chinese AD and IV patients [5,14]. The paradoxical results from case-control and family studies were mainly attributed to population stratification, the presence of a systematic difference in allele frequencies between subpopulations in a population possibly due to different ancestries. Family-based association test is known to be immune to population stratification because this method uses parental genotype data to control for this spurious admixture, which could not be avoided in case-control designs [15,16].

In conclusion, AD patients from none-IV family trios have low probability of carrying *FLG* mutations. The present family samples confirmed the susceptibility of mutation 3321delA to AD in Han Chinese but failed to support the same function for mutation K4671X. The filaggrin expression is influenced by multiple factors. Our investigation of filaggrin expression at both mRNA

Table 4. Analysis of associations between combined common filaggrin gene mutations and atopic dermatitis associated phenotype.

AD probands	Combined *FLG* genotype		
	AA	Aa/aa	P
AD with IV	5	8	0.001
AD without IV	73	14	
AD with Palmar hyperlinearity	16	15	<0.001
AD without Palmar hyperlinearity	61	8	
AD with Keratosis pilaris	0	4	0.002
AD without Keratosis pilaris	78	18	
AD with Dyshidrosis	7	1	0.817
AD without Dyshidrosis	71	21	
AD with Cheilitis	14	7	0.265
AD without Cheilitis	64	15	
AD with Infra-auricular and retroauricular fissuring	20	3	0.237
AD without Infra-auricular and retroauricular fissuring	58	19	

FLG, filaggrin gene; AD, atopic dermatitis; IV, ichthyosis vulgaris.

Table 5. Association analysis of filaggrin mutations with atopic dermatitis in both family and case-control studies.

Results	3321delA		K4671X		3222del4	
	Case-control	family	Case-control	family	Case-control	family
P value	<0.001	0.003	0.002	0.815	0.437	–
T:U	–	12:1	–	10:8	–	–
Odds Ratio	12.28	–	4.53	–	–	–
95% CI	3.35–44.98	–	1.77–11.60	–	–	–
n%(100 probands)	11.0%	–	11.0%	–	1.0%	–
n%(301 controls)	1.0%	–	2.7%	–	0.3%	–

P value represented as ratio of transmitted:untransmitted (T:U) filaggrin gene minor alleles;
CI : confidence interval.

and protein levels demonstrated that K4671X was not a pathogenic mutation.

Materials and Methods

Ethics Statement

The present study was approved by the Medical Ethics Committees of the Shanghai Jiaotong University School of Medicine, China. Written informed consents were given by all the adult participants and carers on the behalf of children participants before enrollment in the study. The present study was conducted in accordance with the principles of the Declaration of Helsinki.

Study Population

A total of 100 unrelated family trios with AD (a total of 300 members with one affected AD proband and both parents) who met the AD criteria of Hanifin and Rajka [17] were recruited. These patients were referred to outpatient dermatological clinics at the Department of Dermatology, Xinhua Hospital affiliated to Shanghai Jiaotong University School of Medicine, China. AD and IV of all 300 subjects were clinically diagnosed by two experienced dermatologists, who also performed a thorough clinical examination and recorded a complete medical history using a standardized questionnaire. All the 100 AD probands also received an overall AD severity grade by SCORAD [18]. The diagnosis of IV was established from clinical features of variable scaling on the extremities, dry skin, palmoplantar hyperlinearity and keratosis pilaris. The DNA samples of 300 subjects were collected. To compare the frequency of *FLG* mutations, DNA samples from 301 normal healthy, unrelated individuals without AD or IV were used as control [9]. In addition, a male adult without AD or IV was selected as the normal control. Two mothers of probands and one male AD patient with mutation K4671X were defined as Patient 1, 2 and 3, respectively. All enrolled individuals were of Chinese Han ancestry.

Skin Biopsy

Skin biopsy was got from the waist of the normal control, the lateral thigh of Patient 1, the medial upper arm of Patient 2 and the abdomen of Patient 3. The skin for biopsy was normal in appearance without any lesions. The amount of skin from the normal control, Patient 2 and 3 was enough for both quantitative real-time RT-PCR and immunohistochemistry. However, skin from Patient 1 was only prepared for immunohistochemistry.

FLG Genotyping

Genomic DNA samples were extracted from peripheral whole blood using TIANamp Blood DNA kits (TIANGEN Biotech, Beijing, China). Using genomic DNA, all the participants in family trios were screened for three *FLG* mutations (3222del4, 3321delA and K4671X) previously identified among the Chinese population[8–9] using an overlapping PCR strategy. A comprehensive sequence of *FLG* was done in the normal control, Patient 1, 2, and 3. Total RNA was extracted from skin samples of the normal control, Patient 2 and 3 using Cell culture and Animal tissue Total RNA extraction and preparation Mini Kit (SLnco, England). Direct sequence analysis of *FLG* cDNA from mRNA expressed in skin samples of Patient 2 and 3 was also performed to screen for the K4671X mutation. PCR primers and conditions were previously described by Sandilands et al. [19] The sequencing of PCR products was conducted on an Applied Biosystems 3730 DNA analyzer (ABI incorporation, Carlsbad, California, USA).

Measurement of mRNA Expression by Quantitative Real-time PCR

The mRNA levels of *FLG* gene were measured by Quantitative Real Time RT-PCR using SYBR Green Realtime PCR Master Mix (Code No:QPK-201, TOYOBO) in a FTC-3000 Real Time PCR machine(Canada, Funglyn). Primer sequences for filaggrin and glyceraldehyde-3-phosphate dehydrogenase were listed in Table 6. All primer sequences were synthesized by Gene Works (Jierui, Shanghai, China). The cycling conditions were at 94°C for 30 s, followed by 40cycles of 20 s at 94°C, 30 s at 61°C and 30 s at 72°C, and finally 1 min at 72°C. Each sample was run in triplicate. The experiments were repeated for three times.

Table 6. Primer sequences for filaggrin and glyceraldehyde-3-phosphate dehydrogenase.

Gene name	Primer sequence (5′ to3′)	Amplicon Size
h-*FLG*-F	CAAATCCTGAAGAATCCAGATGAC	126 bp
h-*FLG*-R	TGCTTGAGCCAACTTGAATACC	
h-*GAPDH*-F	TGAAGGTCGGAGTCAACGGA	225 bp
h-*GAPDH*-R	CCTGGAAGATGGTGATGGGAT	

FLG, filaggrin gene;
GAPDH, glyceraldehyde-3-phosphate dehydrogenase gene.

Immunohistochemistry

Immunohistochemistry was done using the standard ABC technique. The mouse monoclonal antibody filaggrin of Novocastra Laboratories Ltd (Newcastle upon Tyne NE12 8EW, United Kingdom) in a working dilution of 1:50 and the high temperature antigen unmasking technique were used according to the manufacturer's instructions.

Statistical Analysis

All statistics were analyzed with spss 19.0 software package (SPSS Inc., Chicago, Illinois, USA). Descriptive statistics for quantitative and qualitative values were calculated and given as means $\pm$ SD as well as relative frequencies or absolute numbers, respectively. The statistical significance of differences in genotype frequency among analyzed groups and the associations between *FLG* mutations and AD-associated phenotypes were assessed using a Pearson chi-square test, continuity correction, or Fisher's exact test as appropriate. An independent-samples T test was performed to evaluate the association between compound common *FLG* mutations and the SCORAD. The strength of association was estimated by calculating the odds ratio (OR) with a 95% confidence interval (CI). Evidence of associations with AD was evaluated using the classical TDT by McNemar test implemented in SPSS 19.0. The level of statistical significance was established at $\alpha<0.05$. Data for *FLG* mRNA expression were analyzed using the comparative CT method.

Acknowledgments

We thank all subjects for their participation in this study. We thank Prof. Long Yu for his technical support and Mianzhi Yao for critical reading of this manuscript. We also thank Bo Ling, Mei Shi, Huaguo Li, Zhiyong Lu, Ming Yan, Weiqin Yang, Chunyan Mao, Yufang Li, Beibei Zhang, Xiaojuan Pan, Yumin Sun for their support to this study.

Author Contributions

Conceived and designed the experiments: ZRY WQL RHC ML. Performed the experiments: RHC ML XLC JFT AFJ JCG HSQ HY. Analyzed the data: RHC. Contributed reagents/materials/analysis tools: HZ YFG. Wrote the paper: ZRY RHC ML.

References

1. Ching GK, Hon KL, Ng PC, Leung TF (2009) Filaggrin null mutations in childhood atopic dermatitis among the Chinese. Int J Immunogenet 36: 251–4.
2. Smith FJ, Irvine AD, Terron-Kwiatkowski A, Sandilands A, Campbell LE, et al. (2006) Loss-of-function mutations in the gene encoding filaggrin cause ichthyosis vulgaris. Nat Genet 38: 337–42.
3. Zhang X, Liu S, Chen X, Zhou B, Liu D, et al. (2010) Novel and recurrent mutations in the filaggrin gene in Chinese patients with ichthyosis vulgaris. Br J Dermatol 163: 63–9.
4. Bremmer SF, Hanifin JM, Simpson EL (2008) Clinical detection of ichthyosis vulgaris in an atopic dermatitis clinic: implications for allergic respiratory disease and prognosis. J Am Acad Dermatol 59: 72–8.
5. Chen H, Common JE, Haines RL, Balakrishnan A, Brown SJ, et al. (2011) Wide spectrum of filaggrin-null mutations in atopic dermatitis highlights differences between Singaporean Chinese and European populations. Br J Dermatol 165: 106–14.
6. Palmer CN, Irvine AD, Terron-Kwiatkowski A, Zhao Y, Liao H, et al. (2006) Common loss-of-function variants of the epidermal barrier protein filaggrin are a major predisposing factor for atopic dermatitis. Nat Genet 38: 441–6.
7. Weidinger S, Illig T, Baurecht H, Irvine AD, Rodriguez E, et al. (2006) Loss-of-function variations within the filaggrin gene predispose for atopic dermatitis with allergic sensitizations. J Allergy Clin Immunol 118: 214–9.
8. Zhang H, Guo Y, Wang W, Shi M, Chen X, et al. (2011) Mutations in the filaggrin gene in Han Chinese patients with atopic dermatitis. Allergy 66: 420–7.
9. Li M, Liu Q, Liu J, Cheng R, Zhang H, et al. (2012) Mutations analysis in filaggrin gene in northern China patients with atopic dermatitis. J Eur Acad Dermatol doi:10.1111/j.1468-3083. 2011.0443 5.x.
10. Brown SJ, Irvine AD. (2008) Atopic eczema and the filaggrin story. Semin Cutan Med Surg 27: 128–37.
11. Zhang H, Guo Y, Wang W, Yu X, Yao Z (2011) Associations of *FLG* mutations between ichthyosis vulgaris and atopic dermatitis in Han Chinese. Allergy 66: 1253–4.
12. Nemoto-Hasebe I, Akiyama M, Nomura T, Sandilands A, McLean WH, et al. (2009) *FLG* mutation p.Lys4021X in the C-terminal imperfect filaggrin repeat in Japanese patients with atopic eczema. Br J Dermatol 161: 1387–90.
13. Howell MD, Kim BE, Gao P, Grant AV, Boguniewicz M, et al. (2007) Cytokine modulation of atopic dermatitis filaggrin skin expression. J Allergy Clin Immunol 120: 150–5.
14. Hsu CK, Akiyama M, Nemoto-Hasebe I, Nomura T, Sandilands A, et al. (2009) Analysis of Taiwanese ichthyosis vulgaris families further demonstrates differences in *FLG* mutations between European and Asian populations. Br J Dermatol 161: 448–51.
15. Rogers AJ, Celedon JC, Lasky-Su JA, Weiss ST, Raby BA (2007) Filaggrin mutations confer susceptibility to atopic dermatitis but not to asthma. J Allergy Clin Immunol 120: 1332–7.
16. Horvath S, Xu X, Laird NM (2001) The family based association test method: s trategies for studying general genotype–phenotype associations. Eur J Hum Genet 9: 301–6.
17. Hanifin JM, Rajka G (1980) Diagnostic features of atopic eczema. Acta Dermatol Venereol (Stockh) 92: 44–7.
18. (1993) Severity scoring of atopic dermatitis: the SCORAD index. Consensus Report of the European Task Force on Atopic Dermatitis. Dermatology 186: 23–31.
19. Sandilands A, Terron-Kwiatkowski A, Hull PR, O'Regan GM, Clayton TH, et al. (2007) Comprehensive analysis of the gene encoding filaggrin uncovers prevalent and rare mutations in ichthyosis vulgaris and atopic eczema. Nat Genet 39: 650–4.

Permissions

The contributors of this book come from diverse backgrounds, making this book a truly international effort. This book will bring forth new frontiers with its revolutionizing research information and detailed analysis of the nascent developments around the world.

We would like to thank all the contributing authors for lending their expertise to make the book truly unique. They have played a crucial role in the development of this book. Without their invaluable contributions this book wouldn't have been possible. They have made vital efforts to compile up to date information on the varied aspects of this subject to make this book a valuable addition to the collection of many professionals and students.

This book was conceptualized with the vision of imparting up-to-date information and advanced data in this field. To ensure the same, a matchless editorial board was set up. Every individual on the board went through rigorous rounds of assessment to prove their worth. After which they invested a large part of their time researching and compiling the most relevant data for our readers.

The editorial board has been involved in producing this book since its inception. They have spent rigorous hours researching and exploring the diverse topics which have resulted in the successful publishing of this book. They have passed on their knowledge of decades through this book. To expedite this challenging task, the publisher supported the team at every step. A small team of assistant editors was also appointed to further simplify the editing procedure and attain best results for the readers.

Apart from the editorial board, the designing team has also invested a significant amount of their time in understanding the subject and creating the most relevant covers. They scrutinized every image to scout for the most suitable representation of the subject and create an appropriate cover for the book.

The publishing team has been an ardent support to the editorial, designing and production team. Their endless efforts to recruit the best for this project, has resulted in the accomplishment of this book. They are a veteran in the field of academics and their pool of knowledge is as vast as their experience in printing. Their expertise and guidance has proved useful at every step. Their uncompromising quality standards have made this book an exceptional effort. Their encouragement from time to time has been an inspiration for everyone.

The publisher and the editorial board hope that this book will prove to be a valuable piece of knowledge for researchers, students, practitioners and scholars across the globe.

List of Contributors

So-Yeon Lee
Department of Pediatrics, Hallym University College of Medicine, Anyang, Korea

Jinho Yu, Seo Ah Hong, Young-ho Jung, Eun Lee, Song-I Yang and Soo-Jong Hong
Childhood Asthma Atopy Center, Asan Medical Center, Seoul, Korea

Kang-Mo Ahn and Jung Yeon Shim
Department of Pediatrics, Sungkyunkwan University of School of Medicine, Seoul, Korea

Kyung Won Kim
Department of Pediatrics, College of Medicine, Yonsei University, Seoul, Korea

Youn Ho Shin
Department of Pediatrics, CHA University of School of Medicine, Seoul, Korea

Kyung-shin Lee, Ho-Sung Yoo and Mi-Jin Kang
The Asan Institute for Life Science, Seoul, Korea

Ju-hee Seo
Department of Pediatrics, Korea Cancer Center Hospital, Seoul, Korea

Ji-Won Kwon
Department of Pediatrics, Seoul National University Bundang Hospital, Seongnam, Korea

Byoung-Ju Kim, Hyo- Bin Kim and Woo-Kyung Kim
Department of Pediatrics, Inje University College of Medicine, Seoul, Korea

Dae Jin Song
Department of Pediatrics, Korea University Guro Hospital, Seoul, Korea

Gwang Cheon Jang
Department of Pediatrics, National Health Insurance Corporation Ilsan Hospital, Goyang, Korea

Soo-Young Lee
Department of Pediatrics, Ajou University School of Medicine, Suwon, Korea

Ja-Young Kwon
Department of Obstetrics and Gynecology, Yonsei University College of Medicine, Seoul, Korea

Suk-Joo Choi
Department of Obstetrics and Gynecology, Samsung Medical Center, Sungkyunkwan University School of Medicine, Seoul, Korea

Kyung-Ju Lee and Hee Jin Park
Department of Obstetrics and Gynecology, Pochon CHA University College of Medicine, Seoul, Korea

Hye-Sung Won
Department of Obstetrics and Gynecology, Asan Medical Center, University of Ulsan College of Medicine, Seoul, Korea

Hyung-Young Kim
Department of Pediatrics, Kosin University College of Medicine, Busan, Korea

Joanna Ponińska, Graz_yna Kostrzewa and Rafał Płoski
Department of Medical Genetics, Medical University of Warsaw, Warsaw, Poland

Bolesław Samoliński, Aneta Tomaszewska, Filip Raciborski, Piotr Samel-Kowalik, Artur Walkiewicz, Agnieszka Lipiec, Barbara Piekarska, Jarosław Komorowski, Edyta Krzych-Fałta, Andrzej Namysłowski and Jacek Borowicz
Department of Prevention of Environmental Hazards and Allergology, Medical University of Warsaw, Warsaw, Poland

Sławomir Majewski
Department of Dermatology and Venereology, Medical University of Warsaw, Warsaw, Poland

Alexandru D. P. Papoiu, Hong Liang Tey and Hui Wang
Department of Dermatology, Wake Forest University School of Medicine, Winston-Salem, North Carolina, United States of America

Robert C. Coghill
Department of Neurobiology and Anatomy, Wake Forest University School of Medicine, Winston-Salem, North Carolina, United States of America

Gil Yosipovitch
Department of Dermatology, Wake Forest University School of Medicine, Winston-Salem, North Carolina, United States of America
Department of Neurobiology and Anatomy, Wake Forest University School of Medicine, Winston-Salem, North Carolina, United States of America
Department of Regenerative Medicine, Wake Forest University School of Medicine, Winston-Salem, North Carolina, United States of America

Marie Ekbäck, Irene Devenney and Karin Fälth-Magnusson
Division of Pediatrics, Department of Clinical and Experimental Medicine, Faculty of Health Sciences, Linköping University and Department of Pediatrics, County Council of Östergötland, Linköping, Sweden

Michaela Tedner
Pediatric Clinic, Täby, Stockholm, Sweden

Göran Oldaeus
Pediatric Clinic, County Hospital Ryhov, Jönköping, Sweden

Gunilla Norrman
Pediatric Clinic, Hudiksvall, Sweden

Leif Strömberg
Department of Pediatrics in Norrköping, County Council of Östergötland, Norrköping, Sweden

Feng Xu, Shuxian Yan, Fei Li, Kefei Kang and Jinhua Xu
Department of Dermatology, Huashan Hospital, Shanghai Medical College, Fudan University, Shanghai, People's Republic of China

Minqiang Cai
Xinjing Community Health Service Center, Shanghai, People's Republic of China

Weihan Chai
Department of Dermatology, Jiading District Traditional Chinese Medicine Hospital, Shanghai, People's Republic of China

Minmin Wu, Chaowei Fu, Zhuohui Zhao and Haidong Kan
School of Public Health, Key Lab of Public Health Safety of the Ministry of Education, Shanghai Medical College, Fudan University, Shanghai, People's Republic of China

David Wong, Bory Kea and David Fiorentino
Department of Dermatology, Stanford University School of Medicine, Stanford, California, United States of America

Rob Pesich and Patrick Brown
Department of Biochemistry, Stanford University School of Medicine, Stanford, California, United States of America

Brandon W. Higgs, Wei Zhu and Yihong Yao
MedImmune, Translational Sciences, One MedImmune Way, Gaithersburg, Maryland, United States of America

Tomomitsu Hirota and Mayumi Tamari
Laboratory for Respiratory Diseases, Center for Genomic Medicine, The Institute of Physical and Chemical Research (RIKEN), Kanagawa, Japan

Hidehisa Saeki
Department of Dermatology, The Jikei University School of Medicine, Tokyo, Japan

Kaori Tomita
Laboratory for Respiratory Diseases, Center for Genomic Medicine, The Institute of Physical and Chemical Research (RIKEN), Kanagawa, Japan
Division of Otorhinolaryngology Head & Neck Surgery, Department of Sensory and Locomotor Medicine, Faculty of Medical Science, University of Fukui, Matsuoka, Fukui, Japan

Masafumi Sakashita, Takechiyo Yamada and Shigeharu Fujieda
Division of Otorhinolaryngology Head & Neck Surgery, Department of Sensory and Locomotor Medicine, Faculty of Medical Science, University of Fukui, Matsuoka, Fukui, Japan

Shota Tanaka
Laboratory for Respiratory Diseases, Center for Genomic Medicine, The Institute of Physical and Chemical Research (RIKEN), Kanagawa, Japan

Department of Otorhinolaryngology Head and Neck Surgery, University of Yamanashi Faculty of Medicine, Yamanashi, Japan

Kouji Ebe
Takao Hospital, Kyoto, Japan

Akihiko Miyatake
Miyatake Asthma Clinic, Osaka, Japan

Satoru Doi
Department of Pediatric Allergy, Osaka Prefectural Medical Center for Respiratory and Allergic Diseases, Osaka, Japan

Tadao Enomoto
Nonprofit Organization (NPO) Japan Health Promotion Supporting Network, Wakayama, Japan

Nobuyuki Hizawa, Tohru Sakamoto and Hironori Masuko
Division of Respiratory Medicine, Institute of Clinical Medicine, University of Tsukuba, Ibaraki, Japan

Takashi Sasaki, Tamotsu Ebihara and Masayuki Amagai
Department of Dermatology, Keio University School of Medicine, Tokyo, Japan

Hitokazu Esaki, Satoshi Takeuchi and Masutaka Furue
Department of Dermatology, Graduate School of Medical Sciences, Kyushu University, Fukuoka, Japan

Emiko Noguchi
Department of Medical Genetics, Majors of Medical Sciences, Graduate School of Comprehensive Human Sciences, University of Tsukuba, Ibaraki, Japan

Naoyuki Kamatani
Laboratory for International Alliance, Center for Genomic Medicine, The Institute of Physical and Chemical Research (RIKEN), Kanagawa, Japan

Yusuke Nakamura
Laboratory of Molecular Medicine, The Institute of Medical Science, The University of Tokyo, Tokyo, Japan

Michiaki Kubo
Laboratory for Genotyping Development, Center for Genomic Medicine, The Institute of Physical and Chemical Research (RIKEN), Kanagawa, Japan

Erin L. Foster
Department of Molecular Microbiology and Immunology, Oregon Health & Science University, Portland, Oregon, United States of America

Eric L. Simpson
Department of Dermatology, Oregon Health & Science University, Portland, Oregon, United States of America

Lorna J. Fredrikson, James J. Lee and Nancy A. Lee
Department of Biochemistry, Mayo Clinic, Scottsdale, Arizona, United States of America

Allison D. Fryer and David B. Jacoby
Division of Pulmonary and Critical Care, Department of Medicine, Oregon Health & Science University, Portland, Oregon, United States of America

Maria Ekoff, Katarina Lyberg and Gunnar Nilsson
Department of Medicine, Centre for Allergy Research, Karolinska Institutet, Stockholm, Sweden

Maryla Krajewska and John C. Reed
Sanford-Burnham Medical Research Institute, La Jolla, California, United States of America

Monica Arvidsson and Sabina Rak
Department of Respiratory Medicine and Allergology, Sahlgrenska University Hospital, Goteborg, Sweden

Ilkka Harvima
Department of Dermatology, Kuopio University Hospital and University of Eastern Finland, Kuopio, Finland

Tomomitsu Hirota and Mayumi Tamari
Laboratory for Respiratory Diseases, Center for Genomic Medicine, The Institute of Physical and Chemical Research (RIKEN), Kanagawa, Japan

Satoru Doi
Department of Pediatric Allergy, Osaka Prefectural Medical Center for Respiratory and Allergic Diseases, Osaka, Japan

Akihiko Miyatake
Miyatake Asthma Clinic, Osaka, Japan

Tadao Enomoto
NPO Japan Health Promotion Supporting Network, Wakayama, Japan

Kaori Tomita, Masafumi Sakashita, Takechiyo Yamada and Shigeharu Fujieda
Division of Otorhinolaryngology Head and Neck Surgery, University of Fukui, Fukui, Japan

Koji Ebe
Takao Hospital, Kyoto, Japan

Hidehisa Saeki
Department of Dermatology, The Jikei University School of Medicine, Tokyo, Japan

Satoshi Takeuchi and Masutaka Furue
Department of Dermatology, Graduate School of Medical Sciences, Kyushu Universiy, Fukuoka, Japan

Yusuke Nakamura
Laboratory of Molecular Medicine, The Institute of Medical Science, The University of Tokyo, Tokyo, Japan

Wei-Chiao Chen and Yi-Ching Chiu
Department of Medical Genetics, College of Medicine, Kaohsiung Medical University, Kaohsiung, Taiwan

Wei Pin Chang
Department of Healthcare Management, Yuanpei University, HsinChu, Taiwan

Chien-Hui Hong, Hsin-Su Yu and Chih-Hung Lee
Department of Dermatology, Graduate Institute of Medicine, Kaohsiung Medical University, Kaohsiung, Taiwan

Li-Fang Wang
epartment of Dermatology, National Taiwan University College of Medicine, Taipei, Taiwan

Wei-Chiao Chang
Department of Medical Genetics, College of Medicine, Kaohsiung Medical University, Kaohsiung, Taiwan
Cancer Center, Kaohsiung Medical University Hospital, Kaohsiung, Taiwan
Center for Resources, Research, and Development, Kaohsiung Medical University, Kaohsiung, Taiwan

Suh-Hang Hank Juo
Department of Medical Genetics, College of Medicine, Kaohsiung Medical University, Kaohsiung, Taiwan
Department of Medical Research, Kaohsiung Medical University Hospital, Kaohsiung, Taiwan

Edward Hsi
Department of Medical Research, Kaohsiung Medical University Hospital, Kaohsiung, Taiwan

Balvinder Rehal and April Armstrong
Department of Dermatology, University of California Davis, Davis, California, United States of America

Charlotte Giwercman Carson, Liselotte Brydensholt Halkjaer, Signe Marie Jensen and Hans Bisgaard
Copenhagen Prospective Studies on Asthma in Childhood, Health Sciences, University of Copenhagen, Copenhagen University Hospital, Gentofte, Copenhagen, Denmark

Susannah McLean
Allergy and Respiratory Research Group, Centre for Population Health Sciences, The University of Edinburgh, Edinburgh, United Kingdom

Ivette A. G. Deckers and Aziz Sheikh
Allergy and Respiratory Research Group, Centre for Population Health Sciences, The University of Edinburgh, Edinburgh, United Kingdom
CAPHRI, Department of Epidemiology, Maastricht University Medical Centre+, Maastricht, The Netherlands

Sanne Linssen and Monique Mommers
CAPHRI, Department of Epidemiology, Maastricht University Medical Centre+, Maastricht, The Netherlands

C. P. van Schayck
CAPHRI, Department of General Practice, Maastricht University Medical Centre+, Maastricht, The Netherlands

Shin Yong Park, Dipika Gupta and Roman Dziarski
Indiana University School of Medicine–Northwest, Gary, Indiana, United States of America

Chang H. Kim
School of Veterinary Medicine, Purdue University, West Lafayette, Indiana, United States of America

Maiza Campos Ponce
Department of Health Sciences, VU University Amsterdam, Amsterdam, The Netherlands

Suzanne D. van der Werff and Katja Polman
Department of Health Sciences, VU University Amsterdam, Amsterdam, The Netherlands
Department of Biomedical Sciences, Prince Leopold Institute of Tropical Medicine, Antwerp, Belgium

Jos W. R. Twisk
Department of Health Sciences, VU University Amsterdam, Amsterdam, The Netherlands
Department of Epidemiology and Biostatistics, EMGO Institute of Health and Care Research, VU University Medical Center, Amsterdam, The Netherlands

Raquel Junco Díaz and Mariano Bonet Gorbea
National Institute of Hygiene, Epidemiology and Microbiology, Havana, Cuba

Patrick Van der Stuyft
Department of Public Health, Prince Leopold Institute of Tropical Medicine, Antwerp, Belgium
Department of Public Health, Ghent University, Ghent, Belgium

Li Meng, Li Wang, Huayang Tang, Xianfa Tang, Xiaoyun Jiang, Jinhua Zhao, Jing Gao, Bing Li, Xuhui Fu, Yan Chen, Weiyi Yao, Wenying Zhan, Bo Wu, Dawei Duan, Changbing Shen, Hui Cheng, Xianbo Zuo, Sen Yang, Liangdan Sun
Institute of Dermatology and Department of Dermatology, No.1 Hospital, Anhui Medical University, Hefei, Anhui, China
Key Laboratory of Dermatology, Anhui Medical University, Ministry of Education, China, Hefei, Anhui, China
State Key Laboratory Incubation Base of Dermatology, Anhui Medical University, Hefei, Anhui, China

Xuejun Zhang
Institute of Dermatology and Department of Dermatology, No.1 Hospital, Anhui Medical University, Hefei, Anhui, China
Key Laboratory of Dermatology, Anhui Medical University, Ministry of Education, China, Hefei, Anhui, China
State Key Laboratory Incubation Base of Dermatology, Anhui Medical University, Hefei, Anhui, China

Department of Dermatology at No.2 Hospital, Anhui Medical University, Hefei, Anhui, China
Department of Dermatology, Huashan Hospital of Fudan University, Shanghai, China

Charlotte Giwercman Carson and Hans Bisgaard
Copenhagen Prospective Studies on Asthma in Childhood; COPSAC, Health Sciences, University of Copenhagen, Copenhagen University Hospital, Gentofte, Copenhagen, Denmark

Morten Arendt Rasmussen
Faculty of Life Sciences, University of Copenhagen, Frederiksberg, Denmark

Jacob P. Thyssen and Torkil Menné
National Allergy Research Centre, Department of Dermato- Allergology, Copenhagen University Hospital Gentofte, Hellerup, Denmark

John A. Zebala, Aaron D. Schuler and Stuart J. Kahn
Syntrix Biosystems, Inc., Auburn, Washington, United States of America

Alan Mundell
Animal Dermatology Service, Edmonds, Washington, United States of America

Linda Messinger
Veterinary Referral Center of Colorado, Englewood, Colorado, United States of America

Craig E. Griffin
Animal Dermatology Clinic, San Diego, California, United States of America

Stephanie Roll, Thomas Reinhold, Daniel Pach, Benno Brinkhaus and Katja Icke,
Tanja Jäckel and Stefan N. Willich
Institute for Social Medicine, Epidemiology, and Health Economics, Charité University Medical Centre, Berlin, Germany

Doris Staab
Department of Paediatric Pulmonology and Immunology, Charité University Medical Centre, Berlin, Germany

Karl Wegscheider
Department of Medical Biometry and Epidemiology, University Medical Centre, Hamburg-Eppendorf, Germany

Claudia M. Witt
Institute for Social Medicine, Epidemiology, and Health Economics, Charité University Medical Centre, Berlin, Germany
Centre for Integrative Medicine, University of Maryland School of Medicine, Baltimore, Maryland, United States of America

Agne Lidén, Annika Sääf, Elisabeth Ekelund and Magnus Nordenskjö ld
Department of Molecular Medicine and Surgery, Karolinska Institutet, Stockholm, Sweden

Maria Bradley and Mårten C. G. Winge
Department of Molecular Medicine and Surgery, Karolinska Institutet, Stockholm, Sweden
Dermatology Unit, Department of Medicine Solna, Karolinska University Hospital, Stockholm, Sweden

Carl-Fredrik Wahlgren
Dermatology Unit, Department of Medicine Solna, Karolinska University Hospital, Stockholm, Sweden

Ingrid Kockum
Department of Clinical Neurosciences, Karolinska Institutet, Stockholm, Sweden

Elke Rodriguez, Regina Fölster-Holst, Hansjörg Baurecht and Stephan Weidinger
Department of Dermatology, University of Kiel, Kiel, Germany

Andre Franke
Institute of Clinical Molecular Biology, Christian-Albrechts-Universität zu Kiel, Kiel, Germany

Thomas Illig
Research Unit of Molecular Epidemiology, Helmholtz Zentrum München, German Research Center for Environmental Health, Neuherberg, Germany
Hannover Unified Biobank, Hannover Medical School, Hannover, Germany

Maria Tengvall-Linder
Clinical Immunology and Allergy, Department of Medicine Solna, Karolinska Institutet, Stockholm, Sweden

Kim S. Thomas, Elizabeth J. Doney and Hywel C. Williams
Centre of Evidence Based Dermatology, University of Nottingham, King's Meadow Campus, Nottingham, United Kingdom

Masaki Futamura
Centre of Evidence Based Dermatology, University of Nottingham, King's Meadow Campus, Nottingham, United Kingdom
Division of Allergy, National Center for Child Health and Development, Tokyo Japan

Douglas J. C. Grindlay
Centre for Evidence-based Veterinary Medicine, University of Nottingham, Sutton Bonington Campus, Leicestershire, United Kingdom

Donna Torley
Alan Lyell Centre for Dermatology, Southern General Hospital Glasgow, Glasgow, United Kingdom

Ruhong Cheng, Ming Li, Hui Zhang, Yifeng Guo, Xilan Chen, Jianfeng Tao, Aifang Jiang, Jiecheng Gan, Huaishan Qi, Hong Yu and Zhirong Yao
Department of Dermatology, Xinhua Hospital, Shanghai Jiaotong University School of Medicine, Shanghai, China

Wanqing Liao
Department of Dermatology, Changzheng Hospital, The Second Military Medical University, Shanghai, China

Index

CPSIA information can be obtained
at www.ICGtesting.com
Printed in the USA
BVHW02*0448020218
506942BV00003B/29/P